Organ Donation and Transplantation: Issues, Challenges and Clinical Perspectives

Organ Donation and Transplantation: Issues, Challenges and Clinical Perspectives

Editor: Jude Harris

MURPHY & MOORE
www.murphy-moorepublishing.com

www.murphy-moorepublishing.com

MURPHY & MOORE

Cataloging-in-Publication Data

Organ donation and transplantation : issues, challenges and clinical perspectives / edited by Jude Harris.
p. cm.
Includes bibliographical references and index.
ISBN 978-1-63987-416-3
1. Donation of organs, tissues, etc. 2. Transplantation of organs, tissues, etc. 3. Organs (Anatomy). 4. Surgery. I. Harris, Jude.
RD129.5 .O74 2022
617--dc23

Murphy & Moore Publishing,
1 Rockefeller Plaza,
New York City, NY 10020, USA

ISBN 978-1-63987-416-3 (Hardback)

Contents

Preface ... VII

Chapter 1 **Viral Transmission in Organ Transplantation: The Importance of Risk Assessment** ... 1
Cristina Baleriola and William D Rawlinson

Chapter 2 **Family-Centered Care to Improve Family Consent for Organ Donation** ... 24
Maria Grazia Bocci, Alessia Prestifilippo, Ciro D'Alò, Alessandro Barelli, Massimo Antonelli, Emiliano Cingolani, Alessandra Tersali, Alessandra Ionescu Maddalena and Roberta Barelli

Chapter 3 **Living Donor Liver Transplantation for Hepatocellular Carcinoma** ... 40
Chih-Che Lin, Ahmed Mohammed Abdel Aziz Elsarawy and Chao-Long Chen

Chapter 4 **Clinical and Pathological Review of Post Transplant Lymphoproliferative Disorders** ... 66
Seema Naik, Hong Zheng, Kevin Rakszawski, Clare Sample, Jeff Sample and Michael Bayerl

Chapter 5 **Organ Donation and Transplantation: "Life after Death"** ... 79
Kanmani Job and Anooja Antony

Chapter 6 **Procurement of Abdominal Organs in Multi-Organ Donation in Deceased Donor** ... 95
Bulang He, Xiuwu Han and Michael A. Fink

Chapter 7 **Pancreas Transplantation** ... 109
Pedro Ventura-Aguiar, Joana Ferrer-Fábrega and Maria José Ricart

Chapter 8 **The Process of Organ Donation from Non-Living Donors: A Case-Based Journey from Potential Donor Identification to Organ Procurement** ... 139
Alyssa Green, Peter G. Thomas, Rebecca Wilde-Onia, Scott J. Kohler, Joan D. Sweeney, Deborah M. Stahlnecker and Stanislaw P. Stawicki

Chapter 9 **Organ Donation** ... 158
Young-Nam Roh

Chapter 10 **Xenotransplantation** ... 172
Sean Stevens

Chapter 11 **Experimental Brain Death Models in Liver Transplantation** ... 193
Maria Eugenia Cornide-Petronio, Araní Casillas-Ramírez, Mónica B. Jiménez-Castro and Carmen Peralta

Chapter 12 **Cardiovascular Diseases in Patients with Renal Transplantation** ... 210
Daniela Loncar and Selma Hodzic

Chapter 13 **Anaesthesia for Liver Transplantation** 228
Gabriela Droc and Lavinia Jipa

Permissions

List of Contributors

Index

Preface

The process when a person donates an organ and allows it to be transplanted to another person legally, either by consent when the person is alive or by assent of a relative when the person is dead, is referred to as organ transplantation. Organs can be donated for either research or to be transplanted into another person. Common organ transplantations include heart, kidneys, intestines, pancreas, liver, bones, skin, lungs, bone marrow and corneas. Most donations occur after the death of the donor, while some donations, such as a part of liver, kidney or a part of pancreas, can be donated by living donors. This book studies, analyses and upholds the pillars of organ transplantation and its significance. Also included herein is a detailed explanation of the various concepts and applications of organ donation and transplantation. Researchers and students in this field will be assisted by this book.

The information shared in this book is based on empirical researches made by veterans in this field of study. The elaborative information provided in this book will help the readers further their scope of knowledge leading to advancements in this field.

Finally, I would like to thank my fellow researchers who gave constructive feedback and my family members who supported me at every step of my research.

Editor

1

Viral Transmission in Organ Transplantation: The Importance of Risk Assessment

Cristina Baleriola and William D Rawlinson

Abstract

Organ transplantation presents a low but extant risk of allograft transmission of blood-borne viruses (BBV) including human immunodeficiency virus (HIV), hepatitis B virus (HBV), and hepatitis C virus (HCV). Other infections temporarily present in blood are also transmissible from donor to recipient, such as cytomegalovirus (CMV), polyomavirus (BK), Epstein-Barr virus (EBV), and others, where the donor has acute infection at the time of donation. Decisions about accepting organs for transplantation involve a trade-off between the acquisition of good-quality organs, which can confer longer survival time for the recipient, but at the risk of dying from waiting too long from the underlying condition, versus accepting an organ of less quality, but at the risk of potentially acquiring a donor-derived infection (DDI), unless such infection can be ruled out in the donated organ. In this chapter, we describe the different factors contributing to the overall risk of acquiring a BBV infection through the allograft, mechanisms for assessing risk of the donor and the different strategies available to minimize or mitigate the risk. The process is one of risk assessments and risk ameliorations through optimum laboratory and clinical assessment processes, so that transplantation professionals can balance the overall risk against the life-saving and life-enhancing benefits of organ transplantation.

Keywords: blood-borne virus infection through transplantation, donor-derived infections, risk assessment, risk management, risk mitigation

1. Introduction

Organ transplantation currently provides definitive therapy for individuals with end-organ failure. Despite the enormous therapeutic advances in this area, donor-derived infections (DDI)

in the recipient from the donated organ, although rare, have been associated with significant morbidity and mortality [1,2]. These unexpected DDI are often with blood-borne viruses (BBV), including hepatitis B virus (HBV), hepatitis C virus (HCV), and less frequently human immunodeficiency virus (HIV) [3–5]. There are few data available to ascertain the risk of infection in organ transplantation for known and emerging pathogens, as most information comes from events of transmission, which are rare and not always well characterized, with few countries having well-established post-transplant surveillance systems with universal recipient assessment [6].

Due to the scarcity of donor organs, the safety paradigm in solid organ transplantation (SOT) should be based on a risk-benefit trade-off and the decision-making strategy for organ allocation be based on risk management. In this context, it is important to consider that most often the benefits of transplanting the organ outweigh the risk of DDI. Therefore, care should be taken to find the appropriate balance between minimizing the risk of transmission and organ wastage or recipient illness progression [7].

This chapter describes the different factors contributing to the overall risk of acquiring a BBV infection through the allograft, the risk assessment of the donor, and the different strategies available to minimize or mitigate the risk.

2. Donor assessment

Donor assessment often uses a questionnaire based on review of medical and social history to identify donor risks, including those associated with infection with blood-borne pathogens. In Australia, a standard questionnaire is available nationwide to streamline the assessment criteria [8]. The organ donor coordinator must review all potential donor's available medical records to identify evidence of an infectious disease or documentation of established risk behaviors associated with BBV infection. The information should be obtained from a next of kin and/or other person who has an established relationship with the donor (e.g. the donor's general practitioner). Attention to travel history is critical to identify donors at risk of endemic infections [9,10].

- Men who have had sex with another man in the preceding 5 years.
- Intravenous, intramuscular, or subcutaneous injection of drugs in the preceding 5 years.
- Incarceration in the previous 12 months.
- Persons who have had sex in the preceding 12 months with any of the above persons or a person known or suspected to have HIV, HCV, or HBV infection.
- Persons who have engaged in sex in exchange for money or drugs in the preceding 5 years.
- Exposure in preceding 12 months through percutaneous inoculation or open wound.
- Nonsterile tattooing, piercings in the past 12 months.
- Unexplained fever/weight loss/LAD/cough.
- Cocaine snorting.
- Physical concern.

Table 1. Donors with identified risk factors.

Careful physical assessment of the donor's body is conducted by both the organ procurement team and the procuring surgeon. The examination also searches for evidence of underlying disease, such as cirrhosis or other surface manifestations of infections, malignancies or of recent drug use [11]. In the acute donation situation, the appropriate person is not always available to question regarding the donor's risk, and manifestations of BBV can be minimal or non-existent. Thus, optimal donor screening testing is of paramount importance.

3. Prevalence of infection

The prevalence of BBV infection on a given population is particularly important as donor history may fail to uncover donor risk factors and, especially in the case of HBV or HCV, the rate of prevalent disease remains relatively high in 2016 in many countries, even in donors without identified risks. BBV potentially transmitted from donor organ to recipient are prevalent at 2% of the Australian population (**Table 2**) [12], whereas cytomegalovirus (CMV), Epstein–Barr virus (EBV), and polyomavirus (BK) virus are far more common, with prevalence rates of 50–70%, 95% [13], and ~60% [14], respectively.

Virus estimated	Infected population	Prevalence rate (%)	Prevalence rate in high-risk population (%)
HIV	25,700	0.10	2.8
HBV	218,000	0.87	50
HCV	233,525	0.93	50
Total	468,525	1.9	80*

* Some individuals are infected with both HCV and HBV.

Table 2. Prevalence of BBV (HIV-1, HBV, and HCV) in the Australian population.

The prevalence of BBV among potential increased-risk organ donors in our laboratory in the Serology and Virology Division (SAVID), providing testing services to the NSW Organ and Tissue Donation Service was 50% for HBV, 10% for HCV, and 0.1% for HIV-1 [15]. In the United States, the prevalence of HIV and HCV in average-risk donors was reported to be 0.10 and 3.45%, respectively, whereas the prevalence of HIV and HCV among increased risk donors (IRDs) was 0.50 and 18.20%, respectively [16]. Viruses endemic to certain geographical areas or population groups including human T-cell lymphotropic virus 1 (HTLV-1) in the Australian Aboriginal population and HBV in Mediterranean and Asian Countries may be one reason for unexpected positive screening results of average-risk donors or donors without apparent risk factors [17]. The WHO publishes updated prevalence figures of BBV worldwide, which could assist in ascertaining the probability of BBV latent infections [18] and hence background risk of donor infection.

4. Serology/nucleic acid testing results

Donors are routinely screened to identify viral or bacterial infection using serology and nucleic acid testing (NAT) assays. NAT assays detect the presence of specific viral or bacterial RNA/DNA in a patient's blood. The latter is a marker of infectivity of the organ donor when compared with antibody tests, which show previous infection without distinguishing current infection. All BBV serological tests have a 'window period' (WP), which is a time after infection during which the antibody response cannot be detected by the usual testing methods (**Figure 1**). The serological WP varies with the sensitivity of the assay, but generally are 17–22 days for HIV, 38–60 days for HBV, and 70 days for HCV.

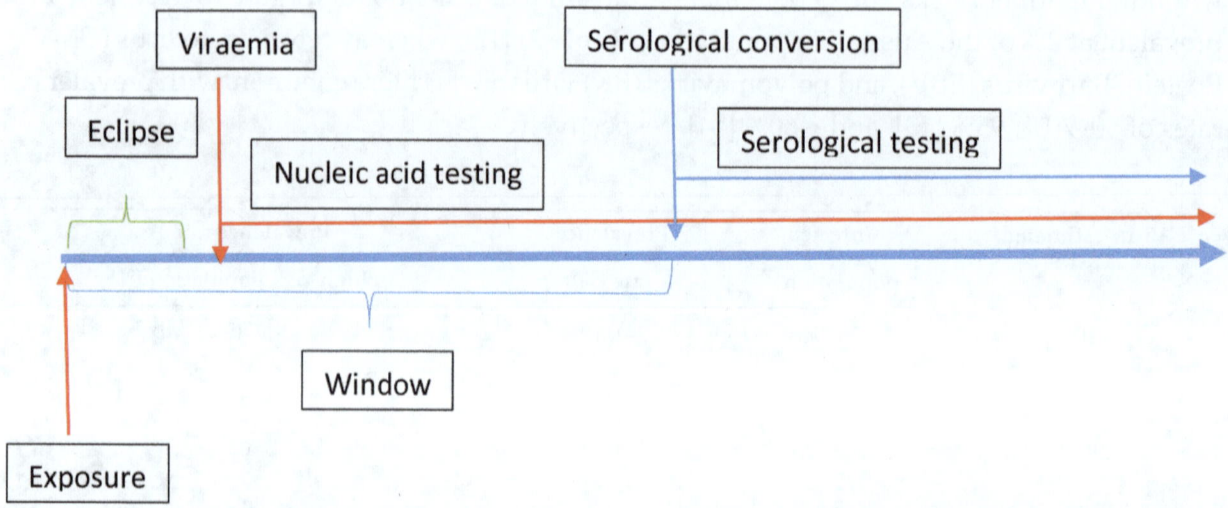

Figure 1. Events taking place after viral exposure.

NAT assays significantly reduce the WP between infection and detection compared with serological testing (6–7 days for HIV, 30–40 days for HBV, and 4–6 days for HCV) (**Figure 2**). Thus, NAT assays also have WP when they are negative following acute infection, therefore a negative NAT assay result does not completely eliminate the possibility of recent infection. In practice, the risk of infection from screened donors has been extremely low, but no screening test that is performed on a donor is entirely capable of reducing risk of transmission to nil, although all efforts are taken to reduce risk of BBV transmission and effectively resulting in extremely low risk.

All potential organ donors (living or deceased) should be tested for antibodies to HIV (anti-HIV 1/2 antigen/antibody combo assay), HCV and HBV. Donors should also be tested for HIV, HCV, and HBV RNA/DNA, whereas increased-risk organ donors should be tested by NAT for HIV, HCV, and HBV prospectively (**Table 3**).

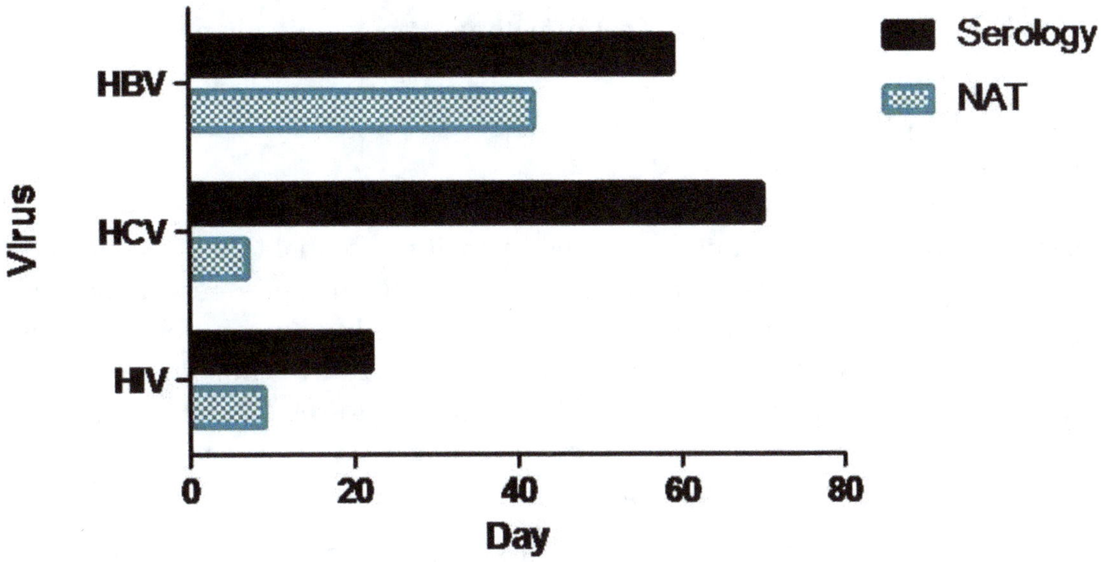

Figure 2. Differences in window periods for serology and NAT for HIV, HCV, and HBV (Data from SAVID).

Serology:	NAT:
• Anti-HIV-1/2	• HIV-1 RNA
• Anti-HCV	• HCV RNA
• Anti-HTLV-I/II	• HBV DNA
• HBsAg	• Prospective in increased risk donors
• Anti-HBc	• Retrospective in average-risk donors
• Anti-HBs	
• Anti-EBV	
• Anti-CMV	
• Syphilis antibody (TPHA)	

Table 3. Mandatory testing for prospective organ donors in Australia.

The WP of an assay has important implications for the risk assessment of a particular donor. The definition of IRD as per the Transplantation Society of Australia and New Zealand guidelines [11] is "where there is concern regarding the donor's risk behavior and it cannot be reliably determined or the behavior may have occurred within the last 2 months". These 2 months cover the NAT WPs for HIV, HCV, and HBV (**Figure 2**).

The arrival of fully automated platforms for triple viral NAT currently in 2016 in Australia by at least two manufacturers opens the possibility of 24-hour access to HBV, HCV, and HIV NAT testing. New technologies, such as the Cobas 6800 system [19] from Roche Molecular Systems and the Panther system [20] from Hologic, are now available with shorter turnaround time (TAT = 3.5 hours), and the possibility of confirmatory testing of initially positive results.

5. Conduct of donor testing

If the specimen sample used for testing has unusual characteristics, such as where donors have had massive blood and/or blood product transfusion, it is essential to indicate to the testing laboratory and the transplanting team the underlying condition of the donor. If the donor has received greater than 50% of blood volume in blood product transfusion, the sample is unsuitable for serology and NAT testing due to dilution of native antibodies by transfused fluids [21]. A pre-transfusion sample should be provided to the laboratory. If this is not possible, NAT-enhanced sensitivity may reduce the frequency of false-negative test results when donor specimens are haemodiluted.

There are significant concerns that the use of assays with higher sensitivity for pathogen detection—such as NAT assays—will result in net organ loss. This is because the majority of positive tests in low-prevalence populations will be false positives [22], and time constrains do not allow confirmatory testing with certain testing platforms. The NAT laboratory at SAVID, Prince of Wales Hospital in Sydney, Australia, has developed screening algorithms using three NAT assays run in parallel for prospective screening of IRD to maximize organ availability by effectively eliminating false-positive results (FPR) [15]. The availability of a 24-hour NAT screening service for organ donors provided diagnosis within 8 hours and enabled the use of organs from donors with positive serology but negative NAT results or donors with false-positive serology results. This algorithm allowed us to perform real-time discrimination of initially reactive results and the use of 35 IRD, which resulted in transplantation of 102 additional organs with safer expansion of the donor pool.

Positive serology or NAT results should be interpreted consistent with current guidelines [10,16] by the accepting teams in consultation with an Infectious Disease Physician.

6. Risk of transmission

The risk of acquisition of a BBV through organ transplantation is related to the efficiency of virus transmission and replication after contact with blood and tissues. Not all BBV are transmitted in the same way, and the result may be related to the type and size of the inoculum, the titre of virus and the immunization status of the recipient. Most of the well-documented transmissions are from blood transfusions but this may correlate with similar level of infectivity from donated organs. In humans, HBV transmission has been reported to be from blood donors in the WP or from donors with occult hepatitis B (OBI) with HBV viral loads of >20 IU/ml [23], whereas donors with an anti-HBs titre of >100 seem to have a protective role to prevent de novo HBV infection [24]. In terms of HIV, a pre-seroconversion donation with a viral load of ≤150 copies of RNA/ml went undetected and resulted in an HIV transmission [25]. Finally, HCV-infected recipients have been reported from donors with a viral load of as low as 182 cp/

ml and even from a donor with undetectable levels of RNA in the transcription-mediated amplification (TMA) assay (limit of detection (LOD) = 9.6 IU/ml)) [26].

In a report by the Canadian Society for Transplantation and Canadian National Transplant Research Program [27], the residual risk to acquire a HIV or HCV infection from transplanted organs of IRD after screening with serology and NAT was calculated (**Table 4**). The group concluded that these donors should screened by serological testing in conjunction with NAT testing for HCV and HIV and hepatitis B surface antigen (HBsAg) or NAT for HBV.

Virus	Risk of WP infection for NAT and ELISA per 10,000	Risk of WP infection for NAT and ELISA expressed as ratio
HIV	0.71	1:14,923
HCV	3.79	1:2,637

Table 4. Risk per 10,000 donors of an HIV or HCV infection occurring during the WP, by enzyme-linked immunosorbent assay (ELISA) and NAT. Assumes a WP of 21 days for ELISA and 7 days for NAT.

7. Organ-specific risks

HBV- and HCV-infected livers produce universally infected HBV- or HCV-naïve recipients, with outcomes determined by factors, such as the viral genotype, the presence or absence of previous immunity and the response to antiviral therapy. On the other hand, a HCV- or HBV-infected donor may be able to donate other organs rather than the liver. As both HBV and HCV can be transmitted via organ donation, especially through liver grafts, a thorough approach is needed for successful management of the recipient, and an emphasis on aggressive immunization and risk mitigation of transplant candidates prior to transplant should be pursued.

Allografts from HBV-infected donors should preferentially be given to recipients who are HBsAg positive, hepatitis B core antibody (anti-HBc) positive, or hepatitis B surface antibody (HBsAb) positive [28]. Transmission of de novo HBV infection to liver grafts recipients from anti-HBc–positive donors has been detected since 1992; however, further studies demonstrated that non-liver allografts from these donors can be safely used [29,30]. Several studies have clearly shown that non-liver organs and tissues from donors who are anti-HBc positive and HBsAg negative can be used with negligible risk, especially if the recipient is protected through vaccination or prior exposure to HBV [31,32].

A different scenario is that of donors with OBI, characterized by persistence of HBV DNA in the liver tissue (and in some cases also in serum) of HBsAg-negative individuals [33], therefore exhibiting undetectable HBsAg in serum and low-level HBV DNA (<200 IU/ml). In HBV, low-prevalence countries, the prevalence of OBI is low (0.1–2.4%) [34], whereas in HBV, high-prevalence countries, the prevalence can range from 7.5 to 16% [35,36].

The molecular bases of OBI appear to be related to the long-lasting persistence in the nuclei of the hepatocytes of the HBV cccDNA, an intermediate form of the virus life cycle that serves as a template for gene transcription [37,38]. The risk of OBI being associated with anti-HBc seropositivity has been demonstrated [39,40], and one of the best sentinel markers for OBI is a positive anti-HBc serology result [41]. Long-standing abnormal results of liver function tests of unknown aetiology in the absence of HBV serological markers and serum HBV DNA may also indicate the presence of HBV DNA in the liver and peripheral blood mononuclear cells [42]. Donors with OBI may transmit HBV infection, especially in orthotopic liver transplantation (OLT), because the hepatocytes are the reservoir of the viral cccDNA. These recipients may develop de novo hepatitis B, particularly when they are HBV naïve [43,44]. Prevention measures include anti-HBV prophylaxis, based on anti-HBs immunoglobulin alone or in combination with lamivudine. These measures, however, cannot completely eliminate HBV transmission because there have been documented reports on the development of OBI in recipients who received an organ from an OBI carrier [44], exhibiting the same viral genomes (including HBV cccDNA) in the transplanted liver.

As already mentioned, HBV-infected donors can be safely used for potential HBV-infected recipients [28] with the use of post-transplantation prophylaxis (hepatitis B immune globulin (HBIg) and nucleoside/nucleotide polymerase inhibitors, such as lamivudine in combination with adefovir, entecavir, or tenofovir) [45–47]. It has also been reported that a titre of HBsAb greater than 100 in the donor has a protective effect [48]. Recipient sero-protection through prior exposure or vaccination is a highly effective way to prevent transmission of HBV through organ transplantation [49]. As some potential organ recipients do not respond well to vaccination and remain unprotected, a priority area is to devise new ways to enhance vaccination responses.

HCV-positive donor organs can also be used in HCV-positive recipients with minimal impact on clinical outcomes [50,51]. Clinical studies have shown that there is no significant difference in survival in HCV-positive recipients who receive either HCV-positive or HCV-negative livers or kidneys [51–55]. Therefore, there needs to be education to enhance uptake of HCV-positive organs in HCV-positive recipients. As first-generation direct acting antivirals (DAAs) offer a significant therapeutic improvement when compared with previous therapies, particularly for patients with HCV genotype-1 infection, this may lead to the use of more HCV-infected organ donors for HCV-infected recipients treated with this highly effective post-transplant prophylaxis [56,57].

8. Use of IRDs

In the United States alone, almost 10,000 individuals die annually while awaiting organ transplantation [58], whereas in Australia, there are almost 3000 individuals in the waiting list. Due to organ scarcity, attempts at expanding the pool of potential donors are necessary, and the criteria for donation are under continuous scrutiny. Recent campaigns globally from organ procurement agencies to expand the donor pool have resulted in use of organs from IRD, who are at greater risk of infection with BBV, including HBV, HCV, and HIV. The use of NAT to screen such IRD has been associated with increased utilization of these organs [10,11,16,27].

The key to using these IRD is to maximize the measures to identify risk factors; particularly ensuring that infectious diseases are not transmitted from donor to recipient in the allograft. A successful strategy to mitigate the overall risk has been to match the allograft to the most appropriate recipient by improved selection and monitoring. In such scenarios, additional consent and recipient screening at regular intervals during the first year after transplant should be performed [10,11,16,27].

We documented in one study that with the use of prospective NAT, 102 additional organs from IRD were used in Australia. These organs would otherwise have been discarded or used with restrictions [15]. This represents 18.8% of all organs transplanted during the study period. Furthermore, the utilization of parallel NAT assays combined with mathematical modeling enabled us to estimate the probability that the combination of results were predictive of true-positive results. Thus, we piloted a methodology for effectively minimizing FPR. This resulted in higher confidence in the NAT results and minimizing the loss of organs secondary to FPR to negligible.

In a Canadian study of 3746 transplants using deceased liver donors [59], it was concluded that over the last decade, there was an increase in the use of older donors and donation after cardiac death (DCD) organs, but recipient survival was not compromised. In Australia, IRDs are routinely used, and this strategy has substantially contributed to an increased use of organs [15]. Furthermore, the acceptance of these organs by the transplantation community has been increased over the years, and from 2013 onwards, the same number of organs was retrieved from IRD and from average-risk donors (**Figure 3**).

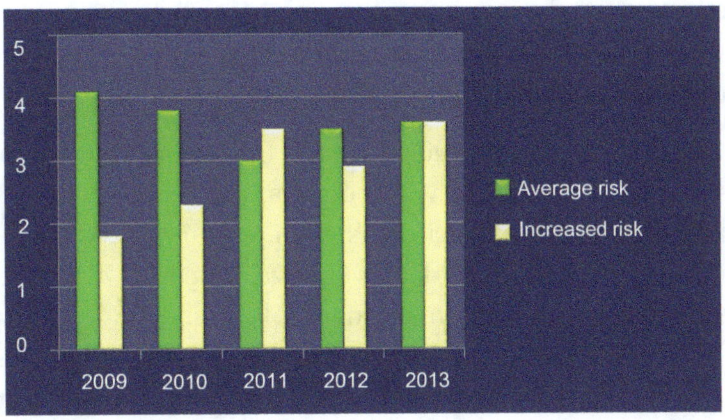

Figure 3. Number of organs retrieved from increased-risk donors vs average-risk donors over the years (data from SAVID).

Final decisions in individual cases about using organs of IRD must acknowledge the recommendations from national and international guidelines, the risk-benefit trade-off in the context of the gravity of recipient's prognosis without transplantation, consideration of all clinical and laboratory assessment parameters and a fully informed consent and risk acceptance by the recipient.

9. Scoring the risk

Decision aids are increasingly being developed to support transplantation teams in making difficult treatment decisions involving trade-offs between provision of a good quality organ with longer survival but longer wait pre-transplant versus accepting an organ of less quality with earlier transplantation but higher risk of shorter survival post-transplantation or post-transplant infections. Furthermore, transplant providers who are helping patients to make treatment decisions may find it difficult to communicate the risks associated with each option in a clear, understandable fashion, particularly for IRD organs, given the complexities of risk assessment.

Scoring systems to indicate recipient's gravity include the Model for End-Stage Liver Disease (MELD) score, which is a scoring system for assessing the severity of chronic liver disease. It was found to be useful in determining prognosis and prioritizing for receipt of a liver transplant [60]. The score was developed by the Organ Procurement and Transplantation network (OPTN)/United Network for Organ Sharing (UNOS) and implemented in February 2002. MELD uses the patient's values for serum bilirubin, serum creatinine, and the international normalized ratio for prothrombin time (INR) to predict survival. It is calculated according to formula [61]. On the other hand, the donor risk index (DRI) by Feng et al. [62] using Organ Procurement and Transplantation Network (OPTN) data was developed as a continuous scoring system that includes donor and transplant parameters that significantly influence outcomes after liver transplantation (LTx). The author undertook a multivariate analysis of a large cohort (20,023 transplants) from the Scientific Registry of Transplant Recipients database. The parameters used were the donor's age, race, height, and cause of death (COD); the split liver donation status; the donation after cardiac death (DCD) status; the type of allocation (local, regional, or national); and the cold ischaemia time.

The DRI was validated in a study conducted by the Eurotransplant region, which aimed to identify its potential use [63]. The study was a database analysis of all 5939 liver transplants involving deceased donors and adult recipients from January 1, 2003, to December 31, 2007, in the Eurotransplant region. Follow-up data were available for 5723 patients with a median follow-up of 2.5 years. The mean DRI was remarkably higher in the Eurotransplant region versus OPTN (1.71 versus 1.45). The results demonstrated that Kaplan-Meier curves per DRI category showed a significant correlation between the DRI and outcomes ($p < 0.001$). A multivariate analysis demonstrated that the DRI was the most significant factor influencing outcomes ($p < 0.001$). Among all donor, transplant, and recipient variables, the DRI was the strongest predictor of outcomes.

In another study [64], it was investigated the impact of the DRI on the outcome of HCV-infected patients undergoing LTx, where the median DRI was 1.3 (range, 0.77–4.27). Increasing DRI was associated with a statistically significant increase in the relative risk (RR) of graft failure and patient death for both HCV (+) and HCV (−) recipients. Finally, Rosemberg et al. [65] using a prospectively collected infection data set, matched liver transplant recipients (and the respective allograft DRI scores) with their specific post-transplant infectious complications. All transplant recipients were organized by DRI score and divided into groups with low-DRI and high-DRI scores. Three hundred and seventy-eight liver transplants were identified, with 189 recipients each in the low-DRI and high-DRI groups. The mean MELD scores were 26.25–0.53 and 24.76–0.55, respectively ($p = 0.052$), and the mean number of infectious complications per patient were 1.60–0.19 and 1.94–0.24, respectively ($p = 0.26$). Logistic regression showed only length of hospital stay and a history of vascular disease as being associated independently with infection, with a trend toward significance for MELD score ($p = 0.13$). The study concluded that although DRI score predicts liver graft survival, infectious complications depended more heavily on recipient factors.

Even though organs from donors with high DRI score correlate with poorer post-transplant survival, the overall contribution of high-DRI grafts to the donor pool and the resultant reduction in wait list mortality make them cost-effective [66].

10. Clinical guidelines

Deciding how to allocate organs for transplantation is a very complex process and raises a number of clinical and ethical issues. Up-to-date guidelines provide an overarching framework to facilitate the decision-making process in clinical robust ways based on previous evidence. In general, transplantation guidelines follow many of the recommendations in place for the selection and microbiological testing of blood donors. However, as in organ donation and transplantation, the logistics are greatly influenced by the need to retain organ viability, the testing of potential donors will be conducted under severe time constraints. In these situations, the testing that needs to be carried out, and the general principles for balancing the risks and benefits are unique to this field.

Some of the most important transplantation guidelines published recently are as follows:

- *PHS Guideline for Reducing Human Immunodeficiency Virus, Hepatitis B Virus, and Hepatitis C Virus Transmission Through Organ Transplantation* was published in the United States in August 2013 [16]. The aim of the guide was to improve organ transplant recipient outcomes by reducing the risk of HIV, HBV, and HCV transmission. The guide is truly comprehensive and based on systematic reviews. It is extremely detailed and specialized and not very practical for the daily use of transplantation professionals.
- Advisory Committee on the Safety of Blood Tissues and Organs (SaBTO) published the *Guidance on the Microbiological Safety of Human Organs, Tissues and Cells Used for Transplantation* in February 2011 in the United Kingdom [67]. The guidance was written by a working group after extensive consultation and is extremely clear, accurate, and user friendly. However, as professionals involved in transplantation need to take real-time decisions that could be life saving for patients, most of the information given in the guidance could have been summarized and presented on tables to facilitate the information to readers.

- The Council of Europe in 2013 published the 5th edition of *the Guide to the Quality and Safety of Organs for Transplantation* [68]. This guideline collates updated information to provide professionals in transplantation with a useful overview of the most recent advancements in the field. The guide has a very comprehensive section on risk of transmission of infectious diseases. However, as pointed out before, the information is too comprehensive and should have been summarized.

- Transplantation Society of Australia and New Zealand (TSANZ) published version 1.4 of the guideline *Organ Transplantation from Deceased Donors: Consensus Statement on Eligibility Criteria and Allocation Protocols* in April 2015 [11]. The guide has only one section related to transmission of infectious agents from donor to recipient with data from HCV and HBV infection risks alone. The information is insufficient as many other real-life situations are not contemplated. Within Australia, the NSW Ministry of Health published the guide *Organ Donation and Transplantation—Managing Risks of Transmission of HIV, HCV and HBV* in 2013 [10]. This is a very useful guide for transplantation professionals.

Ideally, guidelines for transplantation should be comprehensive but presented in a concise manner to facilitate its use to readers, as shown in **Table 5** [69].

Donor status	**Advice**	**References**
Antibody to HIV (+)	Exclude from organ donation	[11,67]
Antibody to HCV (+)	Exclude from organ donation for HCV (−) recipients If used, usually reserve organ for recipient HCV (+) or severely ill recipient. HCV RNA testing should be done and allocated to a donor with a higher HCV viral load	[11,67]
Hepatitis B surface antigen HBsAg (+)	Exclude from organ donation. Use in life-threatening situations with recipient antiviral prophylaxis against HBV	[11,67]
Hepatitis B core antibody IgG (anti-HBc) (+)	Indicates past HBV infection. Organs from anti-HBc (+) of anti-HBs (−) may still be infectious. High risk for transmission with liver donation—generally used with intensive prophylaxis. Non-hepatic organs—small risk of transmission of HBV, and generally used for immunized HBsAb (+) recipients	[11,67,70,71]
Hepatitis B surface antibody Anti-HBs (+)	Anti-HBs >100 IU/l and anti-HBc (+) donations unlikely to be infectious and donation is permitted with the potential exception of livers (see above). HBV DNA NAT should be done and available prior to organ donation HBV DNA (−) indicates suitability for donation, though does not exclude risk of infection from liver. Use in vaccinated recipients and with negative NAT testing if donor vaccination unknown	[11,67,70,71]
Antibody to CMV (+)	Donation permitted. Post-transplant CMV monitoring and preventive strategy based on risk to the recipient	[67]
Antibody to EBV (+)	PCR monitoring of the seronegative or paediatric recipient	[67]

Donor status	Advice	References
RPR (+)	Not a contraindication to donation. Recipients receive standard prophylaxis (benzathine penicillin or ceftriaxone). Ensure administration of adequate antimicrobial therapy and the patient should be monitored for serological evidence of syphilis infection	[11,67,70,71]
Antibody to HTLV I/II (+)	High rate of false-positive results and consistent strategy not available. Some centers exclude from organ donation or use for life-threatening situations, with informed consent	[11,67,71]
Antibody to Toxoplasma IgG (+)	Not a contraindication to donation. Seronegative recipients with a seropositive donor should receive prophylaxis. Cardiac recipients particularly prone to transplant-associated toxoplasmosis	[11,67,71]
Viral encephalitis	Unknown etiology in donor is a contraindication to transplantation (risk of rabies, West Nile Virus or other exotic neurotropic infections). HSV or VZV CNS infection is a contraindication as it may cause systemic infection. HSV encephalitis without evidence of systemic infection treated with antivirals may be used, and antiviral prophylaxis should be used for the recipient. Local HSV/VZV infection treated with adequate antiviral therapy for >7 days organs can be used; if treated <7 days, recipient should receive antiviral prophylaxis (the serological status of the recipient must be known)	[67]

Anti-HBs, hepatitis B surface antibody; IgG, immunoglobulin G; RPR, rapid plasma reagin; VZV, Varicella Zoster virus.

Table 5. Recommendations for organ allocation based on screening data as at 2015 – subject to change with changes in policy.

This kind of format is how the Scandinavian guidelines have been presented and this could be a very useful resource for professionals identifying organ donors, transplant co-ordinators managing the donation process, and transplant physicians responsible for organ allocation [72].

11. Risk stratification and management

Currently, there are two ways in which organ donors are risk stratified in Australia: donors are dichotomized as being either at increased risk (IRD) or without identified risk factors for transmission of infectious diseases. **Figure 4** shows the flowchart for BBV testing and risk stratification in New South Wales (NSW), Australia [10].

In principle, any reactivity in one or more of the mandatory marker assays used for screening donors renders the donor ineligible. However, in life-preserving situations, it is possible to waive this exclusion. The risk-benefit trade-off means that using an IRD should only be considered when the donation is life-preserving. In this situation, the transplant surgeon with the informed consent of the potential recipient should balance the risk of infection against the risk of dying while waiting for another graft. Heart, lung, and liver transplants will almost always fit within this definition because the clinical situation of the recipient is likely to be terminal. However, short-term or intermediate support measures can be employed to avoid the immediate need for transplantation with an organ from an IRD.

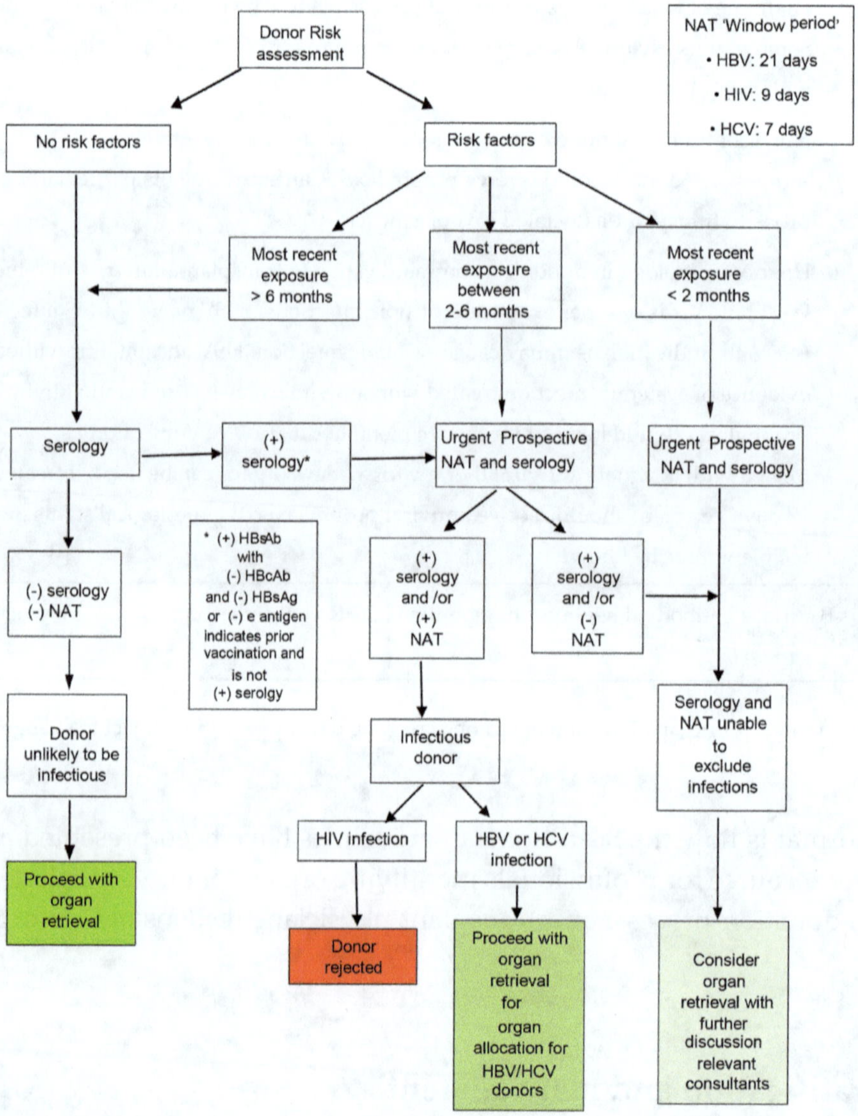

Figure 4. Blood-borne virus testing and risk stratification flowchart (from Organ Donation and Transplantation – Managing Risks of Transmission of HIV, HCV, and HBV). Reproduced with permission from NSW Ministry of Health, 2015.

One strategy when using IRD is matching infection status of donor and recipient. Previous infection, current infection, or immunization may decrease or remove the risk of infection following the use of a transplant from a donor who is known to be infected. Thus, it is appropriate to consider the use of an organ from a donor who is known to be infected, or who is potentially infected with HCV or HBV or a recipient who is also infected with HCV or HBV (i.e. infection match). Another approach involves matching of the immune status of the recipient to the infection status of the donor. For example, a recipient shown to be immune to hepatitis B, naturally or by immunization, is unlikely to suffer re-infection from an HBV-infected donor. In this type of matching, it is essential that the status of the recipient is known with certainty.

Matching the status will also include an assessment of the likelihood of transmitting viral genotypes, which may pose an additional hazard to the already infected recipient, such as using an organ infected with HCV genotype 1 for a non-1 genotype–infected recipient; drug-resistant variants, and immune escape variants. Infectious Disease specialist support should be sought to ensure that appropriate testing has been undertaken to inform the risk assessment and to confirm the recipient's status.

Risk mitigation measures include the use of prophylaxis with antiviral drugs or antibiotics; counseling and discussing with the recipient the potential infection risk and the possibility of disease arising from infection. In addition, a full informed consent and post-transplant surveillance for infection of the recipient with planned interventions should they become necessary in the case of infection transmission should be undertaken.

12. Post-transplant surveillance

The final verification of risk estimates for DDI is carried out using post-transplant surveillance aiming to identify possible donor-derived events and clusters of transmissions. These procedures require careful post-transplant follow-up, diligent clinicians to suspect and report cases and reporting systems to accept and inform investigation of potential transmission reports in a proactive manner. These systems, if universally instituted, could improve investigation of potential clusters of infection, with enhanced rapid detection and improved advice to clinicians. Furthermore, they can be valuable resources for examination of clinical data to establish evidence-based guidelines.

Recent biovigilance initiatives in the United States and Europe have occurred with the aim of developing national surveillance systems for cells, tissues, and organs. In Europe, the Eustite project [73] initiated in 2008 focused especially on inspection, training, and vigilance for tissue banks. The project developed special tools and a system for the classification and reporting of adverse events to all European countries that could be used internationally for biovigilance and surveillance. Subsequently, the tools developed by the Eustite project were streamlined by the WHO, resulting in an educational program designed for organs and tissues through the NOTIFY Project. The vigilance information database collected by the Notify Project is available on the WHO/CNT Global NOTIFY Library website [74]. The library aims to be a comprehensive reference of different types of adverse events and reactions identifying their underlying root causes. The library is regularly maintained and updated and serves as a communication hub for transplantation institutions with international vigilance and surveillance data to enhance donor and recipient safety and for greater public transparency in transplantation. The project also aims to be a reference of internationally terminology for biovigilance of organs, tissues, and cells.

The US program monitoring DDI (the UNOS and the Disease Transmission Advisory Committee (DTAC)) [75] undertakes data collection and dissemination on pre-transplant and post-transplant events and examines and classifies potential donor-derived transmission through transplantation of infection or malignancy. These aim to educate the transplant community and help change policy and improve processes. The membership includes CDC, FDA, transplant centers, transplant infectious disease professionals, laboratory testing personnel, and organ procurement organizations. The OPTN currently requires reporting of donor-derived events. All potential donor-derived transmission events (PDDTE) reported to OPTN/UNOS are reviewed by the DTAC, and real-time reports are available for transplantation professionals.

The ANZDATA [76] registry in Australia and New Zealand is a retrospective reporting system to evaluate data from donors and recipients. Attempts are recently made for timely data collection of key events and the creation of a real-time Web-based system utilization, including historical data for all years and real-time data for the current year grouped by country and state with interactive reports that can be generated at any point of time.

Most of the established surveillance systems are passive, that is laboratories notify positive test results to public health regulators. Thus, only recipients tested are notified. This system is far from ideal as most infections with a BBV do not have symptoms at the time of infection and an infected recipient may not be tested for some time post-transplant. Furthermore, not all notifications are followed up, so a recently infected organ recipient may not be detected even if tested and notified.

Despite the efforts in many countries to gather transplantation data, the main difficulty seems to lie in the absence of dedicated organ donation and transplantation surveillance registries, as usually the transplant team reports back to the organ donation agency and the data are not shared. The transplantation community requires a real-time worldwide surveillance system to identify possible clusters of infections worldwide. This could be achieved through data linkage from already established biovigilance programs. An important aspect of biovigilance systems is to develop data linkages with public health regulators and healthcare providers, so that the integration of databases can be conducted to strengthen responses to potential BBV threats worldwide.

13. Conclusions

The development of national policies for risk assessment and definition of acceptable levels of risk for BBV infection—including specific risk-benefit assessments—is increasing safety, equity and transparency in organ allocation. All decisions related to virological risk assessment need to be supported by up-to-date guidelines, optimal diagnostic testing and ongoing surveillance for DDI post-transplantation. This will continue to result in additional use of organs and continuous improvement of transplantation outcomes.

Acknowledgements

The authors thank the NSW Ministry of Health and the NSW Organ and Tissue Donation Service for the initial establishment and the ongoing support of the NAT organ donor screening program at SAVID.

Author details

Cristina Baleriola[1] and William D Rawlinson[2*]

*Address all correspondence to: w.rawlinson@unsw.edu.au

1 South Eastern Area Laboratory Service, Prince of Wales Hospital, Sydney, Australia

2 South Eastern Area Laboratory Services, Microbiology, Prince of Wales Hospital, Sydney, Australia

References

[1] Palacios G, Druce J, Du L,Tran T, Birch C, Briese T, et al. A new arenavirus in a cluster of fatal transplant associated diseases. N Engl J Med. 2008;358(10):991–998. DOI: 10.1056/NEJMoa073785.

[2] Smith JM, Mcdonald RA. Emerging viral infections in transplantation. Pediatr Transplant. 2006;10(7):838–843. DOI: 10.1111/j.1399-3046.2005.00481.x.

[3] Su WJ, Ho MC, Ni YH, Wu JF, Jeng YM, Chen HL, et al. Clinical course of de novo hepatitis B infection after paediatric liver transplantation. Liver Transpl. 2010;16(2): 215–221. DOI: 10.1002/lt.21980.

[4] Ison MG, Llata E, Conover CS, Friedewald JJ, Gerber SI, Grigoryan A, et al. Transmission of human immunodeficiency virus and hepatitis C virus from an organ donor to four transplant recipients. Am J Transplant. 2011;11(6):1218–1225. DOI: 10.1111/j. 1600-6143.2011.03597.x.

[5] Suryaprasad A, Basavaraju SV, Hocevar SN, Theodoropoulos N, Zuckerman RA, Hayden T, et al. Transmission of hepatitis C virus from organ donors despite nucleic acid test screening. Am J Transplant. 2015;15(7):1827–1835. DOI: 10.1111/ajt.13283.

[6] Weikert BC, Blumberg EA. Viral infection after renal transplantation: surveillance and management. CJASN. 2008;3(Suppl 2):S76–S86. DOI: 10.2215/CJN.02900707.

[7] Duana KI, Englesbeb MJ, Volk ML. Centers for disease control 'high-risk' donors and kidney utilization. Am J Transplant. 2010;10(2):416–420. DOI: 10.1111/j.1600-6143.2009.02931.x.

[8] TSANZ. Confidential Organ Donation Referral Form [Internet]. 2013. Available from: http://www.tsanz.com.au/downloads/Protocols_Appendix1.pdf [Accessed: December 10, 2015.]

[9] Ison MG, Grossi P, the AST Infectious Disease Community of Practice. Donor-derived infections in solid organ transplantation. Am J Transplant. 2013;13(Suppl 4):22–30. DOI: 10.1111/ajt.12095.

[10] NSW Ministry of Health. Organ Donation and Transplantation—Managing the Risk of Transmission of HIV, HCV, and HBV [Internet]. 2013. Available from: http://wwwo.health.nsw.gov.au/policies/pd/2013/pdf/PD2013_029.pdf [Accessed: December 12, 2015].

[11] Donatelife. Consensus Statement on Eligibility Criteria and Allocation Protocols Version 1.4 – 15 April 2015. [Internet]. 2015. Available from: http://www.donatelife.gov.au/sites/default/files/Version%201.4_April%202015.pdf [Accessed: December 13, 2015].

[12] Kirby Institute. HIV/AIDS, Viral Hepatitis and Sexually Transmissible Infections in Australia. Annual Surveillance Report 2013 [Internet]. 2014. Available from: http://kirby.unsw.edu.au/sites/default/files/hiv/resources/2013AnnualSurvReport.pdf [Accessed: December 10, 2015].

[13] Watzinger F, Suda A, Preuner S, Baumgartinger R, Ebner K, Baskova L, et al. Real-time quantitative PCR assays for detection and monitoring of pathogenic human viruses in immunosuppressed pediatric patients. J Clin Microbiol. 2004;42(11):5189–5198. DOI: 10.1128/JCM.42.11.5189-5198.2004.

[14] Druce J, Catton M, Chibo D, Minerds K, Tyssen D, Kostecki R, et al. Utility of a multiplex PCR assay for detecting herpesvirus DNA in clinical samples. J Clin Microbiol. 2002;40(5):1728–1732. DOI: 10.1128/JCM.40.5.1728-1732.2002.

[15] Baleriola C, Tu E, Johal H, Gillis J, Ison M, Law M, et al. Organ donor screening using parallel nucleic acid testing allows assessment of transmission risk and assay results in real time. Transpl Infect Dis. 2012;14(3):278–287. DOI: 10.1111/j.1399-3062.2012.00734.x.

[16] Public Health Service US. PHS Guideline for Reducing Human Immunodeficiency Virus, Hepatitis B Virus and Hepatitis C Virus [Internet]. 2013. Available from: http://www.publichealthreports.org/issueopen.cfm?articleID=2975 [Accessed: December 8, 2015].

[17] Einsiede LI, Spelman T, Goeman E, Cassar O, Arundell M, Gessain A. Clinical associations of human T-lymphotropic virus type 1 infection in an indigenous Australian population. PLOS Negl Trop Dis. 2014;8(1):e2643. DOI: 10.1371/journal.pntd.0002643.

[18] WHO. Global Health Observatory (GHO) Data [Internet]. 2015. Available from: http://www.who.int/gho/en [Accessed: December 4, 2015].

[19] Roche Molecular Systems. Cobas 6800/880 Systems [Internet]. 2015. Available from: http://molecular.roche.com/instruments/Pages/cobas_6800_8800_Systems.aspx [Accessed: December 6, 2015].

[20] Hologic. Panther System [Internet]. 2015. Available from: http://www.hologic.com/products/clinical-diagnostics-and-blood-screening/instrument-systems/panther-system [Accessed: December 3, 2015].

[21] Eastlund T. Hemodilution due to blood loss and transfusion and reliability of cadaver tissue donor infectious disease testing. Cell Tissue Bank. 2000;1(Issue 2):121–127. DOI: 10.1023/A:1010120115451.

[22] Humar A, Morris M, Blumberg E, Freeman R, Preiksaitis J, Kiberd B, et al. Nucleic acid testing (NAT) of organ donors: is the 'best' test the right test? A consensus conference report. Am J Transplant. 2010;10(4):889–899. DOI: 10.1111/j.1600-6143.2009.02992.x.

[23] Gonzalez R, Torres P, Castro E, Barbolla L, Candotti D, Koppelman M, et al. Efficacy of hepatitis B virus (HBV) DNA screening and characterization of acute and occult HBV infections among blood donors from Madrid (Spain). Transfusion. 2010;50(1):221–230. DOI: 10.1111./j.1537-2995.2009.02343.x.

[24] Park JB, Kwon CH, Lee KW, Choi GS, Kim DJ, Seo JM, et al. Hepatitis B virus vaccine switch program for prevention of de novo hepatitis B virus infection in paediatric patients. Transplant Int. 2008;21(4):346–352. DOI: 10.1111/j.1432-2277.2007.00618.x.

[25] Delwart EL, Kalmin ND, Jones TS, Ladd DJ, Foley B, Tobler LH, et al. First report of human immunodeficiency virus transmission via an RNA screened blood donation. Vox Sang. 2004;86(3):171–177. DOI: 10.1111/j.0042-9007.2004.00416.x.

[26] Operskalski EA, Mosley JW, Tobler LH, Feibig EW, Nowicki MJ, Mimms LT, et al. Transfusion-transmitted viruses study. Retrovirus epidemiology donor study. HCV viral load in anti-HCV reactive donors and infectivity in their recipients. Transfusion. 2003;43(10):1433–1441. DOI: 10.1046/j.1537-2995.2003.00475.x.

[27] The CST/CNTRP increased risk donor working group. Guidance on the use of increased risk donors for organ transplantation. Transplantation. 2014;00(00):00. DOI: 10.1097/TP.0000000000000251.

[28] Chung RT, Feng S, Delmonico FL. Approach to the management of allograft recipients following the detection of hepatitis B virus in the prospective organ donor.. Am J Transplant. 2001;1(2):185/191. DOI: 10.1034/ j.1600-6143.2001.10214.x.

[29] Chazouilleres O, Mamish D, Kim M, Carey K, Farrell L, Roberts JP, et al. "Occult" hepatitis B virus as source of infection in liver transplant recipients. Lancet. 1994;343(8890):142–146. DOI: 10.1016/S0140-6736(94)90934-2

[30] Uemoto S, Sugiyama K, Marusawa H, Inomata Y, Asonuma K, Egawa H, et al. Transmission of hepatitis B virus from hepatitis B core antibody-positive donors in living related liver transplants. Transplantation. 1998;65(4):494–499. DOI: 10.1097/00007890-199802270-00007.

[31] Cholongitas E, Papatheodoridis GV, Burroughs AK. Liver grafts from anti-hepatitis B core positive donors: a systematic review. J Hepatol. 2010;52(2):272–279. DOI: 10.1111/j.1477-2574.2011.00399.x.

[32] Ouseph R, Eng M, Ravindra K, Brock GN, Buell JF, Marvin MR. Review of the use of hepatitis B core antibody-positive donors. Transplant Rev (Orlando). 2010;24(4):167–171. DOI: 10.1016/j.trre.2010.05.001.

[33] Raimondo G, Allain J, Brunetto MR, Buendia MA, Chen DS, Colombo M, et al. Statements from the Taormina expert meeting on occult hepatitis B virus infection. J Hepatol. 2008;49(4):652–657. DOI: 10.1016/j.jhep.2008.07.014.

[34] Allain JP. Occult hepatitis B virus infection: implications in transfusion. Vox Sang. 2004;86(2):83–91. DOI: 10.1111/j.0042-9007.2004.00406.x.

[35] Fang Y, Shang QL, Liu JY, Li D, Xu WZ, Teng X, et al. Prevalence of occult hepatitis B virus infection among hepatopathy patients and healthy people in China. J Infect. 2009;58(8):383–388. DOI: 10.1016/j.jinf.2009.02.013.

[36] Kim SM, Lee KS, Park CJ, Lee JY, Kim KH, Park JI, et al. Prevalence of occult HBV infection among subjects with normal serum ALT levels in Korea. J Infect. 2007;54(2): 185–191. DOI: http://dx.doi:org/10.1016/j.jinf.2006.02.002.

[37] Levrero M, Pollicino T, Petersen J, Belloni L, Raimondo G, Dandri M. Control of cccDNA function in hepatitis B virus infection. J Hepatol. 2009;51(3):581–592. DOI: 10.1016/j.jhep.2009.05.022.

[38] Zoulim F. New insight on hepatitis B virus persistence from the study of intrahepatic viral cccDNA. J Hepatol. 2005;42(3):302–308. DOI: http://dx.doi.org/10.1016/j.jhep.2004.12.015.

[39] Ramia S, Mokhbat J, Ramlawi F, El-Zaatari M. Occult hepatitis B virus infection in HIV infected Lebanese patients with isolated antibodies to hepatitis B core antigen. Int J STD AIDS. 2008;19(3):197–199. DOI: 10.1258/ijsa.2007.007200.

[40] Tseliou P, Spiliotakara A, Dimitracopoulos GO, Christofidou M. Detection of hepatitis B virus DNA in blood units with anti-HBc as the only positive serological marker. Haematologia (Budap). 2000;30(3):159–165. DOI: 10.1163/156855900300109152.

[41] Mei SD, Yatsuhashi H, Parquet MC, Hamada R, Fujino T, Matsumoto T, et al. Detection of HBV RNA in peripheral blood mononuclear cells in patients with and without HBsAg by reverse transcription polymerase chain reaction. Hepatol Res. 2000;18(1):19–28. DOI: 10.1016/S1386-6346(99)00081-9.

[42] Zaghloul H, El-Sherbiny W. Detection of occult hepatitis C and hepatitis B virus infections from peripheral blood mononuclear cells. Immunol Invest. 2010;39(3):284–291. DOI: 10.3109/08820131003605820.

[43] Raimondo G, Caccamo G, Filomia R, Pollicino T. Occult hepatitis B infection. Semin Immunopathol. 2013;35(1):39–52. DOI: 10.1007/s00281-012-0327-7.

[44] Cheung CK, Lo CM, Man K, Lau GK. Occult hepatitis B virus infection of donor and recipient origin after liver transplantation despite nucleoside analogue prophylaxis. Liver Transplant. 2010;16(11):1314–1323. DOI: 10.1002/lt.22169.

[45] MacConmara MP, Vachharajani N, Ellen JR, Anderson CD, Lowell JA, Shenoy S, et al. Utilization of hepatitis B core antibody-positive donor liver grafts. HPB (Oxford). 2012;14(1):42–48. DOI: 10.1111/j.1477-2574.2011.00399.x.

[46] Terrault N, Roche B, Samuel D. Management of the hepatitis B virus in the liver transplantation setting: a European and an American perspective. Liver Transpl. 2005;11(7):716–732. DOI: 10.1002/lt.20492.

[47] Suehiro T, Shimada M, Kishikawa K, Shimura T, Soejima Y, Yoshizumi T, et al. Prevention of hepatitis B virus infection from hepatitis B core antibody-positive donor graft using hepatitis B immune globulin and lamivudine in living donor liver transplantation. Liver Int. 2005;25(6):1169–1174. DOI: 10.1111/j.1478-3231.2005.01165.x.

[48] Candotti D, Allain J-P. Transfusion-transmitted hepatitis B infection. J Hepatol. 2009;51(4):798–809. DOI: 10.1016/j.jhep.2009.05.020.

[49] Saab S, Waterman B, Chi AC, Tong MJ. Comparison of different immunoprophylaxis regimens after liver transplantation with hepatitis B core antibody-positive donors: a systematic review. Liver Transpl. 2010;16(3):300–307. DOI: 10.1002/lt.21998.

[50] Northup PG, Argo CK, Nguyen DT, McBride MA, Kumer SC, Schmitt TM, et al. Liver allografts from hepatitis C positive donors can offer good outcomes in hepatitis C positive recipients: a US National Transplant Registry analysis. Transplant Int. 2010;23(10):1038-1044. DOI: 10.1111/j.1432-2277.2010.01092.x.

[51] Kasprzyk T, Kwiatkowski A, Wszola M, Ostrowski K, Danielewicz R, Domagala P, et al. Long-term results of kidney transplantation from HCV-positive donors. Transplant Proc. 2007;39(9):2701–2703. DOI: http://dx.doi.org/10.1016/j.transproceed.2007.09.021.

[52] Fabrizi F, Messa P, Martin P. Current status of renal transplantation from HCV-positive donors. Int J Artif Organs. 2009;32(5):251–261.

[53] Prieto M, Berenguer M, Rayon JM, Cordova J, Arguello L, Carrasco D, et al. High incidence of allograft cirrhosis in hepatitis C virus genotype 1b infection following transplantation: relationship with rejection episodes. Hepatology. 1999;29(1):250–256. DOI: 10.1002/hep.510290122.

[54] Saab S, Ghobrial RM, Ibrahim AB, Kunder G, Durazo F, Han S, et al. Hepatitis C positive grafts may be used in orthotopic liver transplantation: a matched analysis. Am J Transplant. 2003;3(9):1167–1172. DOI: 10.1034/j.1600-6143.2003.00189.x.

[55] Khapra AP, Agarwal K, Fiel MI, Kontorinis N, Hossain S, Emre S, et al. Impact of donor age on survival and fibrosis progression in patients with hepatitis C undergoing liver transplantation using HCV + allografts. Liver Transpl. 2006;12(10):1496–1503. DOI: 10.1002/lt.20849.

[56] Jacobson IM, McHutchinson JG, Dusheiko G, Di Bisceglie AM, Reddy KR, Bzowej NH, et al. Telaprevir for previously untreated chronic hepatitis C virus infection. N Eng J Med. 2011;364(25):2405–2416. DOI: 10.1056/NEJMoa1012912.

[57] Poordad F, McCone JJ, Bacon BR, Bruno S, Manns MP, Sulkowski MS, et al. Boceprevir for untreated chronic HCV genotype 1 infection. N Eng J Med. 2011;364(13):1195–1206. DOI: 10.1056/NEJMoa1010494.

[58] OPTN. Organ Procurement and Transplantation Network [Internet]. 2016 . Available from: http://optn.transplant.hrsa.gov/ [Accessed: January 1, 2016].

[59] Sela N, Croome KP, Chando N, Marotta P, Wall W, Hernandez-Alejandro R. Changing donor characteristics in liver transplantation over the last 10 years in Canada. Liver Transpl. 2013;19(11):1236–1244. DOI: 10.1002/lt.23718.

[60] Kamath PS, Kim WR. The model for end-stage liver disease (MELD). Hepatology. 2007;45(3):797–805. DOI: 10.1002/hep.21563.

[61] UNOS. PELD/MELD Calculator [Internet]. 2015. Available from: https://www.unos.org/wp-content/uploads/unos/MELD_PELD_Calculator_Documentation.pdf [Accessed: December 12, 2015].

[62] Feng S, Goodrich NP, Bragg-Gresham JL, Dykstra DM, Punch JD, DebRoy MA, et al. Characteristics associated with liver graft failure: the concept of a donor risk index. Am J Transplant. 2006;6(4):783–790. DOI: 10.1111/j.1600-6143.2006.01242.x.

[63] Blok JJ, Braat AE, Adam R, Burroughs AK, Putter H, Kooreman NG, et al. Validation of the donor risk index in orthotopic liver transplantation within the Eurotransplant Region. Liver Transpl. 2012;18(1):113–120. DOI: 10.1002/lt.22447.

[64] Maluf DG, Edwards EB, Stravitz RT, Kauffman HM. Impact of the donor risk index on the outcome of hepatitis C virus-positive liver transplant recipients. Liver Transpl. 2009;15(6):592–599. DOI: 10.1002/lt.21699.

[65] Rosemberg LH, Guillen JG, Hranjec T, Stokes JB, Brayman KL, Kumer SC, et al. Donor risk index predicts graft failure reliably but not post-transplant infections. Surg Infect. 2014;15(2):94–98. DOI: 10.1089/sur.2013.035.

[66] Schaubela DE, Guidingerb MK, Bigginsd SW, Kalbfleischa JD, Pomfrete EA, Sharmaf P, et al. Survival benefit-based deceased-donor liver allocation. Am J Transplant. 2009;9(4 Pt 2):970–981. DOI: 10.1111/j.1600-6143.2009.02571.x.

[67] UK Government. Guidance on the Microbiological Safety of human Organs, Tissues and Cells used in Transplantation [Internet]. 2011. Available from: https://www.gov.uk/government/uploads/system/uploads/attachment_data/file/215959/dh_130515.pdf [Accessed: December 3, 2015].

[68] EDQM. Guide to the Quality and Safety of Organs for Transplantation [Internet]. 2013. Available from: https://www.edqm.eu/medias/fichiers/leaflet_on_organ_transplantation_guide_5th_edition.pdf [Accessed: December 5, 2015].

[69] Baleriola C, Webster AC, Rawlinson WD. Characterization and risk of bloodborne virus transmission in organ transplantation: what are the priorities? Future Virol. 2014;9(12): 1049–1060. DOI: 10.2217/FVL.14.94.

[70] Grossi PA, Fishman JA, AST Infectious Disease Community of Practice. Donor-derived infections in solid organ transplant recipients. Am J Transplant. 2009;9(Suppl 4):S19–S26. DOI: 10.1111/j.1600-6143.2009.02889.x.

[71] Fischer SA, Avery RK, AST infectious disease community of practice. Screening of donor and recipient prior to solid organ transplantation. Am J Transplant. 2009;9(Suppl 4):S7–S18. DOI: 10.1111/j.1600-6143.2009.02888.x.

[72] Scandia Transplant. Guidelines for the Prevention of Transmission of Infectious Diseases from Organ Donors to Recipients [Internet]. 2015. Available from: http://www.scandiatransplant.org/organ-allocation/ScandtxInfGuidelines2015incEbola_5.pdf [Accessed: November 15, 2015].

[73] Europa EC. The Eustite Project [Internet]. 2013. Available from: http://ec.europa.eu/chafea/documents/health/conference_27-28_06_2013/EUSTITE [Accessed: November 6, 2015].

[74] Notify Project. Notify Library [Internet]. 2013. Available from: http://www.notifylibrary.org [Accessed: December 12, 2015].

[75] OPTN. Ad Hoc Disease Transmission Advisory Committee (DTAC) [Internet]. 2015. Available from: http://optn.transplant.hrsa.gov/converge/members/committeesDetail.asp?ID=95 [Accessed: December 23, 2015].

[76] ANZOD & ANZDATA. ANZDATA [Internet]. 2015. Available from: http://anzdata.org.au/ [Accessed: December 20, 2015].

2

Family-Centered Care to Improve Family Consent for Organ Donation

Maria Grazia Bocci, Alessia Prestifilippo, Ciro D'Alò, Alessandro Barelli, Massimo Antonelli, Emiliano Cingolani, Alessandra Tersali, Alessandra Ionescu Maddalena and Roberta Barelli

Abstract

The need for organ donation has increased over time, but the shortage of available donors is the major limiting factor in transplantation. Organ donation refusal from relatives of potential donors with brain death significantly reduces organ availability. We report a brief analysis about family conflicts in decision-making and causes for refusing donation; moreover, we describe new family-centered strategies in the intensive care unit (ICU) and our systematic communication approach between medical staff and patients' relatives. In 2016 we conducted a single-center, non-randomized, controlled and before and after study in our ICU, an 18-bed intensive care unit (ICU) of a university hospital. We compared the rate of consent for organ donation before and after the introduction of the new communication approach. The application of a new communication approach between medical staff and relatives of brain-dead patients was associated with a significant increase in the rate of consent to donation. The positive results of the 3-year period 2013–2015 have been confirmed in the 2-year period 2016–2017. Our results highlight the importance of empathy and counselor support of relatives in the ICU.

Keywords: organ donation, patient-centered care, intensive care, family

1. Introduction

The number of donors is inadequate although the need of organ transplant has increased over recent decades [1–4]. Most of the organs available for transplantation come from deceased rather than living donors. Then, patients who have been declared brain death are the largest source of transplantable organs. The consensus rate improvement of solid organ donation from deceased donors is considered one of the main strategies to increase the availability of organs for transplantation. Unfortunately, a low percentage of people register their donation wishes in life. Furthermore the laws concerning individual consent expressed previously in life are dissimilar in different countries; above all, the population's adhesion to the law may not be comparable so that family members are often the only ones that can express consent to organ donation. Although the main factor limiting the number of donations from brain-dead potential donors is the low rate of consent from their families. Furthermore, in the clinical practice, even when the patient has registered their will on the organ donors' registry and there is no legal obligation to obtain consent from the relatives, if a relative denies the consent, organ donation may not proceed [5, 6]. The consensus rate improvement of solid organ donation from deceased donors is considered one of the main strategies to increase the availability of organs for transplantation. They get the bad news about the possibility and then of their loved one's death in a short time. The settings where family members receive this information are intensive care or emergency areas, unfamiliar, unknown and often confusing places. Several studies examined the reason why some potential donors' families refuse consent, while the others analyzed a series of "modifiable" factors related to meeting with the family(s) especially. Kerri Barber et al. in 2006 reported the results of an interesting audit of all deaths in intensive care units (ICUs) from 1 April 2003 to 31 March 2005 regarding 341 intensive care units in 284 hospitals in the United Kingdom [7].

Among the relatives of 2320 potential heart-beating donors who were approached for donation consent, 41% refused. The main reason for refusal is the knowledge of the desire not to donate expressed by the deceased person in life (16%). In the last 20 years different studies have emphasized how privacy and request timing, the involvement in the patient care team that gives information to the family of at least one member of the staff of organ procurement and a care to brain death significance explanation are key factors to improve relationships [8–10]. Furthermore several authors pointed out that religious, cultural and social beliefs play an important role in the family's decision-making process. Besides, concerns on exact time of death and body integrity after death and emotional vulnerability are equally crucial. The process is also influenced by education, income, sex and age of the family members [6, 7, 9, 10]. There are many relationship elements and emotions involved in the donation process. Ignoring family's emotions without taking care of the relational aspects can hamper fully aware choices. De Groot and colleagues in 2015 reported the results of a qualitative research in a group of donors' relatives regarding the decision-making donation process. We reported the main results of this research in this context. The authors confirm how the stressful sudden event, the interaction with unknown people, the difficulty of mourning and making a decision for the loved one whose loss is being wept over are determinant factors in the decision-making process of the family. The occurrence rapidity does not allow us to be aware of the reality we are experiencing and of any decisions that must, in any case, be taken. The potential donors' relatives describe the decision-making process as complex mainly because they had to make a decision on behalf of the deceased (surrogate decision). The conditions that might contribute to this complexity are the feeling of having limited time and a sense of urgency, the feeling of not being competent to decide and a sense of despair and crisis and the need for an agreement between all relatives. The ethical considerations regarding the possibility of helping others, the integrity of the body and life after death reveal the emotions and personal motivations coming into play going beyond the event itself and the immediate and concrete decisions that family members are called to take [11]. Vincent A et al. also reported the common reasons for family refusal: relatives not wishing surgery to the body (concerns regarding disfigurement), feelings that the patient has suffered enough, feeling incompetent regarding the patient's wishes, disagreements among the family group, religious/cultural reasons, dissatisfaction with the health-care staff and process, concerns over delay to the funeral/burial process, inability to accept death, lack of understanding of brain death, concerns regarding integrity of process and the fact that they were emotionally exhausted themselves.

The same authors pointed out that several studies come to the conclusion that following elements could be useful [12]:

1. Guaranteeing the right timing of a request
2. Guaranteeing an appropriate setting
3. Providing emotional support
4. Imparting specific information (e.g. regarding the nature of brain death)
5. Guaranteeing adequate staff training
6. Guaranteeing staff involvement in a planned process of the organ donation request

Italy as a whole is undoubtedly the country that has developed a model similar to the Spanish one. Spain has become a reference point for European and global solid organs donation and transplantation with the highest donation rates. Italy has a cultural and health structure similar to Spain and it is needed to create an organizational structure since the 1999 law [13, 14]. In 1988, the Council of Europe Committee of Experts on Transplantation (SP-CTO) was established. The Committee included more than 30 countries with observatories from Canada, Japan and Israel and was incorporated by the Eastern countries for which it represented the only contact with the great Western countries' transplant referents for many years. The Organización Nacional de Trasplantes (ONT) held the presidency of this Committee for 7 years (1995–2000 and 2003–2005). The majority of the documents you need as a basis for the preparation of the Commission and the European Parliament actions on transplants have been processed in Spain. Following the approval of Article 157 of the Amsterdam Treaty, the European Union has developed the European directives on transplantation, guaranteeing the quality and safety of the tissue and cell organs. In May 2003, the Executive Council of the World Health Organization (WHO) accepted to set up an international group of experts to examine the issues related to transplants, including xenotransplantation. Spain is the promoter of a punctual organization in the field of transplants that Italy has been sharing. In particular, Italy shares with Spain the following key points regarding transplantation.

- The health status of a country or region is also affected by a good functioning of the donation transplantation system. This is conditioned and conditions a good quality health system
- A training program is needed for intensive care and operating theaters' doctors who work with potential and receiving donors

Spain has collaborated very actively organizing different types of courses some of which specifically concern family members' interviews. The proximity between Italy and Spain and the similarity of the language facilitate the collaboration process between the two countries. Italy currently has a three-level (national, regional and hospital) transplant system organization and a training system that follows the Spanish model. Initially, the percentage of refusal to donate was quite high; currently, the percentage of waste is about 30% and it has been stable for some years. We believe we can still do a lot to reduce this waste amount. The WHO provides technical support for the correct development in the field of transplants, promotes international cooperation and continues the examination and collection of global data on allogeneic transplantation safety, quality, efficacy and ethics.

The work strategy adopted to implement donations is based on a process called global base of knowledge about transplant (GKT) defined in resolution WHA57.18. The GKT consists of four lines of work that require progressive development and includes the following aspects:

- GKT1: It includes activities and practices in allogeneic transplants.
- GKT2: It includes allogeneic transplants legislation and organizational systems. The main objective of the registry is to gather information on organs, tissues and cell donation and transplantation activities, as well as information on the legislative and organizational aspects of transplantation all over the world and to make professionals and the general public know them.
- GKT3: It includes response to transplants, risks, survival and surveillance systems, safety aspects and ethical aspects. Creating systems is considered a surveillance priority that guarantees transplants safety, so that any effects and adverse reactions, both in receiving and in living donors, can be communicated to take any necessary measures. From an ethical point of view, it is intended to obtain information on the measures taken from member states to protect the poorest and most vulnerable groups, for example, from organ and tissue trade.
- GKT4: It includes xenotransplantation. Xenotransplantation could be the alternative to the lack of human origin organs and tissues. However, experimental preclinical tests haven't justified human clinical trials yet. Transparency is a fundamental and mandatory requirement for the WHO in donation and transplantation-related practices, as well as in information collected around the world.

To find out more about the world situation regarding organ transplants, we recommend the website [2].

No religious beliefs preclude organ donation; people usually refer to personal conscience. The national frame guarantees quality and safety for the donor and the receiver [15].

With regard to all that was mentioned above, we believe that optimizing the relationship with the potential donors' relatives might represent the main organ procurement strategy. The intensive care setting is the place where this relationship can be created.

The past two decades witnessed an increasing interest in the importance of health-care humanization. The recent guidelines suggest organized interventions and approaches aimed at supporting the families of critical patients. The objectives are twofold: to reduce the impact of serious illness and to prepare family members for decision-making and assistance needs. An international consensus recognized a new definition: "family" and "family-centered care" to identify this approach. The term "family" intends to identify a group of individuals who support the patient and with whom the patient has a significant relationship. "Family-centered care" is a respectful and responsive approach to health-care that meets the needs and values of individual families and is mainly characterized by: family presence in the ICU, family support and communication with family members. Family members will not only be present within the ICU but also actively participate in the care process. It is recommended that validated tools exist to optimize communication quality, medical understanding and reduce family decision-making conflicts, in setting the ICU up. Care practitioners must apply standardized and agreed communication approaches with family members of deceased patients and above all for those who died with brain-death criteria, especially [16]. Seaman J.B. and colleagues in Annals ATS (2017) suggest that the goals of clinician-family communication should be diversified and concern different aspects [17]. We very much share the elements discussed by these authors and we comment on some of them that seem relevant and in line with our choices. First of all, it is about establishing trust. The most important element of the quality of care for seriously ill patients' family members is the condition of trust in the care team. Sharing the decision-making process requires trust in the care team and at the same time allows to achieve a more stable relationship with the family members. Because family members can decide (when they are called on to do so) they must understand what has happened (and what the clinical consequences are), the effect of the choices on the beloved and the risks and benefits of the shared pathway. The second one is providing emotional support. ICU patients' family members have high levels of emotional stress and experience intense negative emotions such as fear and anxiety. These feelings are exacerbated by the communication of the bad news (death or threat of death) and by the decision-making process itself. Research in the neuropsychological field suggests that strong negative emotions such as fear and anxiety do not allow processing information detaching the subject from the reality (as already mentioned above). Therefore, attention to the relationship also allows us to devote a time to recognize emotions and reflect on them. Third element is conveying clinical information. Clinicians should take into account that family members should be informed in a clear, simple and precise manner regarding the diagnosis, prognosis and possibilities of patient treatment. Families need to be involved in the decision-making process. Lack of correct information can lead family members not to take the right decisions for the patient as well as being a source of stress and frustration. The authors confirm the importance of the interdisciplinary team role (involving psychologists, social workers, volunteers, care coordinators and communication facilitator) to improve family satisfaction and decrease psychological symptoms.

2. Our experience and discussion

2.1. New communication approach

Since 2013, as we have recently published, we developed a new communication approach addressed to relatives of patients admitted to the intensive care unit (ICU) ([18], with permission]). It consists of a patient/relative-centered approach, in which doctors, nurses, psychologists and volunteers support relatives throughout the care process. First, they try to acquire information on the family's social and cultural background and adjust the communication accordingly and second, they aim to understand the patient's will, a task that can be challenging in the intensive care context. When the patient first enters the ICU, the physician must give priority to treatment and can only speak briefly to the relatives. He reassures them that there will soon be time to acquire information and ask questions. As soon as the patient's conditions allow an interview with the relatives is performed so as to establish a relationship between the physician and the family. The physician who followed the patient's acute phase, the nurse who is in charge of him or her and a psychotherapist or a psychologist conducts it in a dedicated room. The staff also takes note of the relatives' phone numbers. The following interviews take place in the patient's room. During the first interview, the medical staff harmonizes on the needs and feelings of the family and retraces the patient's history and the recent acute event. This interview also aims to identify the main caregivers and establish the timetable and program for the following days. We applied a well-defined model, which can be divided into several steps:

1. Giving a warm welcome to the patient and his family unit;
2. Identification of the caregiver among the family members;
3. Taking care of the patient and relatives in a multidisciplinary way;
4. Early involvement of a psychotherapist;
5. Communication to the family in the patient's room;
6. Giving information on the patients' clinical conditions by the physician, the nurse and in presence of a psychotherapist and a volunteer;
7. Communication between the family and the psychotherapist and volunteer, with special regard to the family members' emotions and feelings.

2.2. Relationship with donors' families

The changes in the interaction modalities with family members and with the patient, when possible, have been consolidated since 2013 in our ICU; the changes represented a structured intervention. We believe that the new relationship's modalities with the patients' relatives, so far exposed and described in their reliability, have favorably influenced the reduction of opposition to organ donation by the family members of the deceased patient. Our ICU is an 18-bed, multidisciplinary ICU. It is a referral center for acute respiratory failure as well as a trauma center. Relatives of brain-dead patients were approached according to an internal protocol, inspired by NICE guidelines, which temporarily distinguishes two phases: communicating brain death and proposing organ donation. These guidelines deal with delivering the end-of-life communication and developing a supportive relationship with potential beating-heart donors' families [19]. Often, patients who develop brain death did not express their opinion on organ donation during their lifetime. In our ICU all patients and relatives including relatives of brain-dead patients have been approached by the medical staff to establish a relationship since 2013, aiming at making them feel better and understood. The number of acceptances to organ donation in our intensive care was observed before and after the implementation of two major interventions: the opening of the intensive care (project called "OpenICU") to relatives and the introduction of the innovative communication approach mentioned above. Opening ICUs should come about not so much in answer to pressure generated by a growing social awareness, or in simple recognition of a right, but because this policy addresses more comprehensively the issue of respect for the patient, as well as providing more appropriate responses to many needs of both patients and families. It is a decision which requires doctors and nurses to rethink their relationships with patients and their families, which calls for original solutions for each individual situation and which should be subject to periodic checks. Psychotherapists support the relatives in finding a meaning to their experience and to understanding their own reaction and attitude. Further elements could have positively influenced the decline in organ donation, such as:

1. Increased attention to the initial welcome to the patient and his family;
2. The creation of a multidisciplinary team, giving a new value to non-medical figures, such as psychologists and volunteers;
3. The enhancement of giving information in the patient's room.

The Open ICU is realized when the whole team aims to abolish all of the unnecessary limitations at a temporal, physical and relational level. Opening the ward to family members allows patients and their relatives to be actively involved, fueling the healing process through affection and contact with their beloved. Besides, it helps patients to better tolerate hospitalization. When the Open ICU first opened, an innovative concept was introduced: interview with relatives no longer took place in a separate and impersonal "medical staff room." It was moved into the patients' room. This gave the opportunity for relatives to be physically close to their beloved while receiving bad news. This physical nearness soothes the relatives' grief. Being in the patients' room means sharing the environment with him or her: they hear the same sounds, feel the same temperature and see the same colors. The patient, his family and the physician now share the same scene. The relationship is still asymmetrical as the physician decides what to do and is trusted. However, the patient and his family are now considered as central elements of the scene. In fact, during the interview, there is an exchange of information between the physician and the family; the former is open to questions and doubts expressed by relatives, reducing errors related to a subjective interpretation of reality. Rather than speaking to the patient's family, the physician speaks with the patient's family. Conducting the interview in the patient's room also facilitates questions on machines and therapies with which relatives are not familiar. Apart from verbal expressions, body language (which comprehends movements toward or from the patient, facial expressions, position of the relatives in the room) is part of the relationship between physician/nurse and the patient's family. In this regard, the interview taking place in the patient's room recalls the historical role of the doctor, who visited patients at home. Just as in the past, the doctor moves toward the patient. This movement is symbolically meaningful in the relationship. We think it is also important to recognize the emotions of both the family and the physician, who are all involved by seeing the patient while the interview takes place. The physician, the patient and the relatives recreate a family unit, giving more humanity to a very difficult moment that involves communication of the ICU patient's condition.

Besides, there are a few gimmicks that help improve the family's comprehension and memorization of information:

1. Communicate one piece of information at a time, in a specific, accurate and coherent way, "need to be honest, but should aim to mitigate the stress rather than exacerbating the fear and uncertainty";
2. Explain the patient's priorities in that moment;
3. Invite the family member to ask questions;
4. Verify that family members have understood what is explained to them.

The interview with relatives has several functions: it is informative, it is clarifying and it contains the family's emotional reactions. This last one is paramount in an ICU, where patients' deaths or losses of functional capacities can take place unpredictably. Historically, trust in doctors has been an unconditional feeling. During emergencies and critical events, families have no choice but to trust physicians, who are in charge of their relative's lives. Nevertheless, this trust must be respected and preserved because it is no longer unconditional. Nowadays, it is based on the physician's empathy with the relatives' emotions and on giving explanations to their worries and questions. By taking the family's emotions in charge, the physician creates a trustworthy relationship with them and can then make realistic predictions of survival and prognosis with them, also facing the topic of terminal illness. Many patients experience anxiety because of hospitalization and the impending threat to their lives. Similarly, psychotherapists help relatives to decrease their level of anxiety, allowing them to experience the ward as a more "human place," where there is space for relationships with the caregivers, who respond to help requests and throughout which emotions can be shared. The physician respectfully listens to the patient's or relatives' worries, allowing them to elaborate their emotions. At the same time, the physician conveys clear information authoritatively, though in a sensitive and truthful way. This is identified by Castagna as a counseling relationship, through which individuals develop awareness of their experiences and needs. Thanks to such relationship, patients manage to handle a challenging moment of their life by expanding their inner strength, even when reduced by critical illness. By communicating, we improve our shared knowledge, the so-called "common sense," the essential precondition to the existence of a community. Among the multidisciplinary team, a special mention must be addressed to nurses. Nurses are probably the health-care professionals who spend more time with patients. Because of the Open ICU, they often work while relatives are in the room and most of the time not in the presence of physicians. For these reasons, they are in charge of explaining to the relatives what physicians told them during the interview. Their relationship with the patient and with relatives is unique and contributes meaningfully to the care-taking process. Even though they are not professionals, volunteers act as a connection between the world outside the hospital and the ICU. When nurses and physicians are occupied in emergencies or in routine clinical activity, relatives find an important referral in volunteers.

Potential donor patients' family members receive a favorable impact from the host, support and relationship strategies described so far. When brain death is declared, the family is entrusted by the care team to a dedicated team of the organ procurement. Relatives of brain-dead patients were approached according to an internal protocol, inspired by NICE guidelines, which temporarily distinguishes two phases: communicating brain death and proposing organ donation. These guidelines deal with delivering the end-of-life communication and developing a supportive relationship with potential heart-beating donor families.

The end-of-life communication recognized the following seven details:

Suggested locations: doctor's office, conference room, relatives meeting room, no hallways and common areas.

Meeting participants: intensive care specialist in charge of the decedent's care, nurse appointed to provide specific support, physician and nurse in charge of the transplant coordination system, family members wishing to be informed and psychotherapist. It is crucial that both staffs are present during this phase: the medical staff in charge of the patient, which will introduce the transplant coordination system staff.

Environment arrangements: sitting in a circle, if possible, access to phone calls, paper handkerchiefs, glasses and water. Avoid placing writing desks between the speakers and the relatives. Do not behave/act with detachment or indifference: avoid folded arms, fisting and fiddling; do not look away from the interlocutor; do not speak in a formal or distant way.

Delivering the communication (how and when): only after the first observation to assess the patient's death according to the Italian legislation. The assessment declaration is clearly and simply formulated by the intensive care specialist: "The EEG tracing we've just performed reveals the absence of brain electrical activity, there are no reactions to external stimulation, and the patient is not able to breathe autonomously. These circumstances unfortunately describe a death diagnosis. The legal-medical procedure to assess brain death has just started, and it will go on for 6 hours. At the end of the 6 hours, we will stop the artificial respiration procedure that is now keeping the heartbeating." A summary of the patient's clinical and therapeutic history can be added. Verify that relatives understand the meaning of brain death.

Developing a supportive relationship: give the family the appropriate time to react to the communication. Do not try to control or limit their reaction. Let them express rejection, denial, incredulity, anger, violent anger, desperation and so forth.

Medical personnel cope with reactions caused by the end-of-life communication: keep a silent and empathic behavior. Take care of actual necessities such as drinking, making telephone calls and handkerchiefs. Listen empathically to the relatives' memories on the patient's life and on the history of the illness that caused his death (accident dynamics, health-care delays, diagnosis mistakes, disappointed expectations on surgery and treatments, family problems, and so forth). Do not make obvious or inappropriate statements such as: "I'm so sorry for you," "I can understand your pain," "I know you're angry and I understand this," and so forth.

Visiting the bed: the nurse was appointed to support the family or the transplant nurse coordinator introduced themselves and their job. They take the relatives wishing to visit the patient to the patient's bed. Group visits are allowed (according to the size of the patient's room), preferably after the first reactions to the communication of death. The nurse answers to every question about heartbeat after death in a simple way: ".heartbeats and blood pressure are still being monitored because the heart is beating. We are sending oxygen to the heart artificially with a ventilator that is pumping air into the lungs but, unfortunately, there is no brain activity. The patient is not able to breathe autonomously and his chest is still moving just because of the ventilator." The nurse can offer the assistance of a religious person to administer the last rites and pray with the family.

A donation proposal recognized a following four details:

Suggested location: doctor's office, conference room, relatives' meeting room, no hallways and common areas.

Participants: intensive care specialist in charge of the patient's care, nurse appointed to provide specific support, physician and nurse in charge of the transplant coordination system, family members wishing to be informed and psychotherapist.

Environment arrangements: sitting in a circle, if possible, access to phone calls, paper handkerchiefs, glasses and water. Avoid placing writing desks between the speakers and the relatives.

Delivering the communication (how and when): The organ and/or tissue donation proposal follows in all cases the death communication, the bed visit and the last farewell. Before the donation proposal, it is advisable to give a brief summary of the patient's clinical conditions, focusing on the seriousness of initial conditions and prognosis. The donation proposal is communicated in a direct and simple way: "we propose to you an act of solidarity toward people who are in critical conditions. We propose to donate organs of your relative." Provide detailed information on the organ donation process and on its potential benefits. The proposal can be followed by a moment of privacy for the family to discuss and decide.

The Italian Transplant Coordination System monitors, audits and oversees organ donation, harvesting and transplant in our country. The Italian Transplant System controls organ donation, allocation and transplant; it is organized into three levels: National (National Transplant Center), Regional (Regional Transplant Center) and Hospital (Hospital Transplant Center). The Fondazione Agostino Gemelli Hospital Catholic University is one of the major regional hospitals in Italy. As one of the five level-1 regional hospitals in Lazio, it has approximately 1600 beds and 95,000 accesses per year. It is one of the leading centers for identification of patients who have been declared dead with neurological criteria. Our intervention could have a beneficial effect on the rate of consent to organ donation (COD) by the relatives of brain-dead patients. To test this hypothesis, we compared the rate of COD before and after the implementation of the protocol into our ICU [13]. In our work we analyzed the family consent rate (potential and real donors' ratio) before and after the introduction of the new communication protocol. We observed that a consent rate increased from 71% in the pre-intervention period (2007–2012) to 78.4% in the post-intervention period (2013–2015) with a specific increase of 82.75% from 2014 to 2015. In 2017, we observed a consent rate of 78.6% with a steady rise in the number of identified potential donors. At the same time we registered the regional consent rate of 68.1 and 73.1% in 2016 and 2017, respectively. During these periods, no significant variation of organ donation consent has been recorded at a national level. Our center has kept a constant commitment in increasing the observation rates, keeping the opposition to COD rate unvaried at first and then contributing to reduce it significantly. On the whole, the center's opposition rate compared with both national and regional average is significantly lower: 2017: national, 28%; regional: Lazio, 27%; our ICU, 21% (**Figures 1** and **2**).

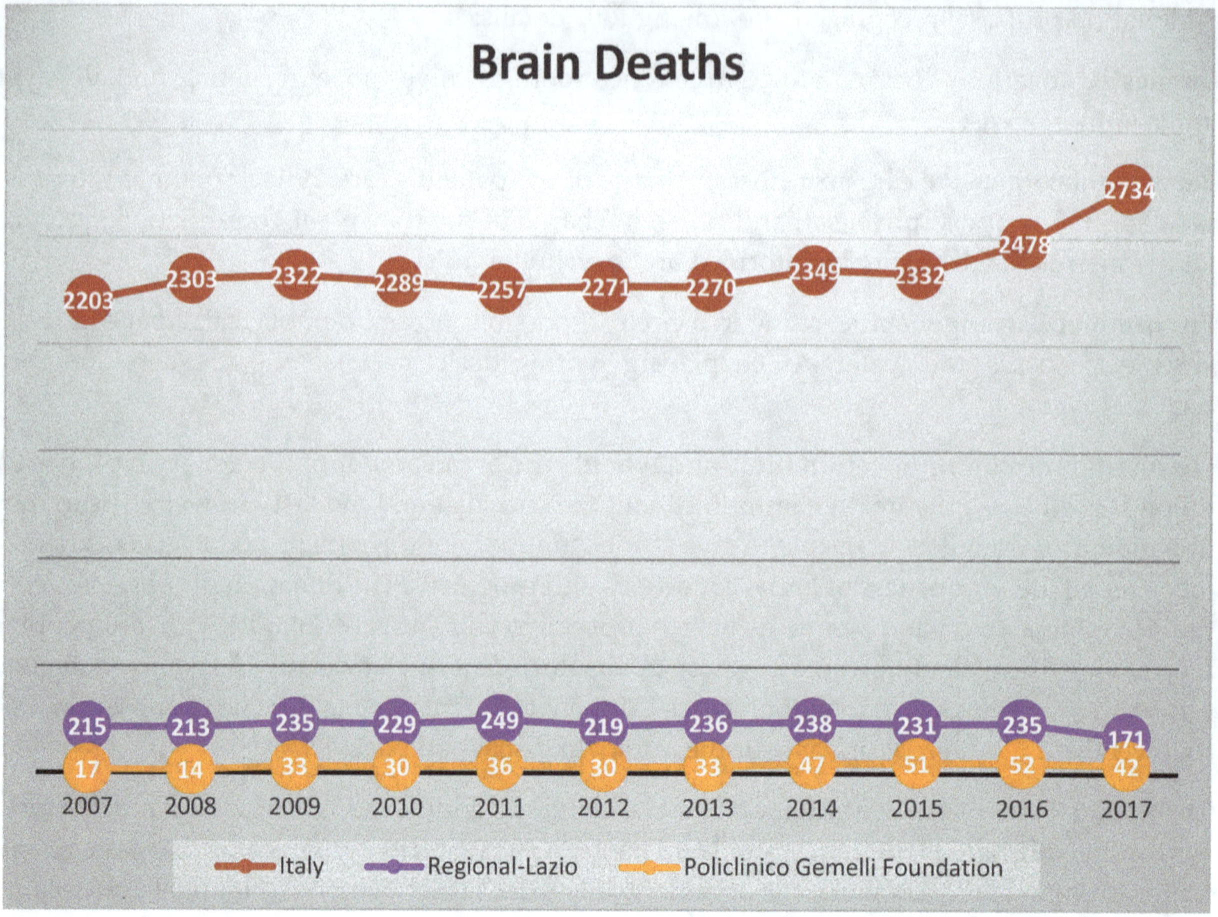

Figure 1. Brain deaths.

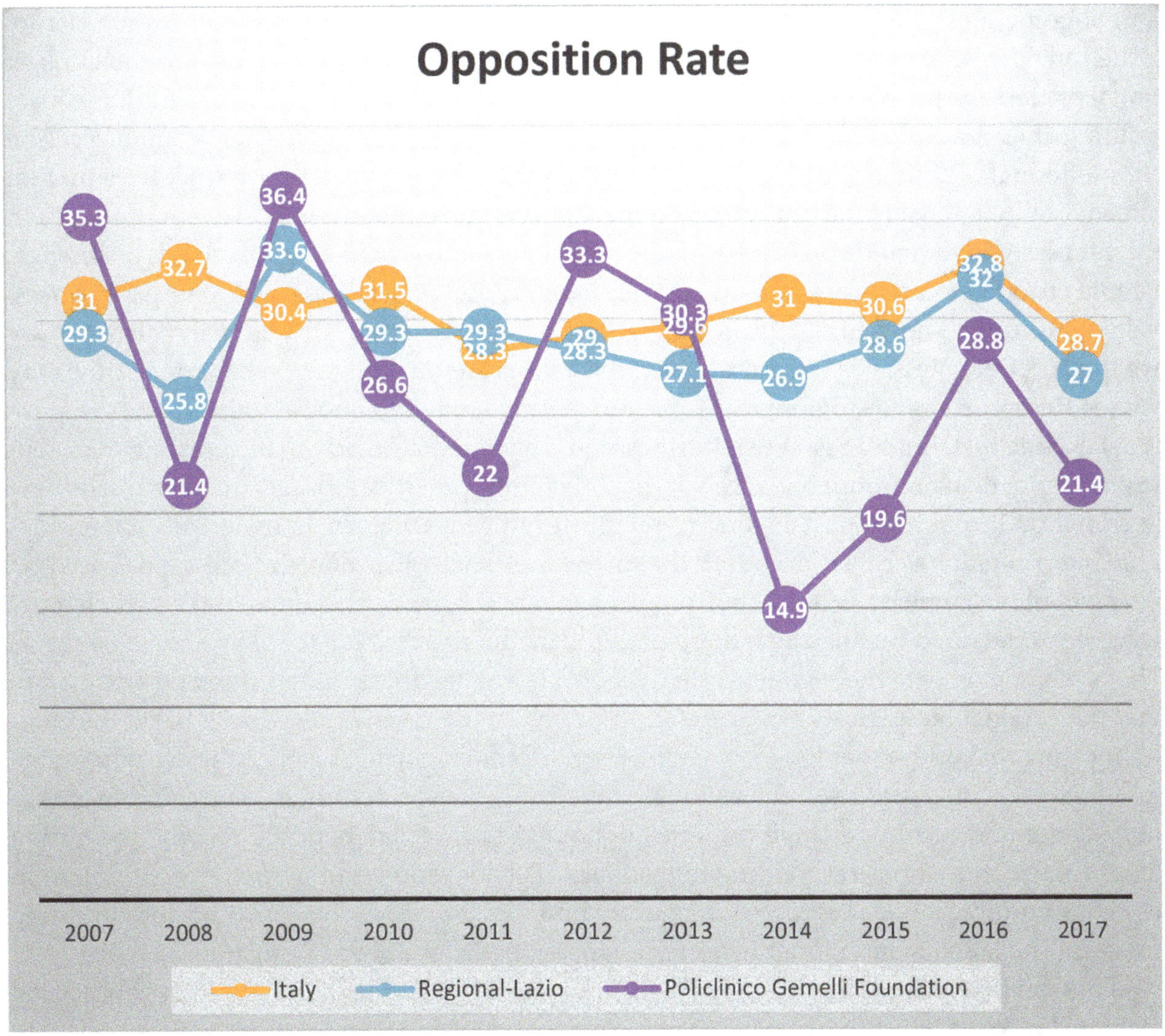

Figure 2. Opposition rates.

In our opinion, in order to suggest behavioral strategies to the care team involved in the assistance of potential donors and their family members, the following factors must be taken into account: family members are facing an acute event and high stress conditions; they may find different nursing teams and different people giving information they first learn about the life-threatening conditions and then about the death of the beloved. In this sudden critical situation, they are asked to take the place of the dear deceased, to make decisions about his body on his behalf. Family members have an extreme difficulty in contacting a condition of understandable reality. This is worsened by the fact of being in an unknown place, with unknown faces managing with emotions and personal convictions. Clinicians in the ICU should use structured approaches to communication including active listening, expression of empathy and considering the importance of explanation care. Communication is the process of sending or receiving messages through verbal and non-verbal means; therefore, an information field may consist of one or more subfields of information items such as thoughts, emotions and ideas. When, among individuals or among an individual and a group, there is a collaborative and ongoing message exchange, aimed to understand each other, the communication is integrated in our social realities and we can define this process as "transactional." In the transactional process the people involved in the act of communicating are actively and simultaneously sending information as well as receiving them. Participants perceive their communication as intentional. The information transfer between them takes place in a particular situation affected by relationship and culture. The speaker and the audience are co-communicators in the process with equal responsibility and power to create, as well as understand, a message. People encode their messages based on their own unique perceptions. Our past experiences, values, attitudes, knowledge, culture and feelings all influence our messages and also the way we interpret the messages of others. These influences are our unique perceptions or the way we see things around us. Before messages can be transmitted to another person or group, we must encode these messages. When the message is encoded it's ready to be transmitted or sent to another person or group. The receiver must then interpret the message, by filtering the new information through his past experiences, culture, attitudes, values, knowledge and feelings. This interpretation is called decoding the message. The receiver decodes messages based on his perceptions, which are different from the sender. The sender needs to make sure that the receiver understood the message; therefore, it is the receiver's job to convey a message back. The receiver's reply to the sender is called feedback. The feedback allows the sender to ensure that the original message was interpreted correctly by the receiver. Feedback helps the communicators make sure that the message has been decoded correctly. Once the cycle has gone full circle, it will repeat itself for as long as the conversation continues. We could even say that sender and receiver change roles throughout the process depending on who is sending the message and who is responding to feedback. The location and the time (the situation) in which communication takes place are relevant and they influence the encoding and decoding process. The latter is paramount in an ICU, where deaths or losses of functional capacities of patients can take place unpredictably. Historically, trust in doctors has been an unconditional feeling. The clinician should know all the elements described that are particularly relevant in the relationship with the potential donors' families. Family members often have difficulty understanding the condition of brain death. Their loved one still has a beating heart and a present breath (although assisted by the machine). The elaboration of death in this condition is not always simple. The doctor also needs to share the consent to the donation as soon as possible with the relatives. A narrative approach can be very useful to create a relationship of trust and support. The critical event causing the current situation is reported as telling a child a story already known. The narrative will describe the growing role of health-care workers who enter the history of the relatives and of the beloved. The care practitioners make supportive statements around non-abandonment and decision-making. We advise to remember the continuous need of feedback and of narrative approach. We also believe it is essential that ICU clinicians receive family-centered communication training as an element of critical care training to improve clinician self-efficacy and family satisfaction. These explanations promote a relationship in the here and now when both health-care practitioners and family members experience a state of stress and intense emotions. Knowing and seeing what is happening to the loved one, feeling part of and understanding the healing process is preferable to the anxiety generated by what is "unknown." Family members are forced by their relative's illness into an unwanted role, which provokes discomfort, dependence and anxiety. The relative is vulnerable and asking for help; the doctor and the nurse, who are experts in medical care, take him or her in charge. Developing a good therapeutic and empathic relationship with the family, taking care of their emotional issues during this process, appears to lead families to opt for donation. The relationship with the care practitioners and family members can allow the creation of a sense of reality of the place and the moment. Then, it can make the relative aware of himself, of the event, of recognizing roles and responsibilities, to give permission to emotions and decision-making power to what is recognized as right and achievable. When considering patients in critical conditions admitted in the ICU, the care-taking process of the medical staff is addressed toward relatives more than toward patients, who continue to receive high-quality care. Clinically speaking, the communication-based relationship has a central role and a positive action on health improvement in the care process [18].

3. Conclusion

Further studies are needed to evaluate the effectiveness of an open intensive care unit and of a new systematic approach to communication between relatives and medical staff to decrease the rate of donation refusals. In our ICU, we applied this new approach based on the introduction of a multidisciplinary team and an increased attention for the patient and his family. In our single-center study, the higher increase in organ donations was registered in the 2014–2015 period, 1 year after the introduction of the new communication approach. This increase was also confirmed in the years following 2015. These results highlight the importance of effective communication with patient's relatives and the need to dedicate attention and time to them, especially in the ICU.

Author details

Maria Grazia Bocci[1], Alessia Prestifilippo[1], Ciro D'Alò[1], Alessandro Barelli[1], Massimo Antonelli[1], Emiliano Cingolani[2], Alessandra Tersali[1], Alessandra Ionescu Maddalena[1]* and Roberta Barelli[1]

*Address all correspondence to: alessandra.ionescu.m@gmail.com

1 Department of Anesthesiology and Intensive Care Medicine, Catholic University of the Sacred Heart, Rome, Italy

2 UOSD Shock and Trauma, San Camillo Forlanini Hospital, Rome, Italy

References

[1] Ministry of Health of the Republic of Italy, National Transplant Centre official website. 2016. http://www.trapianti.salute.gov.it

[2] http://www.transplant-observatory.org

[3] http://www.who.int

[4] Rahmel A. Journalist Workshop on organ donation & transplantation. Introduction to organ donation and transplantation. Frankfurt/Main. Organized by the European Commission, Directorate General for Health and Food Safety. 26 November 2014 – Brussels

[5] Ghorbani F, Khoddami-Vishteh HR, Ghobadi O, et al. Causes of family refusal for organ donation. Transplantation Proceedings. 2011;**43**:405-406. DOI:10.1016/j.transproceed.2011.01.031

[6] Simpkin AL, Robertson LC, Barber VS, Young JD. Modifiable factors influencing relatives' decision to offer organ donation: systematic review. BMJ. 2009;**339**:b991. DOI: 10.1136/bmj.b991

[7] Barber K, Falvey S, Hamilton C, Collett D, Rudge C. Potential for organ donation in the United Kingdom: audit of intensive care records. BMJ. DOI: 10.1136/bmj.38804.658183.55

[8] Franz HG, DeJong W, Wolfe SM, Nathan H, Payne D, Reitsma W, Beasley CJ. Explaining brain death: a critical feature of the donation process. Journal of Transplant Coordination. 1997 Mar;7(1):14-21. PMID: 9188394

[9] Frutos MA, Ruiz P, Requena MV, Daga D. Family refusal in organ donation: Analysis of three patterns. Transplantation Proceedings. 2002;**34**:2513-2514. PMID: 12431506

[10] Siminoff LA, Gordon N, Hewlett J, Arnold RM. Factors influencing families' consent for donation of solid organs for transplantation. JAMA. 2001;**286**:71-77. DOI:10.1001/jama.286.1.71

[11] de Groot J, van Hoek M, Hoedemaekers C, Hoitsma A, Smeets W, Vernooij-Dassen M, van Leeuwen E. Decision making on organ donation: the dilemmas of relatives of potential brain dead donors. BMC Medical Ethics. 2015;**16**:64. DOI: 10.1186/s12910-015-0057-1

[12] Vincent A, Logan L. Consent for organ donation. British Journal of Anaesthesia. 2012; **108**(S1):i80-i87. DOI: 10.1093/bja/aer353

[13] LEGGE 1° aprile 1999, n. 9. Disposizioni in materia di prelievi e di trapianti di organi e di tessuti. Pubblicata nella *Gazzetta Ufficiale* n. 87 del 15 aprile 1999

[14] Gazzetta UN. 80 del 4 Aprile 2008. MINISTERO DELLA SALUTE. DECRETO 11 marzo 2008. Integrazione del decreto 8 aprile 2000 sulla ricezione delle dichiarazioni di volontà dei cittadini circa la donazione di organi a scopo di trapianto

[15] EL MODELO ESPAÑOL de Coordinación y Trasplantes. 2.a Edición. Editor Rafael Matesanz. Grupo Aula Médica, S.L., 2008. ISBN: 978-84-7885-456-1

[16] Davidson JE, Aslakson RA, Long AC, Puntillo KA, Kross EK, Hart J, Cox CE, Wunsch H, Wickline MA, Nunnally ME, Netzer G, Kentish-Barnes N, Sprung CL, Hartog CS, Coombs M, Gerritsen RT, Hopkins RO, Franck LS, Skrobik Y, Kon AA, Scruth EA, Harvey MA, Lewis-Newby M, White DB, Swoboda SM, Cooke CR, Levy MM, Azoulay E, Curtis JR. Guidelines for Family-Centered Care in the Neonatal, Pediatric, and Adult ICU. Critical Care Medicine. 2017 Jan;**45**(1):103-128. DOI: 10.1097/CCM.0000000000002169

[17] Jennifer BS, Robert MA, Leslie PS, Douglas BW. An Integrated Framework for Effective and Efficient Communication with Families in the Adult Intensive Care Unit. Annals of the American Thoracic Society. 2017 Jun;**14**(6):1015-1020. DOI: 10.1513/AnnalsATS.201612-965OI

[18] Bocci MG, D'Alò C, Barelli R, Inguscio S, Prestifilippo A, Di Paolo S, Lochi S, Fanfarillo M, Grieco DL, Maviglia R, Caricato A, Mistraletti G, Pulitanò S, Antonelli M, Sandroni C. Taking Care of Relationships in the Intensive Care Unit: Positive Impact on Family Consent for Organ Donation. Transplantation Proceedings. 2016;**48**:3245-3250. http://dx.doi.org/10.1016/j.transproceed.2016.09.042

[19] NICE Guideline 135: Organ donation for transplantation. www.nice.org.uk/guidance/CG135

3

Living Donor Liver Transplantation for Hepatocellular Carcinoma

Chih-Che Lin,

Ahmed Mohammed Abdel Aziz Elsarawy and

Chao-Long Chen

Abstract

Hepatocellular carcinoma (HCC) is a major worldwide health problem, which is expected to increase steadily due to different underlying liver diseases. Surgical treatment modalities including liver transplantation (LT) or liver resection (LR) are the mainstay options for early cases of HCC. Liver transplantation for well-selected cases provides excellent survival outcomes comparable to nonmalignant indications of LT. Living donor liver transplantation (LDLT) is an alternative option or even the sole one in the current era of organ shortage problem and in some Asian countries where deceased organ donation is markedly reduced due to various reasons. The adoption of LDLT for HCC treatment elicited many dynamic changes and debates to the dilemma of LT as a whole. In this chapter, we focus on different perspectives of LDLT for HCC, including selection criteria evolution, controversial topics, ethical considerations, operative highlights, and other points.

Keywords: hepatocellular carcinoma, living donor, liver, transplantation, criteria, loco-regional therapy

1. Introduction

Hepatocellular carcinoma (HCC) is the sixth most common cancer and the third leading cause of deaths globally. The selection of treatment modalities for HCC is challenging because it depends not only on the stage of tumor and the patient's performance but also on the underlying liver function. Though the staging systems of HCC are clinically useful for treatment allocation, the decision making should be tailored to each patient, taking into account morphological, pathological, and biological tumor criteria. Liver resection (LR) or liver transplantation (LT) can be adopted as a surgical curative therapy for early disease. Ablative therapies such as radiofrequency ablation (RFA) and percutaneous ethanol injection (PEI) can also cure small tumors. Transarterial chemoembolization (TACE), transarterial radio embolization (TARE), and external beam radiation therapy (EBRT) can control locally advanced disease that is no longer amenable to cure [1].

Liver transplantation has been considered theoretically the best treatment for HCC since it cures the cancer and its underlying pathology. Milan criteria (MC) were the cornerstone for LT because patient selection according to them resulted in survival outcome comparable to LT for nonmalignant cases. More cases of HCC were subjected to LT with the changes made in 2002 in western countries when additional points were added to the model for end-stage liver disease (MELD) scoring system for HCC patients that are within MC. However, the protracted waiting list for deceased donor liver transplantation (DDLT) took many patients beyond MC and hence lost their chance of LT [2].

The incorporation of living donor liver transplantation (LDLT) into the treatment roadmaps of HCC not only gave a new horizon to more patients, but also elicited many dynamic scientific debates and opened different perspectives for the field of LT in general and the treatment of HCC in particular. Thanks to the extensive research and experience of many groups working on LDLT, especially the Asian transplantation groups, most LT centers now are achieving excellent results.

Specifically to the treatment of HCC, LDLT has several major advantages including: avoidance of prolonged waiting times, allowing elective timing of transplantation under best circumstances both for the patient and the tumor burden, not consuming the public donor pool that may reduce the chance of LT for nonmalignant cases awaiting transplant, and providing organ replacement therapy in parts of the world where brain death and deceased donation are less commonly accepted [3].

In addition to the conventional hepatitis virus-related HCC, a steadily increasing burden of HCC will be witnessed with the emergence of alcohol-related cirrhosis and nonalcoholic steatohepatitis (NASH) as potential major causes of HCC, adding more burden to the transplantation demands and worsening the worldwide problem of organ shortage. It has been recognized that fine-tuning and timing of liver transplantation for HCC are only possible with live organ donation. For these reasons, the need for implementation and optimization of LDLT program will continue in the near future [4–6].

In the following sections, we will discuss basic concepts, criteria evolution, ethical considerations, and controversial topics regarding LDLT for HCC treatment, some of them are commonplace among LDLT and DDLT. The technical details of the procedure of LDLT in general are beyond the scope of this chapter. However, surgical details that are related to the oncologic outcome of the patients with HCC are highlighted.

2. Current practice of LDLT for HCC

HCC represents more than 90% of primary liver cancers and It has a well-remarked geographic distribution. Around 85% of cases occur in East Asia, sub-Saharan Africa, and Melanesia. The great burden of HCC is most prevalent among the less developed world. In developed regions, the incidence is low, except for Southern Europe where the incidence is significantly higher [7, 8].

By and large, LDLT has emerged as an alternative to DDLT and it is the only option for patients with HCC in many Asian countries, where the problem of organ shortage is commonly faced. It also provides a suitable option for patients exceeding the MC in western countries such as the United States and Europe, and in the absence of legislative regulations and setup for DDLT in some developing countries especially in the Middle East and North Africa [9–11].

At the beginning of this century, it was estimated that LDLT would represent a significant proportion of the patients transplanted with HCC. Unfortunately, the risks of death and major complications for the healthy donors at the early experience (0.3 and 2%, respectively) reduced its practice on a wide scale. With the cumulative experiences over the past two decades, LDLT is now practiced smoothly in centers of excellence with experience of hepatobiliary surgery and transplantation medicine [7, 12].

2.1. Western experience

Since 2002, HCC patients who are within Milan criteria gain additional points under the MELD organ allocation policy. This resulted in shorter waiting time for HCC patients in many regions of the United States, obviating the need for LDLT. In some regions, however, longer waiting times with higher dropout rates support the use of LDLT for cases of HCC within the Milan criteria and in candidates who do not meet criteria for waiting list priority [13].

The situation of LDLT within the western experience can be configured from the 2012 release of European Association of Study of the Liver (EASL) guidelines, that mentioned "Living donor liver transplantation is an alternative option in patients with a waiting list exceeding 6–7 months, and offers a suitable setting to explore extended indications within research programs" [7].

In the United States, approximately 7000 new patients with HCC are put on the waiting list for LT every year, 10–15% of whom die during the waiting period. In Europe and the United States, the dropout rate at various centers ranges between 15 and 35%. From this perspective, LDLT offer a survival advantage to a significant proportion of HCC patients in the western world [14].

2.2. Eastern experience

The liver transplantation setup in Asia differs from that in the West, in the fact that no priority is given to HCC patients. This setup is formulated to avoid the inevitable shift of most of the deceased grafts to the persistently increasing HCC cases on the expense of nonmalignant cases waiting LT. The resultant wait-list lead Asian centers to practice various approaches to cover the needs, including bridging treatment for HCC, salvage transplantation after prior hepatectomy and LDLT for HCC. Shortage of donors in Asian countries is attributed to many factors including cultural and religious beliefs [10, 15].

3. Basic concepts

3.1. Philosophy

The most prominent advantage of LDLT for HCC treatment is the reduction of waiting time on the list for all cases including other etiologies of liver failure with nearly no effect on public donor pool. Living donor liver grafts are dedicated gifts to the recipients and are generally of good quality taking into account that most of living donors are healthy young individuals [15, 16].

The concept of "gifting" allowed LDLT for HCC patients who are beyond MC or any other proposed criteria and opened the door for liberal expansion. This concept is not accepted in the wait list of DDLT in which the procedure is conditioned to the "within criteria" cases only. The concept of "gifting" must not be taken for granted in the case of LDLT. Since the risk of a living donor is taken, selection criteria must be adopted for HCC patients with optimization of the pretransplantation conditions to ensure a high survival outcome. In other words, the readily available willing donor does not justify the ultramajor procedure of transplantation in the absence of a survival benefit for the recipient. In addition, donor safety remains the other pillar of a sound decision of LDLT [17].

3.2. Indications

LDLT is indicated in HCC patients, who are within accepted universal or regional criteria for transplantation. In view of organ scarcity, the indications can be described currently to be result-oriented in terms of overall and recurrence-free survival. Consequently, there is marked variation between different regions and institutions for applied indications. In essence, cases fitting Milan criteria are indicated for LDLT if waiting list would be >7 months or if there is a willing available donor. Milan criteria form the solid base of morphological indications for HCC. As discussed later, LDLT has allowed transplantation for patients who are outside Milan criteria according to the dynamically changing criteria in different institutions [18, 19].

3.3. Contraindications

Likewise, there is heterogeneity in the contraindications between different regions according to criteria limits for patient selection. However, there is a body of evidence that LDLT is absolutely contraindicated in the following conditions: cases of HCC that show major vascular invasion as evidenced by pretransplant imaging, the presence of extrahepatic metastases including suspicious porta hepatis nodal disease and cases with ruptured HCC. Absolute contraindications of LDLT in nonmalignant cases hold true for HCC and include cases with uncontrolled systemic infection or lethal uncontrolled medical comorbidities [20].

4. Terminology

With the implementation of LDLT programs and better understanding of the clinical course and biological nature of HCC, various clinical settings have emerged. In addition, the current progress of the interventional anticancer therapies enforced the armamentarium of the HCC management for all clinical scenarios. The following are different settings rather than different types of LDLT.

4.1. Primary LDLT

It is the procedure of LDLT performed upfront for the treatment of the cancer and underlying primary liver disease. In this setting, no previous liver resection is performed but initial ablative loco-regional therapies like RFA or PEI may have been performed. It is carried out for nonresectable HCC cases fitting the standard Milan criteria, UCSF criteria or other established and justified criteria for individual institutions. According to Barcelona Clinic Liver Cancer (BCLC) guidelines, primary LDLT is conducted for early cases of HCC with poor liver functions that cannot tolerate initial resection or ablation [7].

4.2. Salvage LDLT

In this setting, LT is performed when there is tumor recurrence or deterioration of liver functions after initial hepatectomy. The integral point in salvage LDLT is that it is performed aiming at a similar outcome to nonrecurrent cases. The pretransplant setting in the case of salvage LT after previous hepatectomy differs from that of primary LT in the availability of tissue pathology, so that almost all factors that determine tumor's behavior (grade, the presence or absence of microvascular invasion, the grade of necrosis in response to loco-regional therapy) are determined beforehand. That is why the predictive power of outcome of salvage LT should be more precise. Very importantly, we should consider that patients who have "within criteria" recurrence after hepatectomy, and hence amenable to salvage LT, are not more than 25% in some series. This means that nearly 70% of cases may miss the chance of a curative LT at all. The transplantability at the time of recurrence has been found to be an important variable determining the final outcome [21]. Noteworthy that when salvage LT is considered due to transplantable recurrence, the recurrence pattern should be evaluated before embarking into LT even if the liver functions and tumor burden are amenable to LT. Intrahepatic recurrent tumors after hepatectomy originates from either primary tumor metastases or de novo tumor foci. The interval and histopathological analysis of hepatectomy specimens give a clue to the pattern of recurrence. Tumors recurring in the first 12 months are most likely tumor metastases within the liver, while those arising after 12 months represent newly developed tumor foci. At histopathological analysis of hepatectomy, the presence of satellite nodules and portal vein invasion herald tumor metastases and early recurrence. The transplantation team should not rush to salvage LDLT except after considering the biological aggressiveness of the recurrent tumor and the likelihood of re-recurrence into the implanted neo-liver [22].

4.3. Sequential LDLT and preemptive LDLT

They are new categories with no consensus, performed in some centers within institutional protocols. In preemptive LDLT, cases that underwent initial hepatectomy and showed adverse histopathological criteria like microvascular invasion or satellite tumor nodules are prepared for LDLT without unnecessary waiting for the inevitable expected recurrence [21, 23, 24].

In sequential LDLT, pretransplant loco-regional therapy (LRT) is administered aiming at complete pathological necrosis of the index tumor before LDLT for cases within accepted criteria. Moreover, LDLT is performed after a scheduled short interval due to donor availability. The exact duration of the interval is not yet determined. Some centers perform LDLT after 3 months from the time of pretransplant therapy. This concept developed from the cumulative experience of histopathological assessment of explanted livers and the impact of pathological necrosis on post LT outcomes. HCC patients who achieve pathological necrosis ≥60% have significantly better overall survival and recurrence-free survival [25].

> *The employment of salvage LDLT is sometimes controversial. Some transplant surgeons, in view of certain radiological, pathological and biological hallmarks, don't prefer to wait for the inevitable recurrence or deterioration of patient or liver conditions to occur (preemptive LDLT). Some argue that the readily available donor associated with vigilant surveillance can always tailor the transplantation in the right time for the best outcome (salvage LDLT).*

5. Evolution of selection criteria

Over the previous two decades, criteria of LT had been expanded and modified from morphological and nonmorphological perspectives. Nevertheless, Milan criteria (MC) keep their place as the gold standard for LT. The long-term outcome and prognostic impact of LT within MC had been reproducibly studied with consistent excellent results [19, 26].

5.1. Why the criteria for LDLT had been expanded?

The MC advocated by Mazzaferro et al. [27] in 1996 are considered the base upon which several centers around the world validated their experiences in liver transplantation. These first clear-cut criteria were published in the *New England journal of medicine* as a practice changing and ground breaking progress in HCC treatment. That is because MC provided posttransplant survival rates of 75–95% at 2 years and 70–80% at 5 years in several studies. Indeed, a meta-analysis of published data has confirmed the survival advantage of MC and its association with a low risk of selecting patients with aggressive tumors [19, 27–29].

However, Milan criteria have been expanded and modified steadily for the following reasons:

1. They were considered too restrictive and many reports showed similar outcomes for cases beyond Milan [13, 30].

2. The growing evidence of the clear contribution of nonmorphological tumor characteristics to the outcome of patients after transplantation. So, the static "morphological" Milan criteria were expanded and modified. The other pathological and biological tumor criteria include: micro-vascular invasion, alpha-feto protein (AFP) level, deoxy-gamma carboxy prothrombin (dGCP) level and tumor avidity on PET scan [31–35].

3. The observation of two incorrectly estimated groups: an underestimated group that had been transplanted within MC but showed worse outcome and an overestimated group that was beyond MC and had comparable outcome after LDLT [35, 36].

5.2. Selection criteria according to different centers of excellence (Table 1) [27, 37–45]

Selection criteria of liver transplantation in different series and centers of excellence

Criteria	Parameters	Type of parameters	Over-all survival
Milan	Solitary tumor ≤ 5 cm[T1], up to 3 tumors non >3 cm, no macrovascular invasion	Morphological only	85% (4-year)
UCSF	Solitary HCC ≤ 6.5 cm, or ≤ 3 nodules with the largest lesion ≤ 4.5 cm and a total tumor diameter ≤ 8 cm	Morphological only	75% (5-year)
Modified Milan (Up to 7)	Tumor number + size of the largest tumor (cm) ≤ 7	Morphological only	71% (5-year)
Toronto	Any tumor size or number, if pretransplant tumor biopsy showed no poor differentiation, no major vascular invasion, no extrahepatic disease	Morphological-pathological	72% (5-year)
Kyoto University	≤ 10 tumors, all ≤ 5 cm and the serum level of des. Gama carboxy prothrombin (d.GCP) ≤ 400 mIU/ml	Morphological-biological	87% (5-year)
Kyushu University	HCC ≤ 5 cm and a serum d.GCP ≤ 300 mIU/ml. It had been refined by adding neutrophil to lymphocyte ratio (NLR) >4	Morphological-biological	83% (5-year)
Tokyo University	5-5 rule: HCC not larger than 5 cm and no more than 5 nodules	Morphological only	75% (5-year)
Asan Medical Center	HCC not larger than 5 cm, 6 or fewer nodules without gross vascular invasion	Morphological only	82% (5-year)
Hangzhou	HCC ≥ 8 cm if serum alpha-fetoprotein level ≤ 400 ng/ml and only grade I or II	Morphological, biological, and pathological	72.% (5-year)

Table 1. Different selection criteria for liver transplantation adopted in most of transplantation in the world. Note that the main western criteria (Milan, UCSF, UP to 7) depend largely on morphology. Eastern-based criteria (Kyoto-Kyushu-Hangzhou) had modified by incorporating biological behavior of the tumors. The Toronto criteria are unique in its sole dependence on pretransplant biopsy.

Milan criteria were based on preoperative imaging and validated in many institutions all over the world [27]. In 2001, Yao et al. in the University of California San Francisco (UCSF) expanded the morphological criteria based on pathological assessment of explanted livers and then they prospectively validate their criteria based on pretransplant imaging in 2007 [37, 46]. Though this set of criteria is applied successfully in many regions, it has not been applied on a wide scale because they allow transplantation for large HCCs (6.5 cm, representing a tumor volume of 144 cm^3), which had been associated with worse outcomes in some studies. UCSF criteria (like Milan criteria) also exclude all patients with more than three lesions, some of whom may have the same outcome as those within criteria [47]. The 3- and 5-year survival rates after LDLT based on the UCSF criteria range between 78–96% and 66–90%, respectively, in different centers [28]. This wide variation of survival outcomes may also be attributed to variations of the surgical outcome and early mortality.

It should be emphasized that there are no consensus criteria for LDLT allocation. Each individual institution adopts one of the current criteria, tailoring treatment to their unique patient and general circumstances. Most of centers with high experience in LDLT for HCC currently focus on modification rather than numerical expansion of the number and size of tumors. The incorporation of biological factors (tumor markers, inflammatory markers) or available pathological factors from previous hepatectomy help select best candidates and hence predict the outcome and protect against recurrence [29, 35, 48].

6. Preoperative evaluation

Liver transplantation under optimal circumstances is a clear benefit of LDLT. The procedure can be carried out in a timely fashion after exhaustive assessment of tumor burden by different imaging modalities and biological markers. The tumor burden can then be manipulated by pretransplant therapies using the different loco-regional treatment options. Preoperative evaluation of the donor is not much different from the nonmalignant cases of LDLT except for some additional ethical perspectives as discussed previously. For the recipient, the details of preoperative assessment are beyond the scope of this chapter. However, we consider some important points in the pretransplant setting.

6.1. Imaging

Preoperative imaging of the recipient aims at assessment of tumor burden and suitable metastatic workup, for occult HCC or other cancer types. Dynamic CT or MRI with arterial enhancement is the standard of care according to high level of evidence. Extrahepatic staging should include CT chest and CT or MRI of abdomen and pelvis [12, 23].

The discrepancy between preoperative imaging and real tumor burden in explanted livers had been investigated in many centers. The state-of-the-art imaging modalities are not 100% accurate. CTA and MRI were both accurate to determine whether patients fit within the Milan or UCSF criteria, but CTA was slightly better than MRI to evaluate tumor number and size [49]. In the current era of pretransplant invasive therapies, the liver background became more confusing due to the presence of regenerative nodules, necrotized tumors, and other small tumors [35].

The incidental finding of pulmonary nodule(s) on pretransplant CT warrants appropriate evaluation. Many studies had determined a cutoff point to the size of pulmonary lesion at 5 mm. A lesion < 5 mm is less likely to be malignant and if remained stable or showed regression over a period of 3–6 months, liver transplantation is performed. For a lesion > 5 mm, a biopsy is needed to rule out malignant nature that contraindicates transplantation. If this lesion was the same in repeated images over previous 2 years, the possibility of infection is most likely and management is done accordingly. Video-assisted thoracic surgery (VATS) is perfectly employed for an excision biopsy of these small pulmonary nodules [50].

6.2. Alpha-feto protein (AFP)

This biological tumor marker plays important role in the assessment of tumor burden and aggressiveness although many other markers have been used in clinical practice over the past two decades. The AFP value has its clinical significance either in the preoperative or the posttransplant settings. In addition, the dynamic changes to its value in relation to downstaging therapy had been explored. An important question in the preoperative setting is its role as an exclusion tool, either alone or in combination of other radiological, biological, or pathological markers.

Some studies check the cutoff level above which patients should not undergo LT. At an AFP level >1000 ng/ml, approximately 5% of patients would be excluded from LT with 20% reduction in the rate of HCC recurrence. If a lower cut-off level is applied, this would result in a greater reduction in the recurrence rate but at the expense of excluding many more patients from LT who might not have tumor recurrence and would have benefited from LT. Also, patients who had decline of an initial AFP level >1000 ng/ml after loco-regional therapy had a more favorable prognosis after LT. Alpha feto-protein level <1000 has thus been combined to the UCSF criteria for patient selection in some centers [51].

More recently, a prospective multicenter study has explored the use of a combination of total tumor volume (TTV) ≤ 115 cm^3 and AFP ≤ 400 ng/ml as an exclusion tool from LT in centers with a median waiting time of 8 months. This study took an advantage from a previous observation of the inferior survival outcome of patients who are within MC but have the AFP level ≥400 ng/ml. In this study, patients who were beyond MC but within TTV/AFP had survival outcome similar to cases within MC [29].

Many other biomarkers can be evaluated in the pretransplant setting to predict the posttransplant outcome. A recent study in our center showed that repeated measurement of serum levels of novel biomarkers including fibroblast growth factor-2 (FGF-2), survivin, Ki67, endostatin, and vascular endothelial growth factor (VEGF), before and after LDLT for HCC, could predict HCC recurrence [52].

6.3. Fludro-deoxy glucose-positron emission tomography (FDG-PET) scan

Pretransplant 18F-FDG uptake on PET scan in liver transplant candidates with HCC is a useful additional parameter for the evaluation of tumor biology. Positive preoperative PET scans are significantly associated with an increased risk of posttransplant HCC recurrence and inferior outcome, an observation that relates a positive PET status with the presence of microvascular invasion in explant tumor pathology [31]. In a recent Korean study, the combination of the positive FDG-PET study and AFP level >200 ng/ml could predict tumor recurrence more precisely after LDLT than Milan criteria [35]. More recently, a retrospective study at our center has showed that the combination of UCSF criteria with the FDG-PET status can predict tumor recurrence after LDLT and that tumor recurrence is earlier in cases with positive FDG-PET results. On the basis of the maximal standardized uptake value (SUVmax), high-risk group cases (positive study with $SUV_{max} \geq 5$) had worse recurrence-free survival compared with low-risk cases (positive study with $SUV_{max} < 5$) [53].

6.4. Donor characteristics

In addition to the previously discussed controversy of impact of donor type (living or deceased) on HCC recurrence, other donor factors have been studied. A recent review of the American Scientific Registry of Transplant Recipients (SRTR) that involved 9724 patients revealed that the following donor factors were independently associated with high risk of HCC recurrence after transplantation: high BMI, history of DM, and severe graft steatosis. All the previous factors are evident at the time of organ allocation and must be considered before transplantation [54].

7. Loco-regional therapy (LRT)

The pretransplant therapies are implemented heavily for HCC, being an essential component of HCC treatment algorithms in most of treatment guidelines. Earlier in the treatment of HCC roadmaps, they were considered "bridging" tools to keep the patient chances of LT during the waiting time. Currently, a realized value of LRT is their ability to probe the tumor's internal milieu, acting as a selecting tool based on the degree of tumor's response as an indicator of its aggressiveness. So, adopting such therapies gives the time to observe the tumor's behavior before the ultramajor costly step of liver transplantation [55]. Bypassing such an observation period in the setting of multifocal or locally advanced tumor risks transplanting patients with systemic disease.

7.1. HCC downstaging before liver transplantation

The difference between downstaging and neoadjuvant therapies is that in the former the tumor status is beyond the proposed criteria for transplantation and LRT is administered to reduce the tumor burden and to render the case fit for transplantation. In neoadjuvant therapy, the patient is already within criteria but treatment is given to prevent tumor progression to the "beyond criteria" state while waiting for the donor and to induce tumor necrosis aiming at better long-term outcome [56].

In different series from Asian centers, more than 30% of patients who were beyond Milan/ UCSF criteria were effectively downstaged to the "within criteria" state with a 5-year survival rate similar to the initially fit cases [57, 58]. A meta-analysis explored the effect of downstaging to Milan criteria, and the success rate exceeded 40%. However, the recurrence rate was as high as 16% [59].

TACE and RFA are the main tools of downstaging. TACE mediates its effect by inducing complete pathological necrosis with response rates ranging between 27 and 57%. RFA is used For accessible lesions to induce coagulative necrosis, either alone or in combination with liver resection [60]. In LDLT, timing of transplantation after a period of waiting from the time of LDLT is possible. Most centers wait for a period of 3–6 months to evaluate tumor progression as an indicator of aggressiveness before embarking into LDLT.

Though widely applicable in most HCC guidelines, there are no unified criteria either for selecting cases for downstaging or for determining them as good responders and hence listing them for LT. This fact highlights the wide variation of transplantation criteria among different regions and centers. As a rule of thumb, the criteria to enter a downstaging program should include patients who have well-defined and acceptable chances of good outcomes after transplantation if the downstaging goal is achieved [56]. In our center, not only we apply downstaging for cases beyond UCSF criteria, but also we consider cases with high AFP or high FDG uptake on PET scan for downstaging. In our early experience, patients were downstaged to fit Milan criteria. Our initial results of 35 patients were encouraging with a 5-year survival rate of 90% and those patients are still disease-free up to date, after follow-up of 10 years. Since July 2006, our criteria were extended to UCSF criteria. In our experience of 161 HCC patients, 51 (31.6%) were successfully downstaged to fit the UCSF criteria. The overall 1- and 5-year survival rates for downstaged cases were 94.1 and 92.7%, respectively. The recurrence rate was 9.2%. The survival rates were similar for different pretransplantation downstaging procedures [57].

8. Operative/surgical highlights

The first successful case of liver transplantation in Asia was performed by Chen in 1984 in Chang Gung Memorial Hospital, Taiwan. From the cumulative experience at our center, we would like to emphasize that a sound surgical procedure is mandatory for the best outcome. It has been postulated that the experience of the transplant team is an important factor that independently affects the outcome though the learning curve of liver transplant can be steep and painful in some centers launching an LDLT program. In essence, we prefer not to correct recipient coagulopathy before surgery, because many studies showed no value of preoperative correction. Donor hepatectomy should be accomplished with minimal blood loss, obviating the need for blood transfusion. The routine use of microsurgical procedure is performed in our center for arterial anastomosis as well as biliary reconstruction. Surgical outcome largely affects survival and hence final outcome. Early postoperative vascular complications are the main reasons of graft loss and in-hospital mortality and must be managed vigorously [49, 61–64].

8.1. Timing of donor and recipient surgeries

In nonmalignant cases of LDLT, the recipient surgery is usually begun after the donor surgery commenced till confirmation of feasible biliary anatomy by cholangiography. In the early experience of LDLT for HCC, some surgeons preferred to confirm resectability of the liver containing cancer and the absence of lymph node metastases through a smaller incision before proceeding with graft harvesting from the donor [65, 66]. However, the current imaging modalities surpass this step and allow precise decision in advance. Most experienced centers largely depend on high quality CT or MRI images and the timing is adopted like nonmalignant cases of end-stage liver failure.

8.2. Safety margin

A proper safety margin is an integral part of the sound oncological surgical procedure. Some peripheral lesions may be found in very close proximity to or even adherent to parietal peritoneum, diaphragm, omentum, or less commonly small or large bowl loops. A previous hepatectomy increases the adhesions with the aforementioned structures. It is thus convenient to take a proper safety margin through excision of parts of peritoneum and diaphragmatic muscle. Very infrequently, small or large bowl resection and anastomosis may be required. Re-exploration for additional safety margin after final pathological assessment is a very hazardous procedure for such a frail patient, but may be warranted in some conditions according to institutional experience.

8.3. Management of nodal disease

In a recent review from the International Registry of Hepatic Tumors in Liver Transplantation, the incidence of lymph node metastases in cirrhotic patients with HCC undergoing LT was 6.5%. Hilar lymph node (LN) involvement in cases of HCC constitutes a contraindication for liver transplantation because of dismal prognosis. Recent imaging techniques are able to identify enlarged suspicious lymph nodes in the pretransplant setting. However, the frequent presence of LN enlargement due to chronic inflammation in cases of hepatitis C-induced cirrhosis may make the diagnosis less clear. It is convenient to perform frozen section evaluation for suspicious nodes unexpectedly encountered during recipient operation. The decision to proceed or abort the procedure in the case of inconclusive frozen section analysis or the unavailability of frozen section depends largely on the experience of the transplant team. According to a meta-analysis study, systematic hilar lymphadenectomy during LT for HCC should routinely be undertaken, especially in the context of coexisting hepatitis C or secondary biliary cirrhosis. Some centers recommend harvesting of at least four lymph nodes at the time of liver transplantation but the debate remains open with no available consensus on the extent of such lymphadenectomy [67, 68].

8.4. The middle hepatic vein (MHV)

The MHV is a controversial topic within the LDLT procedure in general. In the case of LDLT for HCC, this issue should be taken more seriously. It has been postulated that the resultant venous congestion from improper management of tributaries of MHV is a possible factor favoring tumor recurrence. Congestion of the graft leads to impediment of portal inflow with subsequent ischemia in the congested region and compensatory accelerated regeneration of the well-drained areas of the graft. Consequently, the cellular changes in response to both processes may enhance tumor recurrence [69].

8.5. IVC management (see Figure 1)

The observation of HCC recurrence after LDLT in the hepatic vena-caval wall has shed light on the possibility of microvascular infiltration with consequent local and distant recurrence. This finding triggered the concept of aggressive en-bloc caval resection and reconstruction during LDLT. This step is also justified by another two facts: first, it prevents a positive margin of latent cancer in caval branches; second, the least amount of manipulation of the native liver with HCC should be employed to avoid and control distant metastasis after LDLT [70].

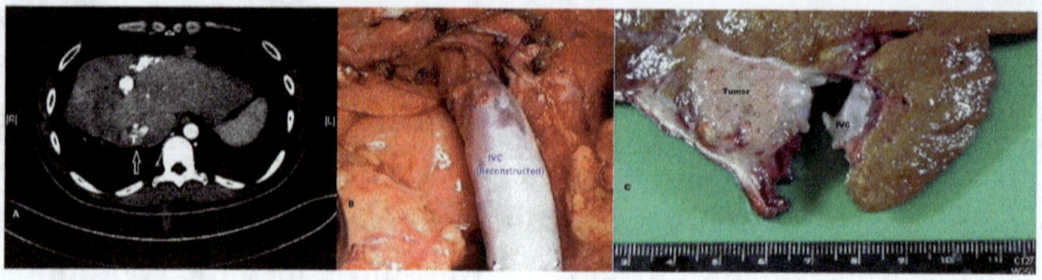

Figure 1. A case of HCC subjected to LDLT. The tumor (T) was intimately adherent to the IVC wall without apparent invasion in pretransplant CT angiography (A; arrow). During the recipient operation, the liver was explanted en-bloc with the IVC segment adjacent to the tumor. Reconstruction of the IVC was carried out using cryo-preserved iliac v. graft (B). Final gross pathology shows no intraluminal transgression by the tumor (C).

8.6. Complications of LDLT of the manipulated liver, i.e., after loco-regional therapy

Extensive adhesions are commonly encountered following previous liver resection in case of salvage liver transplantation. Tough vascular adhesions usually form between a large hepatectomy site and small intestine and omentum. Sharp dissection and meticulous hemostatic control would reduce the difficulty of subsequent transplantation and decrease the incidence of postoperative complications [71]. Laparoscopic liver resection is now performed on a wide scale in many centers. One of the most prominent advantages of laparoscopic initial hepatectomy is the marked reduction of adhesions as evidenced in subsequent liver transplantation in many series thus facilitating the procedure [72].

Intimal dissection (ID) of the recipient hepatic artery has emerged as a grave complication that may occur after TAE or TACE. Intimal dissection if not discovered and managed properly may end up in graft loss. Gentle handling of HA is mandatory during LT to prevent aggravation or precipitation of dissection in the fragile HA. Once this complication is suspected intraoperatively, microscopic assessment is needed for proper decision. Either trimming and discarding the dissected segment or discarding the whole native HA and reconstruction may be considered, hence the importance of microvascular expertise in the LDLT team [73].

9. Ethical considerations

Two main ethical pillars of the decision of LDLT for management of HCC must be considered. First, donor safety and optimizing his or her care is no different in LDLT for HCC compared to that for nonmalignant cases of liver failure. Second, the procedure must provide an acceptable outcome to the recipient compared to DDLT. From the ethical point of view, LDLT is justified, as long as the proposed regional criteria are strictly followed, being MC or any scientifically justified institutional expanded or modified criteria. Noteworthy that there is no consensus about what risk to the living donor might be considered acceptable for a given risk of recurrence [13, 74].

With increased awareness and patient education facilities, the ethical responsibilities regarding patient counseling became more complex. It is not all about the perioperative complications. Recently, ethical considerations took a very different perspective, that is offering LDLT to high-risk patients and excluding others who are low-risk patients based on imaging criteria only. As mentioned earlier, two wrongly estimated groups are revealed: cases within criteria that have aggressive biological behavior and cases beyond criteria with indolent tumors. Two ethical situations subsequently ensued; the first is the risk of recurrence of biologically aggressive tumors even when strict criteria are adhered to, i.e., the underestimated group. The second is about the loss of chance of LT in the other group. The transplantation team should never rush to transplantation in response to family pressure and readily available donor without proper discussion of all that issues [35].

When the partial graft fails for any reason, a special—but very uncommon—ethical situation is encountered because normally it requires an urgent deceased donor retransplantation. It has been established that if LDLT was used in a situation where a deceased donor is contraindicated, such as exceeding the accepted criteria for deceased donation, the patient should not be retransplanted because he/she would not be transplanted initially if on wait-list for DDLT [12, 66]. Finding another living donor must be balanced against the expected outcome of the procedure. There are no clear-cut decisions to such situations and the institutional experience would tailor the right decision.

When talking about salvage LDLT, the patient may be reluctant to undergo the procedure even with the availability of a donor. Some patients may argue that they want to be alive more but do not want to harm anyone. In these circumstances, the transplant team should alert the patient about how long can he/she delay the procedure without a considerable risk of tumor progression or being transferred into the nontransplantable state. A study from Japan revealed that patients who receive downstaging therapy can wait no more than 12 months. However, the exact duration is not determined and the management plan should be tailored to each case [75].

10. Controversial topics

The increasing number of HCC cases, the parallel progress in expertise of LDLT, and the dynamic changes in the selection criteria all enriched the liver transplantation community with many important topics and debates. A lot of studies were carried out to find answers or to reach a consensus in many of these topics. However, the retrospective nature of most studies, the different reporting methodologies and small sample sizes are all flaws that hampered the appearance of high level of evidence to address all topics.

10.1. What is the best treatment option of early HCC? Resection or liver transplantation? Primary or salvage approach?

- The surgical decision can be either LR or LT in 20–25% of cases of HCC amenable for surgery. Liver transplantation is hypothetically superior to resection because it removes the cancer and its underlying pathology. For many patients it is not possible to perform resection because of the tumor size, anatomical location of the tumor, or poor liver function, and liver transplantation is the only surgical option [76]. However, even in many Asian centers which perform LDLT on regular basis, up to 50% of early HCC cases may not have suitable donors or be concerned about the risk to donor. So, many Asian centers adopt the policy of offering LR to patients with resectable tumors with compensated cirrhosis and deferring LT to the salvage setting [13, 23, 77, 78].
- The controversy regarding LR or LT in HCC patients is largely confined to early cases with a well-preserved liver function. There are no randomized controlled trials that addressed this issue through a head-to-head comparison. Given that organ shortage for LT is a persistent challenge worldwide and also the presence of underserved areas with deficient LT programs, the identification of cases that would obtain similar survival outcomes when either submitted to LR or to LT is of paramount importance [79, 80].
- The strategy of offering LR for simultaneously resectable and transplantable cases was based on the observation from many studies that 20–30% of HCC cases that had LR may not witness recurrence for >5 years. In addition, with vigilant surveillance programs, most of recurrent cases would fit into the MC and can be transplanted under optimal conditions due to the availability of the living donor, with no negative impact on the outcome. This obviates many patients the downside of early immunosuppression [5]. In addition, the mortality rate of LR at an experienced center is less than 2–5%, and overall survival rates were comparable to primary LT [4, 24].
- **The Barcelona Clinic Liver Cancer approach**: Resection is the treatment of choice in patients with very early stage HCC and normal bilirubin levels as well as the absence of portal hypertension. If the liver functions are impaired, LT is recommended as a primary treatment approach. In the early stage of HCC, it has been found that the 10-year outcome after LT is superior to LR in view of the latter's well-known higher recurrence risk. So, the choice of primary LT is recommended. The same approach is adopted by the American Association of Study of Liver Disease (AASLD) guidelines that prefer liver resection for very early cases with the optimal liver profile [7, 78, 81, 82].

- A meta-analysis of studies that involved patients within MC revealed a survival advantage for LT over LR [83]. In a more recent meta-analysis that involved 1572 patients in whom both LR and LT are feasible, the authors did not find any survival advantage of LT compared with LR. They concluded—based on low quality evidence—that LR is preferable to LT in patients who are feasible for both options [84].
- Conclusion: the overall survival advantage of LT is unclear, though recurrence-free survival is definitely better with LT. The main drawback for LT—especially LDLT—is the relatively increased mortality in the early postoperative period. In high volume centers where LDLT is performed at high rates, perioperative mortality is reduced significantly. So, a clear overall survival advantage for LT may be evident [85]. For a definite evidence-based conclusion, a randomized controlled trial comparing LT and LR is needed, a condition that is very difficult due to practical and ethical restrictions. Proper patient selection and optimization of criteria according to the pretransplant setting (primary or secondary) would help make a treatment roadmap.

10.2. Living donor or deceased donor for HCC?

One of the most critical controversies in the transplantation field is the possibility of an increased rate of recurrence of HCC after LDLT compared to DDLT.

Several hypotheses have been postulated to figure out this possibility:

- The fast tract effect: due to the shortened waiting time for LDLT, progression of HCC with aggressive tumor biology might not be recognized during such a short-waiting time. This is in contrary to the situation in DDLT, where the long-waiting time can naturally select cases with indolent behavior.
- The growth factors and cytokines released during rapid regeneration of the partial grafts might contribute to tumor progression and recurrence.
- The extensive dissection and mobilization of the liver might increase the feasibility of tumor dissemination through the hepatic vein and increased potential for leaving residual tumor cells.
- The exaggerated vascular inflow associated with small size grafts elicits vast angiogenesis with subsequent carcinogenic effect.
- The less radical hepatectomy in LDLT with the native IVC left in place may constitute a suboptimal oncologic procedure [15, 55, 86–88].

A multi-center study was carried out on the database of China Liver Transplant Registry (CLTR) to highlight this issue. They explored the data of 6860 patients (6471 (DDLT) and 389 LDLT and concluded that both overall survival and recurrence-free survival were comparable between both approaches [89]. In an international consensus conference of liver transplantation (Zurich 2012), it had been stated that no convincing difference in outcome could be identified according to the type of graft, although a higher risk of recurrence was noted in fast-tracked patients. The experts advised an interval of observation for the biological behavior of the tumor to manifest. A period of 3 months had been suggested [12]. Many other groups reported similar recurrence rates after LDLT and DDLT and also similar long-term outcomes [14, 87].

However, others have found significantly higher rates of tumor recurrence after LDLT compared with DDLT for HCC. The Adult to Adult Living Donor Liver transplantation (A2ALL) study reported a significantly higher 3-year tumor recurrence rate after LDLT [15, 88, 90, 91]. One should consider that many studies that reported better outcome of DDLT than LDLT are conducted in the west and some of them were flawed by small sample sizes and the possibility of selection bias since DDLT was applied mostly on cases within Milan criteria only and those beyond Milan criteria are relegated to LDLT [92].

A systematic review and meta-analysis addressed this question (Is the regenerating liver of LDLT a fertile environment for HCC recurrence?). Though no randomized controlled trials were included, they came to a similar conclusion; disease-free survival (DFS) is worse after LDLT compared with DDLT but there was no difference observed in overall survival (OS). In the same meta-analysis, there was a concern that the follow-up periods in the included studies are probably too brief to detect a major impact on survival resulting from differences in disease recurrence. The same study revealed that the overall survival after LDLT vs. DDLT was better —though not statistically significant—in studies from eastern centers compared with studies from western centers. This may reflect differences between these regions in patient selection or case-volumes effects on surgical outcomes [6]. In conclusion, to date there is no definite evidence supporting higher recurrence after LDLT than DDLT [55, 92].

10.3. Pre-LDLT liver biopsy, can the trend be changed?

Because the risk of tumor seeding may be 2–4% along the needle biopsy tract and thus increasing the risk of metastases, liver biopsy should be considered only when there is uncertainty as to the diagnosis. This might occur, for example, in the presence of an HCC arising in the noncirrhotic liver or contradictory clinical, laboratory, and radiological findings [81]. However, a biopsy has the potential problems of sampling error. For example, different nodules may have different grades within the index tumor. It has also been demonstrated that even in a single-needle biopsy, adjacent tumor cells can be of different degrees of differentiation. Nevertheless, if transplantation is planned for HCC beyond the standard criteria, tumor biopsy appears to be a logical approach if there is suspicion of diagnosis [28].

Dubay et al. [44] have provided their experience in the University of Toronto based solely on a liver biopsy before LT. They have no size or number restriction for LT. They concluded that a protocol using a biopsy to exclude poorly differentiated tumors achieved excellent survival rates (70% at 5 years) [44].

10.4. Can we exclude morphological selection criteria in the coming era?

Morphological criteria of HCC describe the appearance, while biological criteria describe the concealed behavior. Ultimately, the behavior of HCC is the final-deciding factor on patient outcome. As shown earlier, modification of morphological criteria is pursued in many studies with the incorporation of biological factors [13]. In a study from Korea, the recipient selection based on pure biological factors was proposed. The group showed that FDG PET positivity with a cutoff point of maximum systemic uptake value (SUV_{max}) of 1.1 combined with the AFP serum level at 400 ng/ml is able—alone—to predict patient outcome more precise than morphological criteria [35]. More studies are needed to explore nonmorphological selection processes.

11. Conclusions

LDLT is a robust treatment pathway for HCC. Indeed, it may be the only pathway in this era of organ shortage especially in some Asian countries. The employment and dynamic application of selection criteria of LDLT for HCC are the cornerstone to acquire the best outcome. The number and size of the tumor(s) are not the only factors to consider for patient selection but some other factors are also present. Most of transplantation centers are combining biological (AFP-tumor avidity in PET scan) and pathological (pretransplant biopsy) factors of the tumors to the morphological factors aiming at refined patient selection for the optimal outcome. In the current era of personalized medicine, treatment of HCC should be tailored according to each individual patient and tumor criteria. A sound oncological surgical procedure is the core of successful LDLT and has its direct impact on the final outcome.

Author details

Chih-Che Lin[1*], Ahmed Mohammed Abdel Aziz Elsarawy[2] and Chao-Long Chen[1]

*Address all correspondence to: immunologylin@gmail.com

1 Department of general surgery and liver transplant center, Chang Gung Memorial Hospital, Kaohsiung, Taiwan

2 Liver transplant center, Chang Gung Memorial Hospital, Kaohsiung, Taiwan

References

[1] Knox JJ, Cleary SP, Dawson LA. Localized and systemic approaches to treating hepatocellular carcinoma. J Clin Oncol. 2015;33(16):1835–44. Available from: http://jco.ascopubs.org/content/33/16/1835.long

[2] Bruix J, Gores GJ, Mazzaferro V. Hepatocellular carcinoma: clinical frontiers and perspectives. Gut. 2014;844–55.

[3] Sonnenday CJ. Recurrent hepatocellular carcinoma after living donor liver transplantation: a preventable problem or an acceptable risk? Ann Surg Oncol. United States; 2010;17:2262–3.

[4] de Villa VH, Lo C-M, Chen C-L. Ethics and rationale of living-donor liver transplantation in Asia. Transplant. 2003;75(3 Suppl):S2–5. Available from: http://www.ncbi.nlm.nih.gov/pubmed/12589129

[5] Chen C-L, Concejero AM. Liver transplantation for hepatocellular carcinoma in the world: the Taiwan experience. J Hepatobil Pancreat Sci. Japan. 2010;17(5):555–8.

[6] Grant RC, Sandhu L, Dixon PR, Greig PD, Grant DR, McGilvray ID. Living vs. deceased donor liver transplantation for hepatocellular carcinoma: a systematic review and meta-analysis. Clin Transplant. Denmark; 2013;27(1):140–7.

[7] Dufour JF, Greten TF, Raymond E, Roskams T, De T, Ducreux M, et al. EASL–EORTC clinical practice guidelines: management of hepatocellular carcinoma. J Hepatol. 2012;56(4):908–43. Available from: http://linkinghub.elsevier.com/retrieve/pii/S0168827811008737

[8] Torre LA, Bray F, Siegel RL, Ferlay J. Global cancer statistics. CA Cancer J Clin. 2015;65(2):87–108.

[9] Shirabe K, Taketomi A, Morita K, Soejima Y, Uchiyama H, Kayashima H, et al. Comparative evaluation of expanded criteria for patients with hepatocellular carcinoma beyond the Milan criteria undergoing living-related donor liver transplantation. Clin Transplant. Denmark; 2011;25(5):E491–8.

[10] Chen C-L, Kabiling CS, Concejero AM. Why does living donor liver transplantation flourish in Asia? Nat Rev Gastroenterol Hepatol. 2013;10(12):746–51. Available from: http://www.ncbi.nlm.nih.gov/pubmed/24100300

[11] Khalaf H, Marwan I, Al-Sebayel M, El-Meteini M, Hosny A, Abdel-Wahab M, et al. Status of liver transplantation in the Arab world. Transplantation. 2014;97(7):722–4. Available from: http://www.ncbi.nlm.nih.gov/pubmed/24603475

[12] Clavien P-A, Lesurtel M, Bossuyt PMM, Gores GJ, Langer B, Perrier A. Recommendations for liver transplantation for hepatocellular carcinoma: an international consensus conference report. Lancet Oncol. England; 2012;13(1):e11–22.

[13] Mazzaferro V, Chun YS, Poon RTP, Schwartz ME, Yao FY, Marsh JW, et al. Liver transplantation for hepatocellular carcinoma. Ann Surg Oncol. United States; 2008;15(4):1001–7.

[14] Bhangui P, Vibert E, Majno P, Salloum C, Andreani P, Zocrato J, et al. Intention-to-treat analysis of liver transplantation for hepatocellular carcinoma: living versus deceased donor transplantation. Hepatology. United States; 2011;53(5):1570–9.

[15] Ng KK, Lo CM. Liver transplantation in Asia: past, present and future. Ann Acad Med Singapore. Singapore; 2009;38(4):310–22.

[16] Chen C, Cheng Y, Yu C, Ou H, Tsang LL, Huang T, et al. Living donor liver transplantation: the Asian perspective. Transplantat. 2014;97 Suppl 8: S3.

[17] Barr ML, Belghiti J, Villamil FG, Pomfret EA, Sutherland DS, Gruessner RW, et al. A report of the vancouver forum on the care of the live organ donor: lung, liver, pancreas, and intestine data and medical guidelines. Transplantat. 2006;81(10):1373–85. Available from: http://content.wkhealth.com/linkback/openurl?sid=WKPTLP:landingpage&an=00007890-200605270-00004

[18] Nadalin S, Bockhorn M, Malagó M, Valentin-Gamazo C, Frilling A, Broelsch CE. Living donor liver transplantation. HPB (Oxford). 2006;8(1):10–21. Available from: http://www.pubmedcentral.nih.gov/articlerender.fcgi?artid=2131378&tool=pmcentrez&rendertype=abstract

[19] Mazzaferro V, Bhoori S, Sposito C, Bongini M, Langer M, Miceli R, et al. Milan criteria in liver transplantation for hepatocellular carcinoma: an evidence-based analysis of 15 years of experience. Liver Transpl. United States; 2011;17 Suppl 2:S44–57.

[20] Farkas S, Hackl C, Schlitt HJ. Overview of the indications and contraindications for liver transplantation. Cold Spring Harb Perspect Med. United States; 2014;4(5).

[21] Majno PE, Sarasin FP, Mentha G, Hadengue A. Primary liver resection and salvage transplantation or primary liver transplantation in patients with single, small hepatocellular carcinoma and preserved liver function: an outcome-oriented decision analysis. Hepatology. United States; 2000;31(4):899–906.

[22] Lee HS, Choi GH, Joo DJ, Kim MS, Choi JS. The clinical behavior of transplantable recurrent hepatocellular carcinoma after curative resection: implications for salvage liver. Transplantation. 2014;2717–24.

[23] Concejero A, Chen C-L, Wang C-C, Wang S-H, Lin C-C, Liu Y-W, et al. Living donor liver transplantation for hepatocellular carcinoma: a single-center experience in Taiwan. Transplantation. United States; 2008;85(3):398–406.

[24] Cherqui D, Laurent A, Alain. Liver resection for transplantable hepatocellular carcinoma. Ann Surg. 2009;250(5). 738–46.

[25] Chan K-M, Yu M-C, Chou H-S, Wu T-J, Lee C-F, Lee W-C. Significance of tumor necrosis for outcome of patients with hepatocellular carcinoma receiving locoregional therapy prior to liver transplantation. Ann Surg Oncol. United States; 2011;18(9):2638–46.

[26] Yoshizumi T, Harimoto N, Itoh S, Okabe H, Kimura K, Uchiyama H, et al. Living donor liver transplantation for hepatocellular carcinoma within milan criteria in the present era. Anticancer Res. Greece; 2016;36(1):439–45.

[27] Mazzaferro V, Regalia E, Doci R, Andreola S, Pulvirenti A, Bozzetti F, et al. Liver transplantation for the treatment of small hepatocellular carcinomas in patients with cirrhosis. N Engl J Med. United States; 1996;334(11):693–9.

[28] Chan SC, Fan ST. Selection of patients of hepatocellular carcinoma beyond the Milan criteria for liver transplantation. Hepatobiliary Surg Nutr. China (Republic: 1949); 2013;2(2):84–8.

[29] Toso C, Meeberg G, Hernandez-Alejandro R, Dufour J-F, Marotta P, Majno P, et al. Total tumor volume and alpha-fetoprotein for selection of transplant candidates with hepatocellular carcinoma: a prospective validation. Hepatology. United States; 2015;62(1):158–65.

[30] Majno P, Mazzaferro V. Living donor liver transplantation for hepatocellular carcinoma exceeding conventional criteria: questions, answers and demands for a common language. Vol. 12, Liver transplantation: official publication of the American Association for the Study of Liver Diseases and the International Liver Transplantation Society. United States; 2006. p. 896–8.

[31] Kornberg A, Freesmeyer M, Barthel E, Jandt K, Katenkamp K, Steenbeck J, et al. 18F-FDG-uptake of hepatocellular carcinoma on PET predicts microvascular tumor invasion in liver transplant patients. Am J Transplant. Denmark; 2009;9(3):592–600.

[32] Hirakawa M, Yoshimitsu K, Irie H, Tajima T, Nishie A, Asayama Y, et al. Performance of radiological methods in diagnosing hepatocellular carcinoma preoperatively in a recipient of living related liver transplantation: comparison with step section histopathology. Jpn J Radiol. Japan; 2011;29(2):129–37.

[33] Piardi T, Gheza F, Ellero B, Woehl-Jaegle ML, Ntourakis D, Cantu M, et al. Number and Tumor Size Are Not Sufficient Criteria to Select Patients for Liver Transplantation for Hepatocellular Carcinoma. Ann Surg Oncol. 2012;19(6):2020–6.

[34] Na GH, Kim DG, Han JH, Kim EY, Lee SH, Hong TH, et al. Inflammatory markers as selection criteria of hepatocellular carcinoma in living-donor liver transplantation. World J Gastroenterol. United States; 2014;20(21):6594–601.

[35] Hong G, Suh K-S, Suh S-W, Yoo T, Kim H, Park M-S, et al. Alpha-fetoprotein and (18)F-FDG positron emission tomography predict tumor recurrence better than Milan criteria in living donor liver transplantation. J Hepatol. Netherlands; 2016;64(4):852–9.

[36] Ito T, Takada Y, Ueda M, Haga H, Maetani Y, Oike F, et al. Expansion of selection criteria for patients with hepatocellular carcinoma in living donor liver transplantation. Liver Transpl. United States; 2007;13(12):1637–44.

[37] Yao FY, Ferrell L, Bass NM, Watson JJ, Bacchetti P, Venook A, et al. Liver transplantation for hepatocellular carcinoma: expansion of the tumor size limits does not adversely impact survival. Hepatology. United States; 2001;33(6):1394–403.

[38] Lee S-G, Hwang S, Moon D-B, Ahn C-S, Kim K-H, Sung K-B, et al. Expanded indication criteria of living donor liver transplantation for hepatocellular carcinoma at one large-volume center. Liver Transpl. United States; 2008;14(7):935–45.

[39] Zheng S-S, Xu X, Wu J, Chen J, Wang W-L, Zhang M, et al. Liver transplantation for hepatocellular carcinoma: Hangzhou experiences. Transplantation. United States; 2008;85(12):1726–32.

[40] Sugawara Y, Tamura S, Makuuchi M. Living donor liver transplantation for hepatocellular carcinoma: Tokyo University series. Dig Dis. Switzerland; 2007;25(4):310–2.

[41] Mazzaferro V, Llovet JM, Miceli R, Bhoori S, Schiavo M, Mariani L, et al. Predicting survival after liver transplantation in patients with hepatocellular carcinoma beyond the Milan criteria: a retrospective, exploratory analysis. Lancet Oncol. 2009;10(1):35–43. Available from: http://dx.doi.org/10.1016/S1470-2045(08)70284-5

[42] Taketomi A, Sanefuji K, Soejima Y, Yoshizumi T, Uhciyama H, Ikegami T, et al. Impact of des-gamma-carboxy prothrombin and tumor size on the recurrence of hepatocellular carcinoma after living donor liver transplantation. Transplantation. United States; 2009;87(4):531–7.

[43] Takada Y, Uemoto S. Liver transplantation for hepatocellular carcinoma: the Kyoto experience. J Hepatobiliary Pancreat Sci. Japan; 2010;17(5):527–32.

[44] DuBay D, Sandroussi C, Sandhu L, Cleary S, Guba M, Cattral MS, et al. Liver transplantation for advanced hepatocellular carcinoma using poor tumor differentiation on biopsy as an exclusion criterion. Ann Surg. United States; 2011;253(1):166–72.

[45] Yoshizumi T, Ikegami T, Toshima T, Harimoto N, Uchiyama H, Soejima Y, et al. Two-step selection criteria for living donor liver transplantation in patients with hepatocellular carcinoma. Transplant Proc. United States; 2013;45(9):3310–3.

[46] Yao FY, Xiao L, Bass NM, Kerlan R, Ascher NL, Roberts JP. Liver transplantation for hepatocellular carcinoma: validation of the UCSF-expanded criteria based on preoperative imaging. Am J Transplant. 2007;7(11):2587–96.

[47] Toso C, Asthana S, Bigam DL, Shapiro AMJ, Kneteman NM. Reassessing selection criteria prior to liver transplantation for hepatocellular carcinoma utilizing the scientific registry of transplant recipients database. Hepatology. 2009;49(3):832–8.

[48] Yang SH, Suh KS, Lee HW, Cho EH, Cho JY, Cho YB, et al. A revised scoring system utilizing serum alphafetoprotein levels to expand candidates for living donor transplantation in hepatocellular carcinoma. Surgery. 2007;141(5):598–609.

[49] Lu C-H, Chen C-L, Cheng Y-F, Huang T-L, Tsang LL-C, Ou H-Y, et al. Correlation between imaging and pathologic findings in explanted livers of hepatocellular carcinoma cases. Transplant Proc. United States; 2010;42(3):830–3.

[50] Wu Y-J, Lin C-C, Lin Y-H, Wang S-H, Lin T-L, Chen C-L, et al. Incidentally small pulmonary nodule in candidates for living donor liver transplantation. Ann Transplant. Poland; 2015;20:734–40.

[51] Hameed B, Mehta N, Sapisochin G, Roberts JP, Yao FY. Alpha-fetoprotein level> 1000 ng/mL as an exclusion criterion for liver transplantation in patients with hepatocellular carcinoma meeting the milan criteria. Liver Transpl. 2014;20(8):945–51.

[52] Chiu KW, Nakano T, Chen KD, Hsu LW, Lai CY, Huang CY, et al. Repeated-measures implication of hepatocellular carcinoma biomarkers in living donor liver transplantation. PLoS One. 2015;10(5):1–12. Available from: <Go to ISI>://WOS:000354916100020

[53] Hsu C-C, Chen C-L, Wang C-C, Lin C-C, Yong C-C, Wang S-H, et al. Combination of FDG-PET and UCSF criteria for predicting HCC recurrence after living donor liver transplantation. Transplantat. 2016 Sep;100(9):1925–32.

[54] Orci LA, Berney T, Majno PE, Lacotte S, Oldani G, Morel P, et al. Donor characteristics and risk of hepatocellular carcinoma recurrence after liver transplantation. Br J Surg. England; 2015;102(10):1250–7.

[55] Park G-C, Song G-W, Moon D-B, Lee S-G. A review of current status of living donor liver transplantation. Hepatobiliary Surg Nutr. China (Republic: 1949); 2016;5(2):107–17.

[56] Toso C, Mentha G, Kneteman NM, Majno P. The place of downstaging for hepatocellular carcinoma. J Hepatol. 2010;52(6):930–6. Available from: http://dx.doi.org/10.1016/j.jhep.2009.12.032

[57] Yu CY, Ou HY, Huang TL, Chen TY, Tsang LLC, Chen CL, et al. Hepatocellular carcinoma downstaging in liver transplantation. Transplant Proc. 2012;44(2):412–4.

[58] Na GH, Kim EY, Hong TH, You YK, Kim DG. Effects of loco regional treatments before living donor liver transplantation on overall survival and recurrence-free survival in South Korean patients with hepatocellular carcinoma. HPB (Oxford). England; 2016;18(1):98–106.

[59] Parikh ND, Waljee AK, Singal AG. Downstaging hepatocellular carcinoma: a systematic review and pooled analysis. Liver Transplant. 2015;21(9):1142–52. Available from: http://www.ncbi.nlm.nih.gov/pubmed/25981135 [cited 2015 Nov 17].

[60] Xu D-W, Wan P, Xia Q. Liver transplantation for hepatocellular carcinoma beyond the Milan criteria: a review. World J Gastroenterol. United States; 2016;22(12):3325–34.

[61] Majeed TA, Wai CT, Rajekar H, Lee KH, Wong SY, Leong SO, et al. Experience of the transplant team is an important factor for posttransplant survival in patients with hepatocellular carcinoma undergoing living-donor liver transplantation. Transplant Proc. United States; 2008;40(8):2507–9.

[62] Chen C-L, Concejero AM. Early post-operative complications in living donor liver transplantation: prevention, detection and management. HBPD INT. China; 2007;6(4): 345–7.

[63] Chen C-L, Concejero AM, Cheng Y-F. More than a quarter of a century of liver transplantation in Kaohsiung Chang Gung Memorial Hospital. Clin Transpl. United States; 2011;213–21.

[64] Jawan B, Wang C-H, Chen C-L, Huang C-J, Cheng K-W, Wu S-C, et al. Review of anesthesia in liver transplantation. Acta Anaesthesiol Taiwanica. Taiwan LLC; 2014;52(4):185–96. Available from: http://linkinghub.elsevier.com/retrieve/pii/S1875459714001088

[65] Nadalin, S., Bockhorn, M., Malagó, M., Valentin-Gamazo, C., Frilling, A., & Broelsch, C. E. (2006). Living donor liver transplantation. *HPB* :8(1), 10–21. http://doi.org/10.1080/13651820500465626.

[66] Abdeldayem HM, editor. Living Donor Liver Transplantation, Liver Transplantation - Technical Issues and Complications. InTech. 2012. Available from: http://www.intechopen.com/books/liver-transplantation-technical-issues-and-complications/living-donor-livertransplantation

[67] Ercolani G, Grazi GL, Ravaioli M, Grigioni WF, Cescon M, Gardini A, et al. The role of lymphadenectomy for liver tumors. Ann Surg. 2004;239(2):202–9.

[68] Sotiropoulos GC, Malago M, Molmenti EP, Losch C, Lang H, Frilling A, et al. Hilar lymph nodes sampling at the time of liver transplantation for hepatocellular carcinoma: to do or not to do? Meta-analysis to determine the impact of hilar lymph nodes metastases on tumor recurrence and survival in patients with hepatocellular carcin. Transpl Int. 2007;20(2):141–6. Available from: http://www.ncbi.nlm.nih.gov/pubmed/17239022\nhttp://onlinelibrary.wiley.com/doi/10.1111/j.1432-2277.2006.00412.x/abstract?systemMessage=Wiley+Online+Library+will+be+disrupted+on+7+July+from+10:00-12:00+BST+(05:00-07:00+EDT)+for+essential+maintenance

[69] Suh S-W, Lee J-M, You T, Choi YR, Yi N-J, Lee K-W, et al. Hepatic venous congestion in living donor grafts in liver transplantation: is there an effect on hepatocellular carcinoma recurrence? Liver Transplant Off Publ Am Assoc Study Liver Dis Int Liver Transplant Soc. United States; 2014;20(7):784–90.

[70] Matsuda H, Sadamori H, Shinoura S, Umeda Y, Yoshida R, Satoh D, et al. Aggressive combined resection of hepatic inferior vena cava, with replacement by a ringed expanded polytetrafluoroethylene graft, in living-donor liver transplantation for hepatocellular carcinoma beyond the Milan criteria. J Hepatobiliary Pancreat Sci. Japan; 2010;17(5):719–24.

[71] Pahari H, Li W-F, Lin T-S, Wang C-C, Yong C-C, Lin T-L, et al. Extensive adhesions in living donor liver transplantation: a retrospective analysis. World J Surg. 2015;40(2): 427–32. Available from: http://link.springer.com/10.1007/s00268-015-3219-x

[72] Memeo R, De'Angelis N, de Blasi V, Cherkaoui Z, Brunetti O, Longo V, et al. Innovative surgical approaches for hepatocellular carcinoma. World J Hepatol. United States; 2016;8(13):591–6.

[73] Lin T-S, Chiang Y-C, Chen C-L, Concejero AM, Cheng Y-F, Wang C-C, et al. Intimal dissection of the hepatic artery following transarterial embolization for hepatocellular carcinoma: an intraoperative problem in adult living donor liver transplantation. Liver Transplant Off Publ Am Assoc Study Liver Dis Int Liver Transplant Soc. United States; 2009;15(11):1553–6.

[74] Pomfret EA, Lodge JPA, Villamil FG, Siegler M. Should we use living donor grafts for patients with hepatocellular carcinoma? Ethical considerations. Liver Transplant Off Publ Am Assoc Study Liver Dis Int Liver Transplant Soc. United States; 2011;17 Suppl 2:S128–32.

[75] Mizuno S, Yokoi H, Shiraki K, Usui M, Sakurai H, Tabata M, et al. Prospective study on the outcome of patients with hepatocellular carcinoma registered for living donor liver transplantation: how long can they wait? Transplantat. United States; 2010;89(6): 650–4.

[76] Taefi a, Abrishami a, Eghtesad B, Sherman M. Surgical resection versus liver transplant for patients with hepatocellular carcinoma (Review). Cochrane Database Syst Rev. 2013;(6).

[77] Ho C, Lee P, Chen C, Ho M. Long-Term outcomes after resection versus transplantation for hepatocellular carcinoma within UCSF criteria. Ann Surg Oncol. 2012;19(3):826–33.

[78] Dai WC, Chan SC, Chok KSH, Cheung TT, Sharr WW, Chan ACY, et al. Good longterm survival after primary living donor liver transplantation for solitary hepatocellular carcinomas up to 8 cm in diameter. HPB (Oxford). England; 2014;16(8):749–57.

[79] Blumgart LH, Jarnagin WR, Belghiti J, Buchler MW, Chapman WC, M.I. D, et al., editors. Liver Transplantation: Indications and General Considerations. In: Blumgart's Surgery of the Liver, Biliary Tract, and Pancreas. 5th ed. Philadelphia: Elsevier; 2012.

[80] Silva MF, Sapisochin G, Strasser SI, Hewa-geeganage S, Chen J, Wigg AJ. Liver resection and transplantation offer similar 5-year survival for Child-Pugh-Turcotte A HCC-patients with a single nodule up to 5 cm: a multicenter, exploratory analysis. Eur J Surg Oncol. 2013;39(4):386–95. Available from: http://dx.doi.org/10.1016/j.ejso.2012.12.011

[81] Bruix J, Sherman M. Management of hepatocellular carcinoma: an update. Hepatol. United States; 2011;53(3):1020–2.

[82] Sapisochin G, Castells L, Dopazo C. Single HCC in cirrhotic patients: liver resection or liver transplantation?? Long-term outcome according to an intention-to-treat basis. Ann Surg Oncol. 2013;20(4):1194–202.

[83] Dhir M, Lyden ER, Smith LM, Are C. Comparison of outcomes of transplantation and resection in patients with early hepatocellular carcinoma: a meta-analysis. Hpb. 2012;14(9):635–45.

[84] Proneth A, Zeman F, Schlitt HJ, Schnitzbauer A. Is resection or transplantation the ideal treatment in patients with hepatocellular carcinoma in cirrhosis if both are possible? A systematic review and metaanalysis. Ann Surg Oncol. 2014;21(9):3096–107. Available from: http://www.ncbi.nlm.nih.gov/pubmed/24866437

[85] Kaido T, Morita S, Tanaka S, Ogawa K, Mori A, Hatano E, et al. Long-term outcomes of hepatic resection versus living donor liver transplantation for hepatocellular carcinoma: a propensity score-matching study. Dis Markers. United States; 2015;2015:425926.

[86] Dionigi R. One Liver for Two: Split and Living Donor Liver Transplantation for Adult and Pediatric Patients. In: Recent Advances in Liver Surgery. Austin, TX: Landes Bioscience; 2009.

[87] Di Sandro S, Slim AO, Giacomoni A, Lauterio A, Mangoni I, Aseni P, et al. Living donor liver transplantation for hepatocellular carcinoma: long-term results compared with deceased donor liver transplantation. Transplant Proc. United States; 2009;41(4):1283–5.

[88] Lee S-G, Moon D-B, Shin H, Kim K-H, Ahn C-S, Ha T-Y, et al. Living donor liver transplantation for hepatocellular carcinoma: current status in Korea. Transplant Proc. United States; 2012;44(2):520–2.

[89] Hu Z, Qian Z, Wu J, Zhou J, Zhang M, Zhou L, et al. Clinical outcomes and risk factors of hepatocellular carcinoma treated by liver transplantation: a multi-centre comparison of living donor and deceased donor transplantation. Clin Res Hepatol Gastroenterol. 2015; 2016 Jun;40(3):315–26

[90] Fisher RA, Kulik LM, Freise CE, Lok ASF, Shearon TH, Brown RSJ, et al. Hepatocellular carcinoma recurrence and death following living and deceased donor liver transplantation. Am J Transplant. Denmark; 2007;7(6):1601–8.

[91] Park M-S, Lee K-W, Suh S-W, You T, Choi Y, Kim H, et al. Living-donor liver transplantation associated with higher incidence of hepatocellular carcinoma recurrence than deceased-donor liver transplantation. Transplant J. 2014;97(1):71–7. Available from: http://content.wkhealth.com/linkback/openurl?sid=WKPTLP:landingpage&an=00007890-201401150-00012

[92] Ninomiya M, Shirabe K, Facciuto ME, Schwartz ME, Florman SS, Yoshizumi T, et al. Comparative study of living and deceased donor liver transplantation as a treatment for hepatocellular carcinoma. J Am Coll Surg. United States; 2015;220(3):297–304.e3.

4

Clinical and Pathological Review of Post Transplant Lymphoproliferative Disorders

Seema Naik, Hong Zheng, Kevin Rakszawski,
Clare Sample, Jeff Sample and Michael Bayerl

Abstract

Posttransplant lymphoproliferative disorder (PTLD) is a rare but potentially serious complication following transplantation with an overall incidence of PTLD of 1–5% in solid organ transplant (SOT) recipients and 1% in hematopoietic stem cell transplant (HSCT) recipients. The clinical and pathological spectrum of PTLD is broad; however, most cases of PTLD occur within the first year after transplantation and are associated with EBV. Clinical features that independently predict rates of response and survival have not been systematically studied for PTLD. Patients whose PTLD expressed CD20 or EBV have shorter intervals to PTLD onset, whereas late-onset cases of PTLD are typically EBV negative. Phenotypic characterization of PTLD reveals potential reliance on EBV or NF-kappaB signaling instead of B-cell receptor signaling, which links PTLD to other subgroups of EBV-related lymphomas, highlighting new potential treatment approaches. PTLD can be a life-threatening post-HSCT complication due to the impact of the patient's underlying disease (malignant or nonmalignant) as well as the type and intensity of the conditioning regimen. EBV-negative PTLD is more often a delayed phenomenon post-HSCT compared to EBV-positive PTLD. Further investigations are needed to better understand the role of EBV in the pathogenesis of different forms of PTLD in the immunosuppressed patients.

Keywords: posttransplant lymphoproliferative disorder (PTLD), Epstein-Barr virus (EBV), immunosuppression (IST)

1. Introduction

PTLD is an uncommon complication of hematopoietic stem cell transplant (HSCT) and solid organ transplant (SOT) with a broad clinical and pathological spectrum ranging from an acute, self-limited illness resembling infectious mononucleosis with histologically innocuous polyclonal lymphoid proliferation to aggressive, life-threatening tumors resembling aggressive lymphomas in immunocompetent individuals. The overall incidence of PTLD is about 1–5% in solid organ transplant (SOT) recipients and 1% in hematopoietic stem cell transplant (HSCT) recipients. Most cases of PTLD occur within the first year after transplantation. Late-onset PTLD, occurring years after transplantation, is often associated with more monoclonal lesions and a worse prognosis [1].

The clinical outcome of untreated aggressive PTLD after HSCT is very poor, suggestive of the biologic heterogeneity between the PTLD and de novo DLBCL. The mortality associated with PTLD induced by EBV infection can be reduced by monitoring EBV by polymerase chain reaction and by preemptively giving rituximab. The prompt initiation of preemptive therapy and early diagnosis of EBV disease are associated with decreased mortality [2, 3].

There is no consensus opinion as to whether a particular subtype of HSCT is associated with increased incidence of PTLD and whether salvage therapy provides survival benefits in patients developing early compared to late PTLD though, empirically, regimens that would reduce EBV-specific T cells, e.g. in vitro or in vivo T-cell purging, are believed to increase the risk of EBV-associated PTLD. Clinical features that independently predict rates of response, progression-free survival, and overall survival have not been systematically studied for PTLD presenting as aggressive non-Hodgkin lymphoma.

From a pathological standpoint, PTLD that represents a spectrum of lymphoid proliferations can be classified as nondestructive, polymorphic, monomorphic, and classical Hodgkin lymphoma types [29] based on morphology, immunophenotype, and clonality. Monomorphic and classical Hodgkin PTLDs are then classified based on their resemblance to de novo in lymphomas in immunocompetent individuals, e.g., diffuse large B-cell lymphoma, Burkitt lymphoma, plasmacytoma, plasma myeloma, peripheral T-cell lymphoma, NOS, hepatosplenic T-cell lymphoma, etc. The majority of monomorphic PTLDs resemble aggressive non-Hodgkin lymphoma, and most indolent lymphomas such as low-grade follicular lymphoma and EBV-negative extranodal marginal zone (MALT) lymphoma are not considered PTLD. However, a small number of EBV+ MALT lymphomas have been reported in the post-transplant setting and are considered a bona fide PTLD [29, 30].

2. PTLD in SOT vs. HSCT

Compared to the general population, the SOT patients have a 30–60-fold increased risk of developing PTLD. Most cases of PTLD occur within the first year after transplantation. EBV DNAemia occurs after transplantation in significantly more SOT recipients than HSCT patients. Correspondingly, more SOT patients also develop PTLD than HSCT patients and also significantly later posttransplant compared to HSCT recipients. The median length of time between transplant and diagnosis of PTLD for SOT patients is 2.8 years versus 121 days for HSCT patients [1, 4].

2.1. PTLD in SOT

In adults, incidence rates range 1–3% in kidney and liver transplants, 1–6% in cardiac transplants, 2–6% in combined heart-lung transplants, 4–10% in lung transplants, and up to 20% in small intestine transplants. The variation in rates among the types of organs transplanted is likely related to the degree and duration of immunosuppression as well as the number of EBV-positive donor lymphocytes in the graft. PTLD is more common in lung and small bowel transplants. Duration of the posttransplant period is important because PTLD is most likely to develop in the first year following transplantation, with an incidence of 224 per 100,000 but falls to 54 per 100,000 in the second year and 31 per 100,000 in the sixth year. PTLD represents a heterogeneous group of non-Hodgkin lymphomas that vary clinically and are ill-defined morphologically [5–8].

2.2. PTLD in HSCT

PTLD develops in approximately 1% of patients post HSCT, among which the majority of cases occur within the first year after allogeneic stem cell transplantation (alloSCT). It is highly related to EBV reactivation. Risk factors that associate with high incidence of EBV-related PTLD include elderly patients (aged ≥50 years at transplantation), T-cell depletion-containing regimens, antithymocyte globulin (ATG) use, and grafts derived from unrelated or HLA-mismatched donors. PTLD can also develop in patients who received autologous stem cell transplants, but the frequency is much lower than alloSCT [9, 10]. PTLD in ASCT cases occurs in younger age group, with shorter duration of onset than solid organ transplantation.

3. Diagnostic markers

3.1. CD20 positivity

The prognostic role of CD20 expression and Epstein–Barr virus (EBV) positivity in PTLD after SOT is poorly understood. In a retrospective study, a total of 45 pediatric SOT patients (28 heart, 11 liver, and 6 kidney) were diagnosed with PTLD 45 months after SOT. Of the 40 evaluable PTLD cases (11 monomorphic, 19 polymorphic, 5 early lesions, and 5 rare subtypes), 32 (80%) had detectable EBV, and 28 (70%) were classified as CD20 (+). Patients whose PTLD expressed CD20 or EBV had shorter intervals between SOT and PTLD onset (28 vs. 64 or 77 months for CD20 and EBV, respectively) ($P < 0.02$). Patients with CD20 (+) tumors had higher 5-year PTLD-related EFS (83.7% vs. 28.6%, $P < 0.001$) and OS (95.8% vs. 56.3%, $P = 0.01$). EBV expression was unrelated to PTLD-related EFS or OS. CD20 expression is thus found to be associated with timing of development of PTLD and predicts survival in pediatric PTLD in SOT [11].

3.2. Other diagnostic markers

Comprehensive phenotypic characterization of PTLD reveals potential reliance on EBV or NF-kappaB signaling instead of B-cell receptor signaling. Several signaling pathways, cells of origin of PTLD, and their relation to viruses were analyzed by immunohistochemistry and in situ hybridization. Most PTLDs are of activated B-cell origin. Two-thirds of cases show an Epstein-Barr virus (EBV) infection of the neoplastic cells. NF-kappaB signaling components are present in the majority of cases, except for EBV-infected cases with latency type III lacking CD19 and upstream B-cell signaling constituents. Proteins involved in B-cell receptor signaling like Bruton tyrosine kinase are seen only present in a minority of cases. Phosphoinositide 3-kinase (PI3K) is found to be expressed in 94% of cases and the druggable PI3K class 1 catalytic subunit p110 in 76%, while other signal transduction proteins are expressed only in occasional cases. Unsupervised cluster analysis has revealed three distinct subgroups: (I) related to EBV infection, mainly latency type III and lacking CD19, upstream B-cell signaling, and NF-kappa constituents; (ii) related to EBV infection with expression of the alternative NF-kappaB pathway compound including RelB, CD10, and FOXP1 or MUM1; and (iii) unrelated to virus infection with expression of the classic NF-kappaB pathway compound p65 [12]. EBV and NF-kappaB are important drivers in PTLD in contrast to B-cell receptor signaling. The main signal transduction pathway is related to PI3K. This links PTLD to other subgroups of EBV-related lymphomas, highlighting also new potential treatment approaches [4].

The diagnosis of PTLD relies on comprehensive morphologic examination, immunophenotyping, genetics, and EBV status. Most of PTLDs are of B-cell origin. EBV plays an important role in the pathogenesis of PTLD. The duration of disease onset is shorter in EBV-positive cases.

3.3. EBV viremia and EBV detection by EBER

The majority of EBV infections that occur after transplantation, especially in adults, are clinically silent reactivations. This leads to a subsequent delay in the diagnosis of PTLD. A positive correlation between the degree of EBV DNAemia and the development of PTLD has significant implications for the importance of monitoring viral load after transplantation. In a study done by Holman et al., the risk of PTLD in viremic patients significantly increased with the peak quantity of EBV DNAemia [2, 13]. Since the occurrence of PTLD is significantly related to the viral load, constant monitoring and quantification of EBV-DNA load are utilized as prognostic markers for the development of PTLD.. In solid organ transplant (SOT) recipients, approximately 50% of patients develop detectable EBV DNAemia, but only a much smaller subset develops PTLD.

3.4. EBV antigens

The broad EBV latency profile (LMP1+/EBNA 2+) is found to be expressed in 59% of EBV (+) PT-DLBCL and is associated with a more elaborated inflammatory response than intermediate latency (LMP1+/EBNA 2-) with a role for innate and tolerogenic immune response in EBV + PT-DLBCL. EBV signature is the most important factor in the pathogenesis of EBV (+) PT-DLBCL [14].

3.5. Genomic profiling of PTLD

Clinical, pathological, and molecular genetic characteristics of PTLD show that EBV-positive and EBV-negative PTLDs have distinct gene expression profiling with clustering related to EBV status than immune status. Except for decreased T-cell signaling, EBV-negative PTLDs are inseparable from EBV-negative IC-DLBCL. In contrast, an EBV viral response signature is clearly shown to segregate EBV (+) PT-DLBCL from EBV (−) PT-DLBCL [14, 16].

3.6. PTLD diagnostic algorithm

Systematic morphological, immunophenotypic, and genetic analysis of each PTLD case should be performed. In DLBCL type, one may apply BCL-6, CD10, and MUM-1 immunostains in order to establish the cell of origin according to the Hans algorithm [17]; but the value of this assignment is not well established in this setting. Based on EBV protein expression, the latency type of EBV infection is defined as LMP1-/EBNA2- (type I, restricted), LMP1+/EBNA2- (type II, intermediate), and LMP1+/EBNA2+ (type III, broad). The stromal infiltrate can be estimated semiquantitatively based on the ratio of tumor cells and stromal cells in the entire tissue section. In situ hybridization: EBER (EBV-encoded RNA) in situ hybridization is considered the standard for diagnosis of EBV infection and should be performed in all PTLD cases. PTLD cases are defined as EBV (+) if EBER was expressed in all tumor cells in which RNA was preserved [14].

4. EBV-positive PTLD vs. EBV-negative PTLD

Epstein-Barr virus-positive (EBV (+)) and EBV-negative (EBV (−)) PT-DLBCL have distinct gene expression profiles, and the transcriptomic profile of EBV (−) PT-DLBCL is similar to that of DLBCL in immunocompetent individuals (IC-DLBCL) and supports the hypothesis that EBV (−) PT-DLBCL are de novo lymphomas. EBV (+) and EBV (−) PT-DLBCL have distinct aCGH profiles and shared only one recurrent imbalance. EBV (−) PT-DLBCL, however, display at least ten aberrations recurrent in IC-DLBCL, among which characteristic gain of 3/3q and 18q and loss of 6q23/TNFAIP3 as well as 9p21/CDKN2A. The most prevalent aberration in EBV (+) PT-DLBCL is due to gain/amplification of 9p24.1 targeting PDCD1LG2/PDL2. FOXP1 oncogene and the tumor suppressor CDKNA2 implicated in EBV (−) DLBCL do not play a critical role in the pathogenesis of EBV (+) PT-DLBCL [14].

5. Nondestructive vs. monomorphic PTLD

Destructive PTLD, which has typically not correlated with other specific risk factors, has recently been shown to be associated with older recipient age and prolonged receipt of calcineurin inhibitors. Furthermore, recent data has contributed to and, in some instances, shed light on previous debate concerning the role of viruses other than EBV and the level of HLA mismatch as risk factors for PTLD [15]. Gene association studies focusing on key cytokines and their receptors have identified several polymorphisms that may prove useful to identify patients at risk, with distinction for early nondestructive and late occurring monomorphic PTLD.

6. Monomorphic PTLD vs. polymorphic PTLD

The term PTLD represents a spectrum of B-cell hyperproliferative states that can be classified as nondestructive PTLD, polymorphic PTLD, monomorphic PTLD, and classical Hodgkin lymphoma, all of which may be associated with Epstein–Barr virus (EBV).

Nondestructive lesions are classified as reactive plasmacytic hyperplasia, florid follicular hyperplasia, and infectious mononucleosis-like PTLD. These lesions are frequently associated with an acute illness similar to mononucleosis, with polyclonal B-cell proliferation, but without evidence of malignant transformation by definition, the lymphoid architecture is preserved.

Polymorphic PTLDs are polyclonal or monoclonal lymphoid infiltrates with evidence of destructive growth patterns including necrosis, destruction of underlying lymphoid architecture, and nuclear atypia. However, polymorphic PTLD does not otherwise meet all criteria for B-cell or T-/NK-cell lymphomas as characterized in immunocompetent patients [1].

Monomorphic PTLDs are monoclonal lymphoid proliferations. Monomorphic PTLD most commonly resembles aggressive B-cell lymphomas such as Burkitt lymphoma/high-grade B-cell lymphoma or diffuse large B-cell lymphoma (DLBCL), as seen in immunocompetent patients. Likewise, classical Hodgkin-like lymphoma variably resembles those observed in immunocompetent patients. Small B-cell lymphomas such as follicular lymphoma, small lymphocytic lymphoma, and EBV-negative marginal zone lymphomas that occur in the post-transplant setting are not characterized as PTLD. A small group of EBV+ MALT lymphoma is now recognized as *bona fide* PTLD [30].

7. Pediatric PTLD

PTLD occurs more commonly in pediatric patients than in adults. The higher incidence in children is thought to result from being EBV-naïve recipients. PTLDs can arise during post-transplant period after both myeloablative and nonmyeloablative allogeneic hematopoietic cell transplantation. EBV is frequently expressed in PTLD in patients with both HSCT and SOT. Posttransplant lymphoproliferative disorder (PTLD) has been associated with high mortality, but recent anecdotal survival appears better. NAPRTCS registry had 235 registered PTLD cases from 1988 to 2010 which showed that survival has improved with more recent PTLDs in children following kidney transplants [6, 18].

8. Role of immunosuppression (IST)

The degree and duration of immunosuppression play a major role in the development of PTLD. Cytotoxic T cells provide a defense mechanism against EBV-infected B cells in immunocompetent individuals. However, when T-cell function is impaired, this defense mechanism is lost, therefore promoting the development of PTLD.

8.1. ATG and PTLD

In vivo T-cell depletion (TCD) with antithymocyte globulin (ATG) or alemtuzumab (AL) is commonly used in HSCT. TCD facilitates engraftment and reduces the incidence and severity of graft-versus-host disease (GvHD). As reduced intensity conditioning (RIC) and matched unrelated donor transplants (MUD) are now being performed more frequently, ATG and AL have become integral components of preparative regimens. Although ATG and AL provide safer T-cell depletion, delayed T-cell reconstitution following TCD accounts for infectious complications and increased mortality.

EBV PTLD is predominantly derived from donor B cells before reconstitution of the EBV-specific cytotoxic T lymphocyte (CTL) response. It can, however, occur later in the most severely immunocompromised patients with additional risk factors such as donor and recipient mismatch, graft manipulation with T-cell depletion, as well as the degree and duration of immunosuppression.

In a study by Buyck et al., an overall incidence of 6.3% for EBV PTLD was reported in 89 patients with severe aplastic anemia. A marked increase in the incidence (13.3%) was noted in patients exposed to ATG, with 5 of 43 patients developing EBV PTLD [19].

9. Other rare subtypes of PTLD

Although the majority of monomorphic PTLDs fall into the category of diffuse large B-cell lymphoma, other types of lymphoma may also occur. These include plasma cell myeloma, classical Hodgkin lymphoma, or HL-like PTLD, EBV+ MALT lymphoma as well as various T-cell lymphomas with or without EBV infection.

9.1. Burkitt PTLD

A variety of lymphomas can develop as PTLD, although some types appear infrequently and remain poorly understood. PTLD-Burkitt lymphomas behave aggressively and require intensive chemotherapeutic intervention. These display the typical histological features of Burkitt lymphoma but are markedly positive for EBV. While BL-PTLD is a rare entity, it is a discrete form of PTLD with a high EBV expression and should be treated as a high-grade lymphoma. BL-PTLD historically represents a small, but significant, proportion of PTLD cases. BL-PTLD represents 15% of PTLD patients for pediatric heart, lung, and heart-lung transplants from

1982 to 2009, with a 1.1% overall incidence among pediatric transplant heart-lung recipients, 14% of our pediatric renal PTLD patients, 1.6% among kidney recipients, and 0.71% pediatric liver-transplant recipients, as reported in a single institution study. BL-PTLD is a more aggressive type of PTLD and does not respond to a trial of decreased immunosuppression like P-PTLD and some M-PTLDs. BL-PTLD does require cessation of conventional immunosuppression during treatment with multiagent lymphoma-specific chemotherapy. Bone marrow involvement remains a poor prognostic factor, despite the use of lymphoma-specific chemotherapy in these cases [20–24].

BL after organ transplantation is often found in extra-nodal sites; it involves the central nervous system more frequently than it does in immunocompetent patients. In 70% of BL occurring after organ transplantation, genes or gene products related to EBV can be demonstrated within the tumor cells. The EBV status of the tumor is of important prognostic significance: EBV-positive BL occurring in organ transplant patients usually responds well to reduction or cessation of immunosuppressive therapy; in some cases permanent complete remissions can be achieved even without chemotherapy. In contrast, patients with EBV-negative BL have a very poor prognosis and rarely respond even to aggressive chemotherapy protocols [23].

9.2. T cell PTLD

The etiology of posttransplant T-cell lymphomas remains unclear. Similarities with posttransplant B-cell proliferations are the predominant extranodal presentation and the finding that the time of occurrence is influenced by the type of immunosuppression. In contrast with posttransplant B-cell proliferations, only a minority of the cases are associated with EBV. Most tumors appear to be monoclonal. Prognosis is generally poor, but tumor presentation with localized disease might have a somewhat better prognosis. Ambiguity about the pathogenesis of T-PTLD and the lack of accepted diagnostic criteria may contribute to the rarity and inconsistent characterization of T-PTLD in the literature. While there is a general impression that T-PTLD is very difficult to cure, several recently reported cases demonstrate that these tumors can be very treatment responsive with the use of different chemotherapy regimens than those typically used to treat B-PTLD, such as the intensive ALL-type treatments we employed, and/or the use of different strategies for immunosuppression. Most T-PTLDs are not EBV-driven; thus, reduction of immunosuppression may not be effective as a sole treatment strategy and may be less critical for management of T-PTLD than it is in EBV-driven B-PTLDs.

T-PTLD cases may sometimes exhibit a bimodal response to therapy, with initial eradication of the bulk nodal disease with regimens typically used to treat ALL but persistence of low-level clonal T cells in the marrow, CSF, and lung. Due to small patient numbers, different strategies of treatment may be needed compared to B-lineage PTLD [25, 26].

9.3. HL-PTLD

PTLD that resembles Hodgkin lymphoma (HL-PTLD) has been reported infrequently. These cases have variable numbers of Reed-Sternberg-like (RS-like) cells and highlight differences in the phenotype that may distinguish these from true Hodgkin lymphoma (HD). These occur 8 months to 13 years following transplant. The large cells of HL-PTLD are pleomorphic B cells that react strongly for CD20 and/or CD79a and express CD30 but are usually negative for CD15 and have few mitoses. They are positive for EBV early RNA (EBER) using an EBER-1 probe, as are some of the background small lymphocytes. HD-PTLD is managed by withdrawal of immunosuppression and variably treated with rituximab to chemotherapy [27]. HL-PTLD and HD appear to be two related but immunophenotypically and biologically distinct forms of lymphoproliferation in posttransplant patients and may require different protocols for their management [27, 28]. Overall survival at 2 and 5 years was 86% with 81% of patients surviving event-free. Rituximab monotherapy has not been shown to lead to long-term remission, but treatment with classical HL chemotherapy is effective and tolerable. New treatment modalities such as CD30-targeted or EBV-specific agents may diminish toxicity.

10. DLBCL vs. PTLD

Within the PT-DLBCL series, EBV (+) cases were different from EBV (−) cases. The fact that all EBV (+) PT-DLBCL cases are of activated B-cell (ABC) origin whereas 45% EBV (−) PT-DLBCL cases were of GCB origin might contribute to the observed difference in survival. Overall, EBV (−) PT-DLBCL was similar to DLBCL arising in immunocompetent individuals regarding median age at diagnosis (63 versus 65 years). The amount of stromal infiltration was significantly higher in IC-DLBCL than PT-DLBCL (12/13 and 12/33 cases contained ≥15% stroma, respectively, $P = 0.0012$). Geographical necrosis was almost exclusively observed in EBV (+) PT-DLBCL (46%), compared to EBV (−) PT-DLBCL (11%). In contrast, there was no obvious difference in the absolute amount of stromal infiltration between both groups. IDO1 was variably expressed in the tumor and/or stromal cells of 7/22 EBV(+) PT-DLBCL. The Epstein–Barr virus broad latency profile (LMP1+/EBNA2+) was most frequently expressed in PT-DLBCL ($n = 13/22$; 59%) and associated with a more elaborate inflammatory response than intermediate latency (LMP1+/EBNA2−).

11. Therapy and prevention of PTLD

Prevention of PTLD involves limiting the duration and degree of immunosuppression while still maintaining the adequacy of the donor graft. Achieving a balance of reduction in immunosuppression and preventing graft rejection or graft-versus-host disease can be challenging.

Antiviral prophylaxis may also play a role in preventing PTLD, though data are scarce, particularly in SOT recipients. The use of antivirals such as acyclovir, valganciclovir, and ganciclovir is common for HSV, CMV, and EBV prophylaxis, though utilization varies according to institutional guidelines and protocols.

Many transplant centers will preemptively reduce immunosuppression and/or administer the anti-CD20 agent rituximab when EBV reactivation (i.e., ≥1000 EBV genome equivalents per mL) has occurred in the posttransplant setting.

11.1. Treatment of nondestructive lesions

Reduction of immunosuppression is typically recommended for patients with early lesions. If there is residual disease or reduction in immunosuppression is not tolerated or allowable due to concerns regarding the donor graft, rituximab may be utilized.

11.2. Treatment of polymorphic PTLD

A combination of reduction in immunosuppression and rituximab is recommended for patients with polymorphic PTLD.

11.3. Treatment of monomorphic PTLD

For patients with monomorphic PTLD, treatment involves rituximab alone or in combination with systemic chemotherapy, in addition to reduction in immunosuppression. Single-agent rituximab may be utilized in patients with minimal PTLD-related symptoms or low disease burden or if poor performance status or other medical comorbidities preclude the use of systemic chemotherapy. The most commonly employed chemotherapy regimen is R-CHOP (rituximab plus cyclophosphamide, doxorubicin, vincristine, and prednisone); rituximab is omitted in cases of CD20-negative PTLD.

11.4. Conclusion(s)

PTLD can be a life-threatening post-HSCT complication due to the impact of the patient's underlying disease (malignant or nonmalignant) as well as the type and intensity of the transplant conditioning regimen. EBV-negative PTLD is a delayed phenomenon post-HSCT as compared to EBV-positive PTLD. Biomarkers that measure the extent of immunosuppression may have a role in avoiding PTLD and other posttransplant complications. Further investigations are needed to better understand the role of EBV infection in the pathogenesis of the different forms of PTLD in the immunosuppressed patients.

Author details

Seema Naik[1*], Hong Zheng[1], Kevin Rakszawski[1], Clare Sample[2], Jeff Sample[2] and Michael Bayerl[3]

*Address all correspondence to: snaik@pennstatehealth.psu.edu

1 Department of Medicine, Division of Hematology/Oncology, Penn State Cancer Institute, Milton S. Hershey Medical Center, Hershey, PA, USA

2 Department of Immunology, Penn State College of Medicine, Milton S. Hershey Medical Center, Hershey, PA, USA

3 Department of Pathology, Penn State College of Medicine, Milton S. Hershey Medical Center, Hershey, PA, USA

References

[1] Carbone A, Gloghini A, Dotti G. EBV-associated lymphoproliferative disorders: Classification and treatment. The Oncologist. 2008;**13**(5):577-585

[2] Clave E, Agbalika F, Bajzik V, Peffault de Latour R, Trillard M, Rabian C, et al. Epstein-Barr virus (EBV) reactivation in allogeneic stem-cell transplantation: Relationship between viral load, EBV-specific T-cell reconstitution and rituximab therapy. Transplantation. 2004;**77**(1):76-84

[3] Coppoletta S, Tedone E, Galano B, Soracco M, Raiola AM, Lamparelli T, et al. Rituximab treatment for Epstein-Barr virus DNAemia after alternative-donor hematopoietic stem cell transplantation. Biology of Blood and Marrow Transplantation. 2011;**17**(6):901-907

[4] Ghobrial IM, Habermann TM, Ristow KM, Ansell SM, Macon W, Geyer SM, et al. Prognostic factors in patients with post-transplant lymphoproliferative disorders (PTLD) in the rituximab era. Leukemia & Lymphoma. 2005;**46**(2):191-196

[5] Dharnidharka VR, Lamb KE, Gregg JA, Meier-Kriesche HU. Associations between EBV serostatus and organ transplant type in PTLD risk: An analysis of the SRTR National Registry Data in the United States. American Journal of Transplantation. 2012;**12**(4): 976-983

[6] Dharnidharka VR, Martz KL, Stablein DM, Benfield MR. Improved survival with recent post-transplant Lymphoproliferative disorder (PTLD) in children with kidney transplants. American Journal of Transplantation. 2011;**11**(4):751-758

[7] Manez R, Breinig MK, Linden P, Kusne S, Torre-Cisneros J, Wilson J, et al. Factors associated with the development of post-transplant lymphoproliferative disease (PTLD) in Epstein-Barr virus (EBV)-seronegative adult liver transplant recipients. Transplant International. 1994;**7**(Suppl 1):S235-S237

[8] Khedmat H, Characteristics TS. Prognosis of post-transplant lymphoproliferative disorders within renal allograft: Report from the PTLD.Int. survey. Annals of Transplantation. 2010;**15**(3):80-86

[9] Rasche L, Kapp M, Einsele H, Mielke S. EBV-induced post transplant lymphoproliferative disorders: A persisting challenge in allogeneic hematopoetic SCT. Bone Marrow Transplantation. 2014;**49**(2):163-167

[10] Sanz J, Andreu R. Epstein-Barr virus-associated posttransplant lymphoproliferative disorder after allogeneic stem cell transplantation. Current Opinion in Oncology. 2014; **26**(6):677-683

[11] Orjuela MA, Alobeid B, Liu X, Siebert AL, Kott ER, Addonizio LJ, et al. CD20 expression predicts survival in paediatric post-transplant lymphoproliferative disease (PTLD) following solid organ transplantation. British Journal of Haematology. 2011;**152**(6): 733-742

[12] Menter T, Dickenmann M, Juskevicius D, Steiger J, Dirnhofer S, Tzankov A. Comprehensive phenotypic characterization of PTLD reveals potential reliance on EBV or NF-kappaB signalling instead of B-cell receptor signalling. Hematological Oncology. 2017;**35**(2):187-197

[13] Kinch A, Oberg G, Arvidson J, Falk KI, Linde A, Pauksens K. Post-transplant lymphoproliferative disease and other Epstein-Barr virus diseases in allogeneic haematopoietic stem cell transplantation after introduction of monitoring of viral load by polymerase chain reaction. Scandinavian Journal of Infectious Diseases. 2007;**39**(3):235-244

[14] Craig FE, Johnson LR, Harvey SA, Nalesnik MA, Luo JH, Bhattacharya SD, et al. Gene expression profiling of Epstein-Barr virus-positive and -negative monomorphic B-cell posttransplant lymphoproliferative disorders. Diagnostic Molecular Pathology. 2007;**16**(3):158-168

[15] Styczynski J, Reusser P, Einsele H, de la Camara R, Cordonnier C, Ward KN, et al. Management of HSV, VZV and EBV infections in patients with hematological malignancies and after SCT: Guidelines from the second European conference on infections in Leukemia. Bone Marrow Transplantation. 2009;**43**(10):757-770

[16] Morscio J, Dierickx D, Ferreiro JF, Herreman A, Van Loo P, Bittoun E, et al. Gene expression profiling reveals clear differences between EBV-positive and EBV-negative posttransplant lymphoproliferative disorders. American Journal of Transplantation. 2013;**13**(5):1305-1316

[17] Hans CP, Weisenburger DD, Greiner TC, Gascoyne RD, Delabie J, Ott G, et al. Confirmation of the molecular classification of diffuse large B-cell lymphoma by immunohistochemistry using a tissue microarray. Blood. 2004;**103**(1):275-282

[18] Cohen J, Gandhi M, Naik P, Cubitt D, Rao K, Thaker U, et al. Increased incidence of EBV-related disease following paediatric stem cell transplantation with reduced-intensity conditioning. British Journal of Haematology. 2005;**129**(2):229-239

[19] Buyck HC, Ball S, Junagade P, Marsh J, Chakrabarti S. Prior immunosuppressive therapy with antithymocyte globulin increases the risk of EBV-related lymphoproliferative disorder following Allo-SCT for acquired aplastic anaemia. Bone Marrow Transplantation. 2009;**43**(10):813-816

[20] Bellan C, Lazzi S, Hummel M, Palummo N, de Santi M, Amato T, et al. Immunoglobulin gene analysis reveals 2 distinct cells of origin for EBV-positive and EBV-negative Burkitt lymphomas. Blood. 2005;**106**(3):1031-1036

[21] Lohrisch CA, Nevill TJ, Barnett MJ, Hogge DE, Connors JM, Keown PA, et al. Development of a biologically distinct EBV-related lymphoproliferative disorder following autologous bone marrow transplantation for an EBV-negative post-renal allograft Burkitt's lymphoma. Leukemia & Lymphoma. 2000;**39**(1-2):195-201

[22] Navari M, Fuligni F, Laginestra MA, Etebari M, Ambrosio MR, Sapienza MR, et al. Molecular signature of Epstein Barr virus-positive Burkitt lymphoma and post-transplant lymphoproliferative disorder suggest different roles for Epstein Barr virus. Frontiers in Microbiology. 2014;**5**:728

[23] Picarsic J, Jaffe R, Mazariegos G, Webber SA, Ellis D, Green MD, et al. Post-transplant Burkitt lymphoma is a more aggressive and distinct form of post-transplant lymphoproliferative disorder. Cancer. 2011;**117**(19):4540-4550

[24] Razzouk BI, Srinivas S, Sample CE, Singh V, Sixbey JW. Epstein-Barr virus DNA recombination and loss in sporadic Burkitt's lymphoma. The Journal of Infectious Diseases. 1996;**173**(3):529-535

[25] Waller EK, Ziemianska M, Bangs CD, et al. Characterization of posttransplant lymphomas that express T-cell-associated markers: Immunophenotypes, molecular genetics, cytogenetics, and hetero-transplantation in severe combined immunodeficient mice. Blood. 1993;**82**:247-261

[26] van Gorp J, Doornewaard H, Verdonck LF, et al. Posttransplant T-cell lymphoma. Report of three cases and a review of the literature. Cancer. 1994;**73**:3064-3072

[27] Kampers J, Orjuela-Grimm M, Schober T, et al. Classical Hodgkin lymphoma-type PTLD after solid organ transplantation in children: a report on 17 patients treated according to subsequent GPOH-HD treatment schedules. Leuk Lymphoma. 2017 Mar;**58**(3):633-638

[28] Ranganathan S, Webber S, Ahuja S, Jaffe R. Hodgkin-like posttransplant lymphoproliferative disorder in children: Does it differ from posttransplant Hodgkin lymphoma? Pediatric and Developmental Pathology. 2004 Jul-Aug;**7**(4):348-360

[29] Swerdlow SH, Campo E, Harris NL, et al. WHO Classification of Tumours of Haematopoietic and Lymphoid Tissues. Revised Ed 4th ed. Lyon, France: IARC Press; 2018

[30] Gibson SE, Swerdlow SH, Craig FE, Surti U, Cook JR, Nalesnik MA, Lowe C, Wood KM, Bacon CM. EBV-positive extranodal marginal zone lymphoma of mucosa-associated lymphoid tissue in the posttransplant setting: A distinct type of posttransplant lymphoproliferative disorder? The American Journal of Surgical Pathology. 2011 Jun;**35**(6): 807-815

5

Organ Donation and Transplantation: "Life after Death"

Kanmani Job and Anooja Antony

Abstract

Organ donation is defined as giving an organ or part of an organ to be transplanted into another person. Organ transplantation is the only option to save lives in patients affected by terminal organ failures and improve their quality of life. However, there is a disparity exists between the supply and demand of donated organs, leads to a loss of many lives. The number of organ transplantation have gradually increased in the last two decades and provide excellent results in children and young adults, and are challenging by the growing proportion of elderly transplant patients with co morbidity. The results of organ transplantation continue to improve, as a consequence of the innovations and the improvements in peri-operative management. This chapter describes organ donation and transplantation and its trends and challenges.

Keywords: organ donation, motivation, psychosocial

1. Introduction

Organ donation is defined as giving an organ or part of an organ to be transplanted into another person. Organ transplantation is the only option to save lives in patients affected by terminal organ failures and improve their quality of life. However, there is a disparity exists between the supply and demand of donated organs, leads to a loss of many lives. The number of organ transplantation have gradually increased in the last two decades and provide excellent results in children and young adults, and are challenging by the growing proportion of elderly transplant patients with co morbidity. The results of organ transplantation continue to improve, as a consequence of the innovations and the improvements in peri-operative management.

Organ transplantation currently depends on the availability of human organs. Their scarcity means that there is a waiting list of almost 63,000 in the European Union, and over 100,000 people in the United States according to the recent survey. The process of obtaining organs for donation and transplantation purely depends on the resources of health services and by health professionals' performance in potential donor identification and management tasks. However, in accordance with the current legislation it is mainly subjected to a personal or family decision, strongly mediated by psychosocial processes. Therefore, the need to analyze and intervene both in the practices of the professionals involved in the process of organ generation and in the attitudes of the general population need to stressed and addressed [1–5].

2. Organ transplantation and organ donation: an overview

Organ transplantation involves the surgical implantation of an organ or section of an organ into a person whose own organ is failing. The donor organ may come from both deceased individual as well as from a living donor. The patients psychological and behavior aspect as well their emotional response and mental health and adherence to medical regimen should be assessed before and after organ transplantation. The living donor's psychological response towards organ donation (most commonly for kidney and liver segment transplantation) is an important aspect to consider in the transplantation process.

Organ donation is defined as "giving an organ or part of an organ to be transplanted into another person" (Organ procurement of Transplant Network (OPTN), 2015), organ donation has the potential to save lives. The organs donated from one single donor can save up to eight lives. Organ transplantation may be one of the options left to sustain someone's life. However, the disparity that exists between the supply and demand of donated organs, leads to a loss of many lives. Based on recent OPTN data, approximately 21 people will die each day while waiting for a transplant in the United States (US). Currently, 123, 358 people are awaiting organs and on the transplant list in the US with this number growing and the number of donated organs declining.

Asian Indians are more likely to have higher rates of having obesity and diabetes when compared with other Asian subgroups which make them at an increased risk of needing a donated organ [35]. These conditions can lead one to develop coronary artery disease and hypertension which then can lead to chronic kidney disease and other chronic illnesses. Patients who suffer from chronic kidney disease need regular dialysis which can ultimately lead them to organ transplantation to improve one's quality of life. Also, conditions such as diabetes and obesity can be detrimental to one's life and can lead to fatty liver disease which can lead to chronic liver disease requiring liver transplantation if the liver decompensates.

The development of organ transplantation in the second half of the 20th century has been a remarkable achievement. Recently; organ transplantation is one of the most effective options for those with an end-stage organ failure. Its success has been basically dependent on public awareness, support and active participation. Without these factors, the efficiency of organ transplantation and the consequent saving or extension of lives would have undoubtedly suffered adversely.

The number of patients in need of organ transplantation has increased at a rapid pace; in contrast, the number of available organs has increased only slightly. Expanded criteria for donor selection, such as older age, have resulted in more people who meet the criteria for brain death becoming organ donors although fewer organs are transplanted from each donor. Improvements in automobile and highway safety, as well as increased enforcement of gun control laws, have also contributed to a plateau in the number of young, healthy donors. Public education efforts that encourage organ donation may be effective in getting more people to sign organ donor cards, but most individuals who do so will never be in a position to become organ donors.

Faced with increasing numbers of patients who need transplantation, deaths on the waiting list, and a fixed number of available organs, some transplant programs are working to increase the number of transplants from living donors. Although living donation has always been an option for some types of transplants, many programs have been reluctant to promote it, as living donation requires invasive surgery on a healthy person with associated risks of morbidity and mortality. For example, since dialysis is an option for patients with end-stage renal disease, surgery on a healthy donor may be difficult to justify, despite the dialysis patient's diminished quality of life.

The most important in organ donation is to maximize the psychological status and well-being of the donors before and after transplantation has become the foremost goal of all transplantation centres. The psychological issues that mainly concern with the living organ donation includes prevention of psychological harm, ensuring the donors are fully informed and decide to donate without coercion, monitoring donor psychosocial outcomes are intimately linked to the factors that historically served as barriers to use of organs from living donors. These barriers can be overcome by the motivating of the public and creating awareness and responsibility among oneself.

Organs that can be transplanted from the living donor includes one kidney, part of intestine, pancreas, islets of Langerhans, bone, part of liver, one testis, bone marrow and blood. The organ that can be transplanted from the deceased donor are heart, kidney, pancreas, stomach, hand, skin, blood vessels, lungs, liver, intestine, testis, cornea and heart valve.

Types of organ donation

1. **Autograft:** Transplanting a person's tissues from one site and use it in another site of his body and is called autograft. For example, removal of skin from the legs and using it for damaged skin face or other exposed part.

2. **Allograft:** Transplant of an organ between two genetically non identical individuals, it is called allograft. Due to the genetic difference, the donor's organ will be treated as foreign by the recipient and will try to destroy it. This is called s rejection.

3. **Isograft:** Transplant of organ/tissue from a donor to genetically identical recipient is called isograft. There will not be any immune response hence no transplant rejection.

4. **Xenograft:** Transplantation of organ/tissues forms one species to another species. For example, the heart valve of pig is transplanted successfully to human.

5. **Split transplant:** An organ like liver retrieved from the deceased donor can be divided between two recipients, usually an adult and a child.

6. **Domino transplant:** When the lungs are to be transplanted, surgically it is easier to replace them along with the heart. If the recipient's original heart is healthy, it can be transplanted into another recipient in the need of one.

7. **ABO incompatible transplantation:** The immune system of young children aged below 12 months might have developed fully. They can receive organs from incompatible donors.

Types of donors

1. **Live donors:** A living person, mentally and physically healthy can donate one of a paired organ, part of an organ or a tissue. The organs donated are kidneys, part of live, one of the lung, part of small intestine, skin, bone marrow, one of the testis and one of the ovaries. Live donor can either be related or unrelated.

2. **Unrelated donors:** For altruistic reasons, a person can donate one of his organs to an unrelated donor. According to TOHO act, the unrelated donor should be known to the recipient and have some obligation to him. It has to be established that there is no monetary transaction between them. But in many other countries, even a stranger can donate one of his organs to a needy person on altruistic grounds.

3. **Deceased donors:** Organs are harvested from brain dead person whose respiration and circulation are maintained artificially. Brain dead has to be certified by a team of doctors nominated by Government I every organ retrieval centers.

4. **Paired exchange:** When a living donor is not compatible with the related recipient, but may be compatible for another recipient. That second recipient related donor is compatible to the first recipient, then permission can be granted for transplantation. The surgery for all four donors and recipient are conducted simultaneously and anonymity is kept until after the transplant.

5. **Spousal donation:** A spouse can donate an organ to the partner. It has to be recorded that the couple is legally married.

3. Current scenario: trends

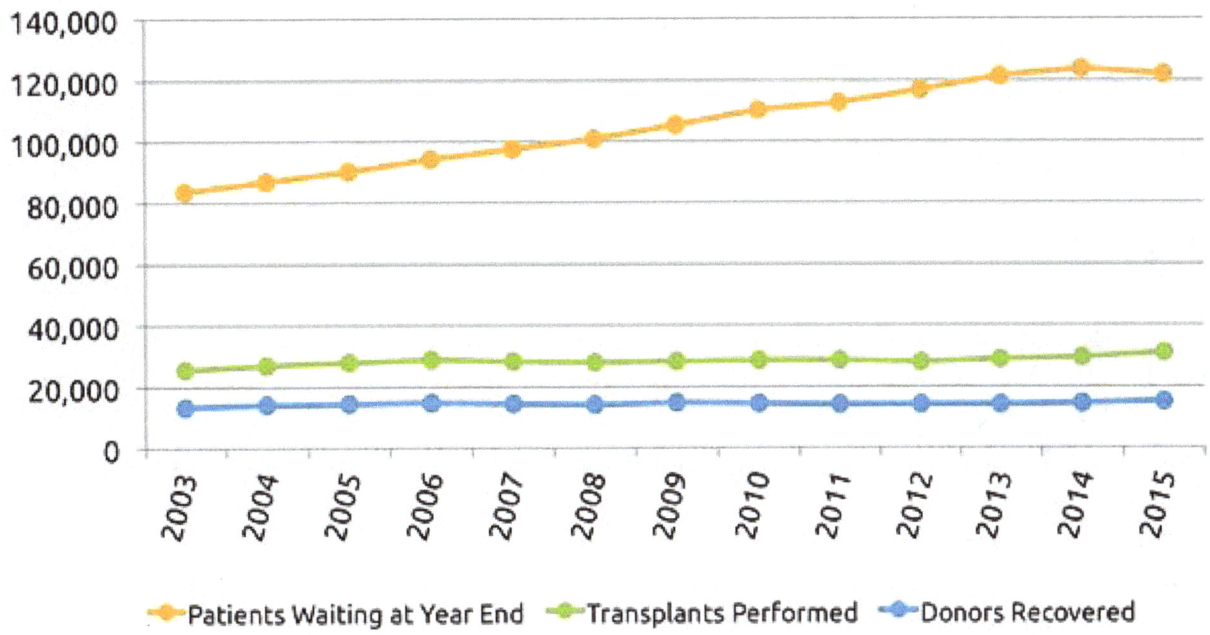

Despite advances in medicine and technology, and increased awareness of organ donation and transplantation, the gap between supply and demand continues to widen. Each year, the number of people in the waiting list is increasing in both donor and transplant. The donation statistics according to OPTN Annual report shows that in 2016, total of 41,335 organs were donated. It can be either deceased or living and four out of five donations came from deceased donors and four out of ten from living donors. According to the report by OTPN 2018, 115,033 people need life-saving organ transplant, of those 74,926 people are the active waiting list candidates.

The real reason behind a living person's interest in donating one's organ is important to determine but it is often difficult. Now days, money has become the motivation for donation. The relationships also have played a great role in increasing donation rates. The shortage of available organs can be reduced if; people choose to donate their organs after they die. If more people did that the issue regarding organ shortage can be minimized.

The trend is expected to accelerate each year. Many organ procurement and the Joint Commission on Accreditation of Healthcare Organizations actively participate to increase the donation rates. The organizations take various to steps against traditional social taboos.

The approach, known as "donation after cardiac death" (DCD), usually involves patients who have suffered brain damage, such as from a car accident or a stroke. After family members have made the difficult decision to discontinue a ventilator or other life-sustaining treatment, organ-bank representatives talk to them about donation. Sometimes, the donor is suffering from an incurable disease also end up with the decision of organ donation.

According to U.S Department of Health and Human Services, more than 1,23,000 men, women and children currently needed life-saving organ transplants every 10 minutes and another name is added to the national organ transplant waiting list. In 2014, more than 8500 deceased donors made possible approximately 24,000 organ transplants. In addition, there were nearly 6000 transplants from living donors. In India, nationally with a population of 1.2 billion people, the statistics stands 0.08 persons as organ donor populations. Mrithasanjeevani, Kerala network of organ sharing which began in 2012, also states that the need for organ transplantation is high as the patients in waiting list is increasing day by day who requires organ transplantation.

The need for organ has gone up substantially all over the world. India also suffers from acute organ shortage with little to no solution for this issue. It is estimated that every year 1.5 lakh people suffer from renal failure out of which only 3000 people get donors. Similarly, every year around 2 lakh people die of liver failure or cancer and rarely get any help in the form of organ donors. It is the same for heart patients, for every 50,000 heart attack patients there are only 15 hearts available for transplant. Therefore, there is an urgent need for widespread campaigns to spread awareness about organ donation in India and to bridge the gap between supply and demand. The numbers that are mentioned here are estimates and real numbers could be far more than this, it is scary because this means very few people get relief and get a second chance in life.

The main reasons for organ shortage in India are mainly ignorance and lack of knowledge. People are not well informed enough about the benefits of organ donation. Today social media and so many other forums can promote the positives of organ donation and how it will save so many lives if more people register themselves for organ donation. The reason for organ shortage is myth and superstition. Many people do not want to donate their organs even after death because of so many myths and superstition they are instilled with. People with existing medical condition or old people, who wish to donate, do not donate thinking they are not fit or eligible. Almost everyone can donate some part or the other unless you have any extreme medical condition.

The need for organ donation is necessary because out of the 1.5 lakh people who need kidney in India only 3000 people receive them, only 1 out of 30 people receive kidney and 90% of people in the waiting list die without getting any donor. Around 70% liver transplants are dependent on a live donor but 30% dependent on cadaver (corpse) donations. Hence, there is an urgent need to increase the organ donation rates and give a person a second chance in their life.

4. Challenges in organ donation

As far as the challenges concerned it includes mainly donor's motives for donation, the predominant ways in which donors arrive at the decision to donate, and the donors' psychological status and its relationship to their fitness as donors.

4.1. Pre-donation challenges

4.1.1. Donor's motives

Most donors are likely to be motivated by multiple factors. These factors include intrinsic factors (e.g., desires to relieve the suffering of another or to act in according to the religious convictions) and extrinsic factors (e.g., the social pressures or perceived norms) that may operate simultaneously. The particular combination of motivational forces will also differ depending on whether and how the donor is related to the recipient.

Among living related donors, it has long been assumed that family members or emotional partners are motivated primarily for saving the lives of their loved ones. Such motives are indeed the most commonly expressed feelings, as noted in a variety of studies over the past 30 years. Among nondirected living donors (individuals donating to unrelated patients whom the donors did not select)(NDLDs), it was identified as the altruistic/humanitarian motives, along with beliefs that the donor's self-worth would be improved, and feelings of moral and religious obligation or self- identity.

4.1.2. Donor's decision-making

The motivation for the organ donation is purely on the donor's decision of organ donation and it may be influenced by many factors including the relationship to the recipients. Decision-making swiftness may indicate the type of decision being made. There appear to be two decision-making approaches that include the moral decision making and the rational decision making. "Moral decision-making" involves awareness that one's actions can affect another; ascription of responsibility to oneself; acceptance of the social/moral norm governing the behavior; and taking action consistent with that norm. Because moral decision-making does not involve the costs and benefits of a given behavior but, instead, is based on perceived norms governing that behavior, it is likely to lead to non- deliberative, instantaneous decisions. In contrast, "rational" decision-making includes various steps that focus on gathering relevant information, evaluating alternatives, selecting an alternative, and implementing the decision.

4.1.3. Support

It includes mainly the assessment of the donor's available physical, financial and emotional support. It is necessary to identify whether the donor have someone to provide care in the recovery period, have sufficient financial support and so on. This important to avoid distress if the donor develops any complications. Finally, does the donor have the support of significant others for being a donor, or is he or she choosing to donate over the objections of persons who have a legitimate interest in the outcome of an autonomous decision.

4.1.4. Family attitudes toward donation

Spouse and family attitudes about donation should also be explored. Collateral interviews with significant others is necessary, especially those who will be providing tangible support to the donor during the recovery period, should be conducted whenever possible. Conflicts between potential donors and significant others should be addressed and, ideally, resolved prior to surgery itself in order to avoid conflicts later. Family members should provide a good understanding of the donor's wishes and motives, even if they agree to disagree to the donor's decision.

4.1.5. Behavioral and psychological health

The behavioral and psychological health of the donor should also be considered before donation. It is important to identify donor's lifestyle is sufficiently healthy to reduce unnecessary risk for both donor and recipient. Many potential donors may have some unhealthy behaviors, such as moderate obesity or smoking. It is necessary to identify that there is sufficient time for the donor to reduce risks (e.g., lose weight, stop smoking). Moreover, it needs to be taken care of that the donor is emotionally stable to cope with stresses which may come up before, during, and after the donation. Hence it is important to identify psychological and behavioral status of the donor or else it may affect the quality of life.

4.1.6. Donor-recipient relationship

The relationship between the donor and recipient is a complex matter. Even when both parties are agree for donation and transplant, family dynamics may be complicated, and other family members may assertively involve themselves in the decision-making process. The donor may have unrealizable expectations that transplant will alter his or her relationship with the recipient. The health care team should not expect an ideal relationship in which all interactions between donor and recipient are harmonious. However, obvious tensions and overt psychological issues should be addressed. Joint interviews, involving both donor and recipient, should be avoided early in the evaluation process in order to preserve privacy and give the potential donor the opportunity to express reservations or "opt out" gracefully.

4.1.7. Diversity issues

Non directed donors may have diversity concerns that may affect the organ donation. The potential donors should be assessed for comfort with donation to recipients of different genders, races, religions, sexual orientations, nationalities, ages, underlying diseases, and lifestyles. Donors who express objections, fears, or concerns about who might receive their organ may need to be deferred until they can receive counseling.

4.1.8. Psychological status of potential donors

The potential donor's psychological status is of greatest concern for donation and transplantation. Concerns have been particularly high in case of unrelated donation (either directed to a specific patient, or NDLD): the willingness or desire to donate to a stranger has been historically viewed with suspicion and as likely to reflect significant psychopathology. There is no doubt that some potential donors will be psychologically poor candidates to serve as donors.

4.1.9. Post-donation challenges

The donors' perceptions of their physical functional, psychological, and social well-being were found to be either nonsignificantly different from or significantly better than levels reported in the general population. The post challenges mainly includes recipient death or graft loss, donor medical complications, donor history of mood or other psychiatric problems, and poor donor relationships with recipient or family. The other factor is that it may affect the donor's quality of life if any complication arises.

The post transplantation challenges are many which include minimizing rejection risks, immunosuppression, organ shortage, handling of the stressors of transplantation, psychosocial adaptation and psychological disorders and so on.

4.1.10. Minimizing rejection risks

The twin conditions of antibody sensitization and antibody-mediated rejection remain challenging and frustrating to treat. The recent drugs which are used to desensitize patients or reverse antibody-mediated rejection, especially chronic antibody mediated rejection is totally unsatisfactory. Development of therapies those are more effective and less toxic should be made available. Recent regimens used for antibody desensitization and reversal of antibody-mediated rejection include plasmapheresis, immunoglobulin (IVIG), and rituximab, an anti-chimeric, anti-CD20 antibody. Recently, the proteasome inhibitor Velcade has also been reported to reverse refractory antibody rejection. Eculizumab, a humanized anti-C5 monoclonal antibody appears to protect the renal allograft despite the presence of donor-specific antibodies (DSA). None of these agents have been tested in rigorous studies.

4.1.11. Immunosuppression

This is one of the major challenges after organ transplantation. Many studies have suggested that most of the late graft loss occurs because of immunologic reasons, frequently antibody-mediated. So the approach of minimizing immunosuppression is necessary with the present drugs to reduce toxicities may actually be helpful in the long-term survival of the graft. The toxicities are minimized by allowing more grafts to be rejected by immune mechanisms. Hence, development of effective agents that lack long-term toxicities so that we can maintain optimum immunosuppression over the long-term.

4.1.12. Stressors after transplantation

In the perioperative period, the focus is on the patient's physical recovery, with possible rejection episodes and other medical complications causing anxiety and emotional strain. Within the first days after transplantation, a postoperative delirium can occur. The patient can present with symptoms of mental confusion, language disturbances, and occasional hallucinations and delusions are often a frightening experience to patients and their families. Acute brain dysfunction can occur in intensive care patients and patients after surgery. The corticosteroids which are administered for immunosuppression cause these problems. Some of the patients experience problems in accepting the new organ from another individual and suffer with feeling of guilt towards the donor which, in turn, can increase psychological stress and nonadherence [6–11].

In the long-term postoperative period, medication side effects and associated comorbidities become central stressors impeding patient's life quality. Most common comorbidities seen are infections, diabetes mellitus, hypertension, lipometabolic disorders, adipositas, cardiovascular diseases, oncological diseases, osteoporosis, and chronic kidney failure [12, 13]. Furthermore, psychiatric symptoms (e.g., depression, anxiety, agitation, psychosis) and neurological symptoms (e.g., sleep disturbances, cognitive impairment, delirium) can occur as neurotoxic side effects in patients receiving immunosuppressive drugs.

Faced with the multiple health risks, patients often continue to experience anxiety and worries regarding possible retransplantation, serious comorbidities, and death. Even patients in good physical health are confronted with severe challenges, for example, regaining their previously lost or restricted social roles as family members and partners (including sexual activity) and returning to work or taking up other meaningful activities. Financial constraints and legal disputes with health or pension insurance agencies constitute other possible sources of psychological strain.

5. Psychosocial adaptation and psychological disorders

After the transplantation, the psychosocial burden more severe in preoperative period than postoperative period. Nevertheless, patients themselves have to demonstrate considerable coping skills. In the best case, transplant patients learn to adapt to their new situation, often by reevaluating life goals and by focusing on more positive consequences, for example, personal growth. On the other hand, unsuccessful readjustment can lower the quality of life and psychiatric morbidity. The most common psychological disorders among patients before and after transplantation are affective and anxiety disorders.

The literature review shows that prevalence of depression in 20–25% of cases before and after kidney transplantation. Less information is available concerning patients receiving other organs. Prior to and following lung transplantation, depression seems to be prevalent in approximately 30% of patients. Hence these show that the depression is a major challenge after transplantation. These issues can be reduced by personal and social resources (resilience factors), that is, favorable coping skills, self-efficacy, sense of coherence, optimism, and social support.

6. Factors affecting donor's motivation

There are many factors affecting donor's motivation which includes feelings of love and responsibility, spiritual motives, and greater success rate of organ donation.

6.1. Feelings of love and responsibility

Motives for donating organ to their relative patients were that they tended to do something for their loved ones. In fact, they feel responsible for their problems. They do not treat others' problems with indifference and attempted to do whatever they could for resolving the problems experienced by transplant recipients. It is considered as their own responsibilities to help them to get rid of their problems. The feel like they are the ones who need to support their patients.

6.2. Close and constant companionship

Another factor affecting the participants' feeling of responsibility for donation to their family members was close and constant companionship with recipients. This close and constant companionship made the participants to clearly understand the recipients' conditions and hence, it had resulted in their decision on organ donation in order to alleviate recipients' problems. This close and constant companionship with patients help family members understand patients' problems well and increase their degree of commitment to do something for patient's pain and discomfort. They also noted that this had made them experience deeper shared emotions with their patients and hence, required them to feel responsible for minimizing their patient's problems.

6.3. Inability to tolerate recipient's discomfort

Another motive for organ donation was one's difficulty in tolerating recipient's discomfort. Love for their sick family members had made the participants feel responsible and decide on doing something for solving their patient's problems. Their patient's pain, suffering and discomfort cause a great inconvenience and irritation which lead them to the decision of organ donation. They hoped that organ donation alleviate their patient's problems [14–34, 36].

6.4. Spiritual motives for donation

Religious beliefs played a significant role in motivating to organ donation. Some of them believed that donation was a way for expiating their past sins. They referred to faith in God, reliance on Him, and hope for a successful transplant as the important motives for organ donation. Some of them even accused themselves of causing their family members to develop organ failure and believed that donation was a way for alleviating their feelings of guilt. Such a practice was particularly common among the parents of sick children. Some of them considered donation as a God-approved practice, and noted that God has helped them donate their organs. They noted that they donated their organs for gratifying God and believed that he sees it and help them in all bad situations.

6.5. Greater success rate of organ transplantation

The category is the greater success of organ transplantation. In other words, obtaining information and realizing the greater benefits of organ transplantation had motivated the participants to opt for organ donation. Some of them reported that they had never thought about donation until obtaining information from their patient's physicians. However, after obtaining adequate information, they had made an irreversible decision about organ donation. Accordingly, a major motive for organ donation was the lower likelihood of organ rejection.

7. Measures to overcome challenges for organ donation

The decisions regarding organ donation based on the personal beliefs (religious, cultural, family, social and body integrity) levels of knowledge about organ donation and previous interaction with the health care team. Many maintained positive attitudes to organ donation despite significant reservations about the organ donation process. Resistance to organ donation found to be less in the case of living donation for family.

There are some religious beliefs that can have both positive and negative influences, these often stemmed from uncertainty or misrepresentation of religious edicts. One solution would be to actively engage religious leaders in the transplant community, especially when it has been reported that, across the major religions, there are very few cases where organ donation can be seen to be inconsistent with religious beliefs. Religious leaders should be made available in hospitals and other transplantation setting to assist families in making decisions regarding organ donation and potentially to remove the misperceptions. Staff members who are involved in approaching families to request consent for donation should be part of the awareness programs and resources about religious concerns. Similarly, cultural sensitivity to issues such as apprehensiveness to discuss death among certain groups or individuals and the importance to many of death rituals may improve dialog regarding organ donation.

Studies have shown that engaging some minority groups in the health care system and creating a sense of belonging and ownership can improve compliance with organ donation. As a consequence, more efforts should be made to create positive interactions within the health care team members, especially for minority groups, to improve the organ donation rates. Although many of the studies have showed that higher socio-economic status and education were associated with a stronger willingness to be an organ donor. Some of the strong reservations held, even among those with generally positive views towards donation, such as concerns that agreeing to donation would discourage doctors from caring so much about saving their lives in case of an emergency or that it would result in the premature removal of their organs or indeed prevent them from having an open coffin at their funerals, are examples of very real barriers that can be readily addressed through information. Through a proper awareness and motivation the donation rates can be improved which can save many lives.

7.1. Psychological care

Psychological consultation is essential for all disease stages enabling patients to better cope with their extraordinarily stressful situation. A need for psychological care was found in up to 50% of transplant patients. Educational and supportive therapies are of utmost importance but also cognitive-behavioral interventions including relaxation techniques can also be considered. Less common methods like hypnotherapy and "Quality of Life Therapy" have also been utilized for overcoming the challenges.

Moreover, family members as well as caregivers of transplant patients show increased psychological strain before and after transplantation. Family counseling, and psychotherapeutic support, can help reduce psychological strain, thus also maintaining the valuable social support provided by care givers and family members of the transplant patient. Henceforth, the family and care givers should also be considered in psychosocial evaluation to overcome the problems.

7.2. Alternative methods to increase donation

In view of ethical, legal and political issues, it was deemed important to obtain some opinion about alternative methods to increase organ donation rates. Financial incentives were given to increase organ donation. Many in both donor and non-donor groups were given a reasonable incentive. Education and dissemination of information about donation and transplantation was important to increase organ donation rates. There was nearly universal agreement that implied consent (presumed consent) should not be tried. The use of financial incentives was not markedly opposed (some accepted the idea of funeral expense reimbursement), although there was not strong support either. In general, methods to increase organ donation had not been well thought out by either donors or nondonors indicating, perhaps, that the assumption of altruism or motivation is the best way to increase the donation rates.

8. Responsibilities of nurses in organ donation and transplantation

Organ and tissue transplant nurses need comprehensive and scientific knowledge. They include the evaluation and management of deceased donors, transplant recipients, potential donors or live donors, teaching and counseling of transplant recipients and live donors related to self-care management, healthy life and a peaceful death when this is imminent. This is important in order to improve the posttransplant quality of life.

Nurses have important role in the development of a successful transplantation program. They are key members of the team that works to deliver care to patients and relatives, through the use of technological, logistic and human resources, with a view to coordination, care, education and research on organ and tissue donation and transplantation. Therefore, the nurses need adequate knowledge on the principles of good ethical principles and should have resources available for them to assess patient's risks and social issues related to organ transplants and donation. The researchers hope that the future studies will encourage further researches on the role and responsibilities of nurses.

9. Conclusion

The organ donation decision is a complex one, based strongly on personal beliefs. There are some factors, such as religious and cultural beliefs, that are seemingly intractable and are often cited as reasons for a refusal to donate. In this chapter, it is shown that these have often been found to be tied in with more complex issues such as a distrust of the medical system, misunderstandings about religious stances and ignorance about the donation process. Interventions to better engage the community, including disadvantaged and minority groups, to foster trust and provide information represent promising opportunities of promoting organ donation in the future.

Donor motives directly contribute to their decision to donate, is not uniform and is influenced by multiple factors. Majority of the donors were relationship oriented donor, whose major motives were desires to relieve the suffering & save the life of their loving ones. Creating awareness to the organ donation will directly influence the donor motives and willingness. By deriving the motives many more intervention to improve the willingness to be a living organ donor can be evolved. Recruitment of living donors represents a medical and moral responsibility. The possibility of organ removal from healthy donor to a recipient needs great inner motivation. Saving one's life is divine.

The psycho social assessment must be made as a routine part of the nursing process. These assessments are meant to identify patients at risk for poor outcomes, provide guidelines for their management and improve the post-transplant quality of life [6]. "Because donated organs are a severely limited resource, the best potential, recipients should be identified. The probability of a good outcome must be highly emphasized to achieve the maximum benefit for all transplants" (OPTN/UNOS Ethics committee General Considerations in Assessment for Transplant Candidacy White paper-2010).

Author details

Kanmani Job* and Anooja Antony

*Address all correspondence to: kanmanijob@aims.amrita.edu

Amrita College of Nursing, Amrita Vishwa Vidyapeetham, Kochi, India

References

[1] United Network for Organ Sharing. 1999 Annual Report of the U. S. Scientific Registry of Transplant Recipients and the Organ Procurement and Transplantation Network.: Transplant Data 1989–1998. Richmond, Va: US Department of Health and Human Services, Health Research Services Administration, Office of Sponsored Projects, Division of Transportation, and United Network for Organ Sharing; 2000

[2] Alexander JW, Zola JC. Expanding the donor pool: Use of marginal donors for solid organ transplantation. Clinical Transplantation. 1996;**10**:1-19

[3] Kumar A, Mandhani A, Verma BS, et al. Expanding the living related donor pool in renal transplantation: Use of marginal donors. Journal of Urology. 2000a;**163**:33-36

[4] Mandal AK, Kalligonis AN, Ratner LE. Expanded criteria donors: Attempts to increase the renal donor transplant pool. Advances in Renal Replacement Therapy. 2000a;**7**:117-113

[5] Simmons RG et al. Gift of Life: The Social and Psychological Impact of Organ Transplantation. NY: Wiley; 1977. Reprinted with additions, Brunswick, NJ: Transaction Books, 1987

[6] Corley MC et al. Attitude, self-image, and quality of life of living kidney donors. Nephrology Nursing Journal. 2000;**27**(1):43-52

[7] Goldman LS. Liver transplantation using living donors: Preliminary donor psychiatric outcomes. Psychsomatics. 1993;**34**(3):235-240

[8] Pradel FG et al. Exploring donors' and recipients' attitudes about living donor kidney transplantation. Progress in Transplantation. 2003;**13**(3):203-210

[9] Fellner CH. Renal transplantation and the living donor. Decision and consequences. Psychother Psychosomat. 1976/77;**27**:139-143

[10] Toronyi E et al. Attitudes of donors towards organ transplantation in living related kidney transplantations. Transplant International. 1998;**11**(Suppl 1):S481-S483

[11] Henderson AJZ et al. The living anonymous kidney donor: Lunatic or saint? American Journal of Transplantation. 2003;**3**:203-213

[12] Jacobs CL et al. Twenty-two nondirected kidney donors: An update on a single center's experience. American Journal of Transplantation. 2004;**4**:1110-1116

[13] Matas AJ et al. Nondirected donation of kidneys from living donors. The New England Journal of Medicine. 2000;**343**(6):433-436

[14] Olbrisch ME et al. Psychological, Social and Behavioral Characteristics of Living Donor Candidates for Adult Liver Transplantation. Biennial Meeting on Psychiatric, Psychosocial and Ethical Issues in Organ Transplantation. Santa Monica, CA; February, 2005

[15] Crowley-Matoka M et al. Long-term quality of life issues among adult-to-pediatric living donors: A qualitative exploration. American Journal of Transplantation. 2004;**4**:744-750

[16] Karliova M et al. Living-related liver transplantation from the view of the donor: A 1-year follow-up survey. Transplantation. 2002;**73**(11):1799-1804

[17] De Graaf Olson W, Bogetti-Dumlao A. Living donors' perception of their quality of health after donation. Progress in Transplantation. 2001;**11**(2):108-115

[18] Beavers KL et al. The living donor experience: Donor health assessment and outcomes after living donor liver transplantation. Liver Transplant. 2001;**7**(11):943-947

[19] Lennerling A et al. Becoming a living kidney donor. Transplantation. 2003;**76**:1243-1247

[20] Pradel FG. Exploring donor's and receipient's attitudes about living door kidney transplantation. Progress in Transplantation. 2003;**13**(3):203-210

[21] Smith MD. Living related kidney donors. A multicenter study of donor education, socioeconomic adjustment and rehabilitation. American Journal of Kidney Diseases. 1986;**8**(4): 223-233

[22] Jacobs CL. Expanding living donor options. Minnesota Medicine. 2001;**84**:46-48

[23] Switzer GE. Understaning donor;s motivations. A study of unrelated bone arrow donors. Social Science & Medicine. 1999;**45**(1):137-147

[24] Rosenthal JT. Expanded criteria for cadaver organ donation in renal transplant. The Urologic Clinics of North America. 1994;**21**:283-292

[25] Shiel AGR. Transplantation and society. In: Ginns LC, Cosimi A, Morris PJ, editors. Transplantation. Malden, MA: Blackwell Science; 1999. pp. 897-913

[26] Callender CO, Bay AS, Miles PV, Yeager CL. A national minority organ/tissue transplant education program: The first step in the evolution of a national minority strategy and minority transplant equity in the USA. Transplantation Proceedings. 1995;**27**:1441-1443

[27] Surman OS et al. Live organ donation: Social context, clinical encounter, and the psychology of communication. Psychosomatics. 2005;**46**:1-6

[28] Papachristou C et al. Motivation for living-donor liver transplantation from the donor's perspective: An in-depth qualitative research study. Transplantation. 2004;**78**:1506-1514

[29] Haljamäe U. Remaining experiences of living kidney donors more than 3 yr after early recipient graft loss. Clinical Transplantation. 2003;**17**:503-510

[30] Hamburger J, Crosnier J. Moral and ethical problems in transplantation. Rapaport F, Daussert J. Human Transplantation. NY: Grune & Stratton; 1968. pp. 68

[31] Sadler HH et al. The living, genetically unrelated, kidney donor. Seminars in Psychiatry. 1971;**3**:86-101

[32] Walter M et al. Psychosocial outcome of living donors after living donor liver transplantation: A pilot study. Clinical Transplantation. 2002;**16**:339-344

[33] Fukunishi I et al. Psychiatric disorders before and after living-related transplantation. Psychosomatics. 2001;**42**(4):337-343

[34] Crowley-Matoka M, Switzer G. Nondirected living donation: A survey of current trends and practices. Transplantation. 2005;**79**(5):515-519

[35] Boparai J, Davila H, Chandalia M. Cardiovascular disease in Asian Indians living in the United States. Current Cardiovascular Risk Reports. 2011;**5**:240-245

[36] Ji WR, Frederick B, Hsin CY. Trends in prevalence of Type 2 diabetes in Asians Versus Whites results from the United States National Health Interview Survey 1997-2008. Diabetes Care. Feb 2011;**34**(2):353-357

6

Procurement of Abdominal Organs in Multi-Organ Donation in Deceased Donor

Bulang He, Xiuwu Han and Michael A. Fink

Abstract

Organ procurement is an essential step for organ transplantation, from which a quality organ is received for subsequent transplantation. As the demand for organ transplantation continues to grow, multi-organ donation including the heart, lung, live, pancreas, kidneys, and small intestine from one potential donor is always a priority to meet the demand. The donor is generally rigorously assessed for suitability of organ donation prior to proceeding to organ procurement. The quality of the organ from multi-organ procurement is usually satisfactory without jeopardizing its transplantation. In this chapter, the surgical technique for procurement of the organs from the abdomen is described. Some alternative techniques have also been discussed. Some pictures are inserted to facilitate understanding of the surgical procedure.

Keywords: abdomen, multi-organ procurement, liver, pancreas, small intestine, kidney

1. Introduction

Organ transplantation is a definitive treatment for patients with end stage of organ failure. It is one of the greatest advancements in medicine in the twentieth century. Organ transplant is a life-saving treatment and improves the quality of life. Organ donation and procurement are essential steps for performance of the organ transplantation. Organ donors are classified as live organ donors, donation after brain death (DBD), and donation after circulatory death (DCD). Rigorous assessment of a potential donor is mandatory prior to proceeding organ procurement. For DBD and DCD donors, procurement of multi-organs is always the priority to ultimately benefit multiple recipients without jeopardizing the graft function [1, 2].

The surgical technique for abdominal multi-organ procurement is based on the anatomy and has been evolved over the decades as a result of the increased demand for organ transplantation [2–5]. In this chapter, the surgical technique is described with some pictures inserted to facilitate understanding of the progress of the surgery.

2. Preparation in theater

It is mandatory for the surgeon in charge to check the documents: certification of brain death of the donor, the consent form for organ and tissue donation, signature of the hospital delegation, and the patient serology test. The team time-out should be carried out. The communication is confirmed between the surgeon and anesthetist for administration of medications at various stages. One dose of intravenous antibiotics is given intravenously, as well as 1 g of methylprednisolone prior to surgery. One dose of mannitol 20 g is given after completion of abdominal dissection. Heparin 25,000 IU is administered following cardiac team dissection prior to the cold perfusion.

If the pancreas is retrieved for organ transplantation, 100 ml of half-strength betadine (5%) is injected through the nasogastric tube that is then clamped off during procedure to retain betadine solution in the duodenum.

Preparation and drape: under sterile condition, the surgical area from the lower part of the chin to the proximal one-third of the thigh is prepared. The hairs are shaved. The dressing and central venous catheter or femoral catheter is reorganized to ensure the surgical field is clean and neat for preparation and drape.

3. Surgical procedure

3.1. Dissection of the organs with normal circulation (warm dissection)

3.1.1. Open of the abdomen and chest

An incision is made from suprasternal notch to the point just above the symphysis pubis (**Figure 1**). The abdominal cavity is entered first, and a Balfour retractor is placed to have adequate exposure of the abdomen (**Figure 2**). The round ligament of the liver is divided and tied as well as the falciform ligament of the liver. Examination of intra-abdominal organs is carried out to exclude potential malignant disease. The quality of the liver is usually assessed at this stage, and liver biopsy should be taken if any concern is raised. The biopsy is taken by using F18 Trucut needle from the left and right lobe. An additional wedge biopsy is also taken for the frozen section and histopathology examination. Following that, the soft tissue over the sternum is cut opened by diathermy along the line for sternotomy. A tunnel is created behind the sternum by insertion of a pair of long Metzenbaum scissors to ensure that the posterior side of the sternum is clean from soft tissue attachment. The sternum is sawed open with bone wax applied to the cut surface. Hemostasis is reassured by using diathermy to all active bleeders. A sternal retractor is placed to open the chest. The pleura and pericardium are remained intact at this stage (**Figure 2**). If the donor had previous sternotomy for cardiac surgery, then the wires

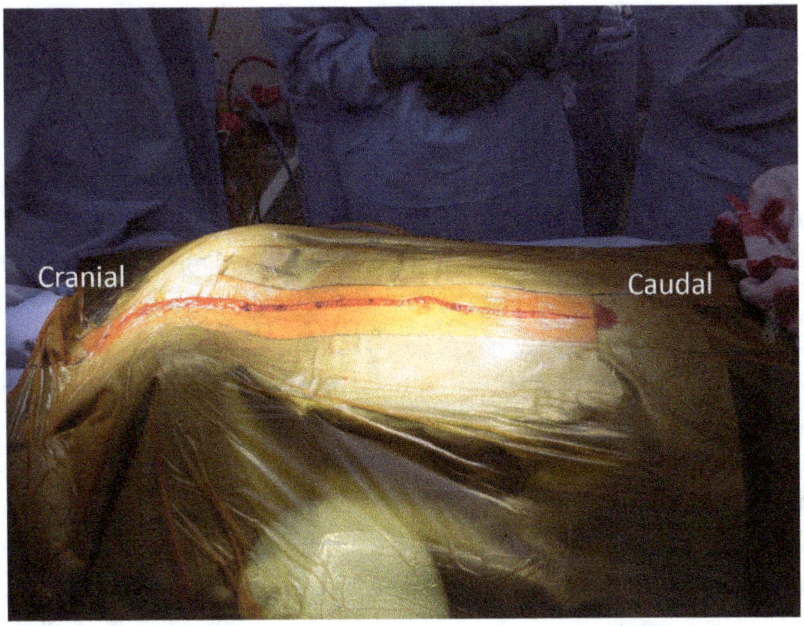

Figure 1. Incision for multi-organ procurement.

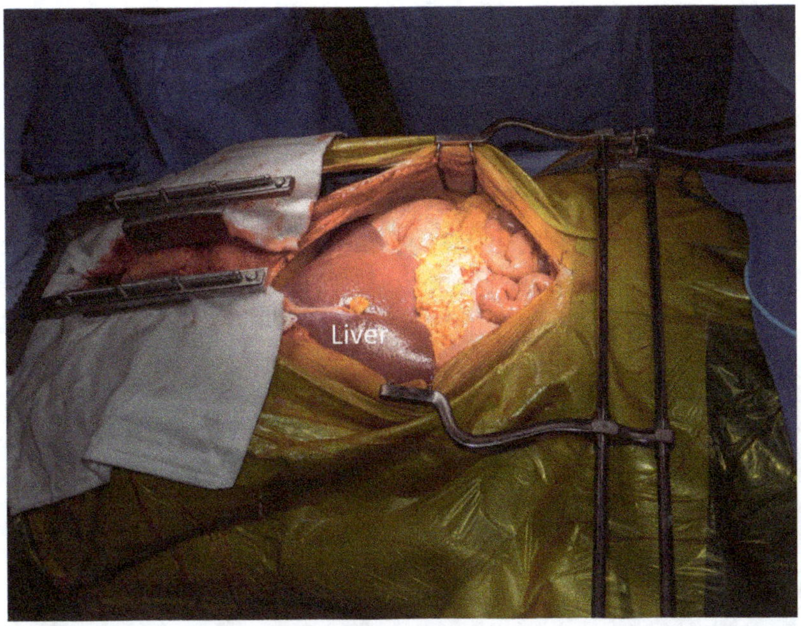

Figure 2. Retractors placed for exposure of abdominal organs.

over the sternum are removed, and a resternotomy saw is used for precise cut with caution. A surgical pack is placed over the chest wound to give the cardiothoracic team a nice clean field for subsequent heart and lung dissection. Now, the concentration is directed to the dissection of abdominal organs.

3.1.2. Dissection of the distal aorta

The retro peritoneum is incised along the white line of Toldt from the cecum to the hepatic flexure. The dissection is continued along the retroperitoneal avascular plane superiorly and medially to mobilize and retract ascending colon medially. The right ureter is easily identified and preserved with the surrounding tissue. The dissection is continued by a Cattell-Braasch and Kocher maneuver. The inferior duodenal fold is divided allowing broad exposure of the inferior vena cava (IVC) and aorta (**Figure 3**). The left renal vein should be well visualized at this stage, and superior mesentery artery is palpated at its origin from the aorta. The distal segment of the aorta is dissected, and inferior mesentery artery is ligated and divided allowing the distal segment of aorta exposed adequately. A size 2 Dacron tie is placed around the aorta at the level proximal to the bifurcation of the common iliac arteries, which is used for ligation of distal aorta prior to cold perfusion (**Figure 4**). The second size 2 Dacron tie is placed around the aorta a few centimeters proximally that is used for tying the cannula after its insertion to the aorta for cold perfusion. At this stage, the inferior mesentery vein (IMV) is readily visualized along the edge of dissected mesentery of sigmoid colon lateral to the proximal jejunum. If the portal system perfusion is required, then a segment of IMV can be dissected, and a 2/0 tie is encircled for cannula placement at later stage immediately prior to aorta cannula insertion (**Figure 4**). Currently, most transplant units do not perform in situ portal perfusion but give 500 ml of cold UW perfusion to the portal vein on the back table when packing the liver.

3.1.3. Dissection of the liver

Following dissection of the aorta, the attention is directed to the liver. The left triangle ligament of the liver is divided to free the left lobe of the liver. The hepato-gastric ligament is divided, but it is usually checked for left accessory hepatic artery that usually arises from the left gastric artery. It should be preserved if present. The common bile duct is identified and transected at the level close to the duodenum (**Figure 5**). The portal vein is then visualized. At this stage, it is usually checked whether there is a right accessory or replacement of hepatic artery posteriorly to the portal vein by palpation via the omentum of foramen (Winslow). It

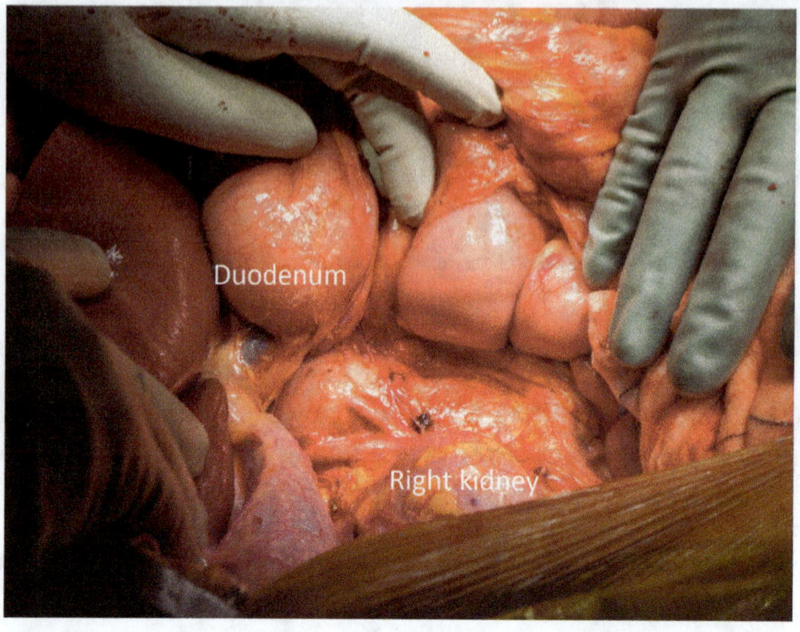

Figure 3. Cattell-Braasch and Kocher maneuver for exposure of retroperitoneal structure.

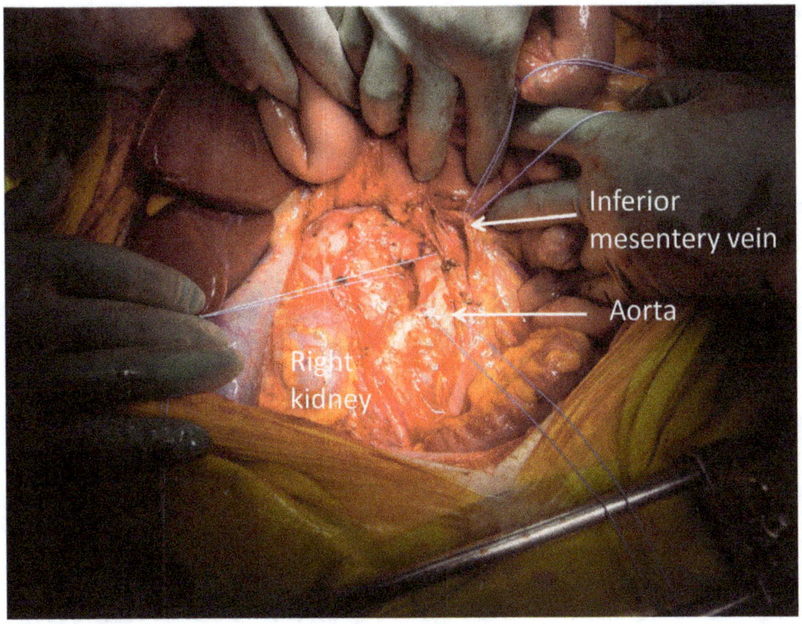

Figure 4. The distal aorta and inferior mesentery vein dissected.

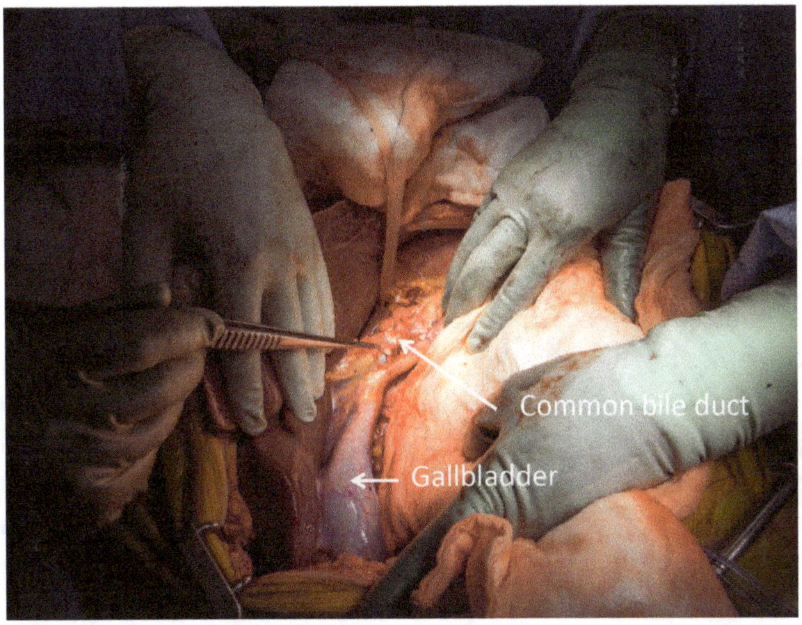

Figure 5. Transection of the common bile duct.

usually arises from the superior mesentery artery. The hepato-duodenal ligament is divided. The right gastric artery and veins are tied and divided. The proper hepatic artery as well as the gastroduodenal artery is identified. A short length of gastroduodenal artery is dissected (**Figure 6**). Dissection of proper hepatic artery is continued toward celiac trunk. Then, the splenic artery and left gastric artery is seen, and a short segment is dissected, respectively, which is readily for transection after cold perfusion during procurement. The left gastric vein may be encountered, which is ligated and divided. The liver dissection is now completed.

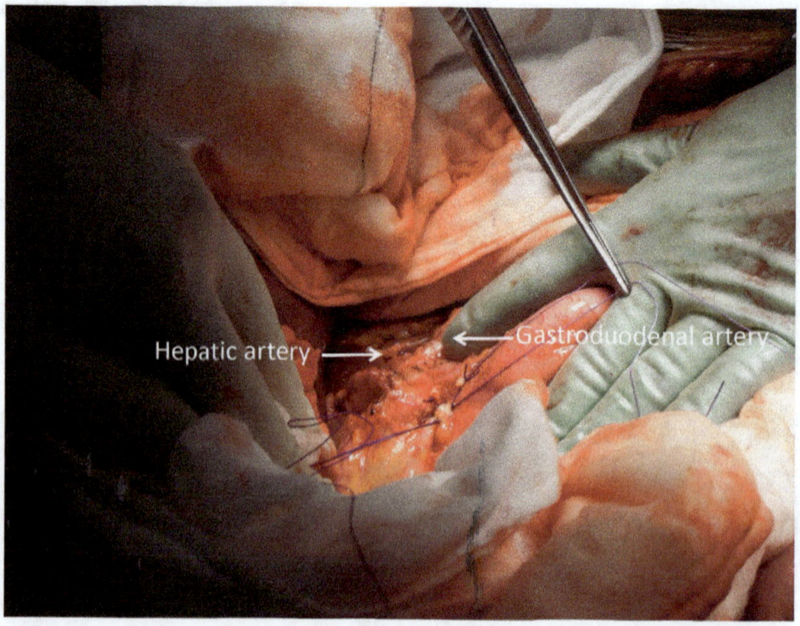

Figure 6. The proper hepatic artery and gastroduodenal artery dissected.

3.1.4. Pancreas dissection

The superior edge of the pancreas is partly exposed after dissection of proper hepatic artery. Then, the gastrocolic ligament is divided and ligated between the stomach and transverse colon. So, the anterior surface of the pancreas is visualized. The division is continued along the greater curvature of the stomach to its fundus, and gastrosplenic ligament is divided. The texture of the pancreas is properly assessed for suitability of transplantation. The spleen is always remained with the pancreas for procurement as a handle to prevent manipulation over the pancreas and reduce the risk of pancreatitis. The transverse mesocolon is divided as well as splenic-colon ligament on the left and duodenocolic ligament on the right side, and the inferior edge of the pancreas is exposed. The dissection is continued along the sigmoid colon and ascending colon allowing the colon retracted inferiorly or outside of the abdomen (this part of dissection can be done after cold perfusion). The superior mesentery vein (SMV) and superior mesentery artery (SMA) are identified inferiorly to the pancreas and anteriorly to the third part of the duodenum, which are slung with a 2/0 Vicryl tie, respectively, and subsequently tied and divided during pancreas procurement after cold perfusion.

3.1.5. Dissection of the small intestine

In rare circumstance, procurement of the small intestine may be required as part of multi-organ donation. In such case, the abdominal multi-organ procurement should be performed by the team who performs intestinal transplantation. After the laparotomy, the intestine is examined and wrapped in a surgical pack. The entire large intestine is dissected and placed caudally outside of the abdomen. The ileal branches of the ileocolic artery are preserved. Proximally, the small intestine is divided at the jejunum 5–10 cm post Treitz, and distally the small intestine is divided near the ileocecal valve by GIA stapler. A mark suture is placed at the jejunal end for orientation of the intestinal graft at transplantation. The small intestine is lifting upward, and the mesentery is dissected posteriorly along the avascular retroperitoneal attachments. A short segment of the superior mesentery artery and vein is dissected inferiorly to the pancreas and anteriorly to the fourth part of the duodenum by dividing some small arterial branches or venous tributaries. Care must be taken to avoid injury to the inferior pancreaticoduodenal artery, which arises proximal to the origin of the middle colic artery and supplies pancreas head [6, 7].

3.1.6. Dissection of the aorta under the diaphragm

The last dissection before the cold perfusion is to dissect supra celiac aorta under the diaphragm. The hepato-esophagus ligament is divided, and the esophagus is retracted left laterally. The aorta pulse is palpated, and the overlayer crus is divided to expose the aorta. A thin fascia layer is incised, and the aorta is freed from the surrounding attachment. A nylon type is slung over this segment of the aorta that is subsequently tied when the cold perfusion is commenced to limit the perfusion to the abdominal organs (**Figure 7**). Care must be taken not to injure the aorta in particular when trying to free the posterior part of the aorta for bringing through the nylon type. This part can be done later if the risk of bleeding is predicted. Alternatively, the segment of thoracic aorta in the left chest can be dissected and slung with a nylon type.

At this stage the warm dissection to the multi-abdominal organs is completed. The gallbladder is incised open and flushed with normal saline until the outflow at the common bile duct becomes clear. The cardiothoracic team is informed for scrubbing and proceeds to heart-lung dissection.

3.1.7. Insertion of the perfusion cannula into the aorta for cold perfusion (in situ cooling of the organs)

A cold perfusion line is set up at this stage, and a large cannula is connected to the perfusion line. The air bubbles are removed from the line.

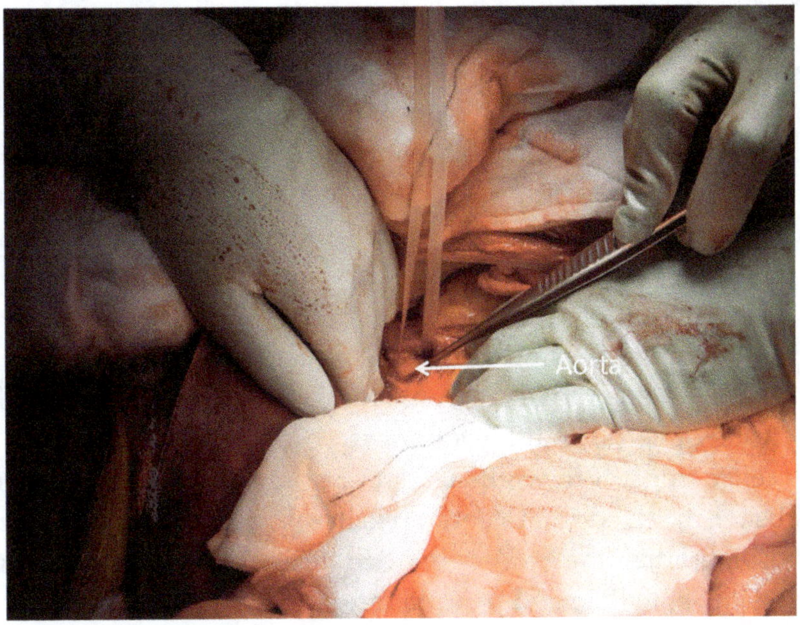

Figure 7. A segment of the aorta under the diaphragm dissected and slung with a nylon tape.

After heart-lung dissection, Heparin 25,000 IU is given intravenously. The distal part of the aorta is tied by pre placed Dacron tie just above the bifurcation of the common iliac arteries. A vascular clamp is placed onto the aorta about 5 cm proximally to this tie to block the blood flow to this segment of the aorta where an arteriotomy is made. The cannula is inserted via arteriotomy and is tied by a pre placed Dacron tie. The cannula is secured and the vascular clamp is removed. At this point, the cold perfusion is commenced simultaneously with cardiothoracic perfusion. The IVC is divided just below the right atrium above the diaphragm for draining the blood and perfusion fluid. Attention is made to leave adequate length of IVC with the liver at suprahepatic end. Alternatively, incision of IVC can be made at the lower part just proximal to the level of confluence of common iliac veins. A suction tube can be placed into the vena cava for adequate drainage of the perfusion fluid. At least, three sets of suction line are used to have proper evacuation of the blood and fluid during perfusion period. At the same time, the ice slush is poured into the abdominal cavity over the liver, pancreas, kidney, and intestine for immediate topical cooling of the organs. Usually, 2 L of Hartman fluid is used for initial flush of the blood followed by 4 L of UW preservation solution. The organs are checked in the meantime to ensure that the progression of perfusion is adequate. The in situ cold perfusion takes about 20 min.

3.2. Procurement of abdominal organs (cold procurement)

3.2.1. Procurement of the small intestine

After completion of the cold perfusion, the small intestine is harvested first. The superior mesentery artery and vein are divided below the origin of inferior pancreaticoduodenal artery, and the entire small intestine is removed and placed in ice-slush filled basin for package and transportation. The bowel contents are remained in the intestine and are managed at the time of transplantation. The small intestine can be harvested en bloc with liver and pancreas, and separation is performed on the back table [6, 7].

3.2.2. Procurement of the liver

Following procurement of the heart and lung by cardiothoracic team, the liver is taken first for the abdominal organs if the small intestine is not for procurement. The gastroduodenal artery is tied and divided. The portal vein is divided at the level of 1 cm proximal to the junction of splenic vein and superior mesentery vein if the pancreas is retrieved for transplantation. Otherwise, the division can be at the level of the confluence of splenic vein and SMV. The splenic artery is divided 0.5 cm from its origin arising from the celiac trunk as well as left gastric artery. However, if the left accessory hepatic artery is present arising from the left gastric artery, then the left gastric artery is preserved on the celiac trunk for its continuity to the left hepatic accessory artery. Along the celiac trunk, the celiac complex and lymphatic tissues are divided at the left side of aorta, and the aorta is exposed. An aortic patch is excised around the ostium of the celiac trunk. If the right accessory or replacement hepatic artery is present, then the SMA is better included in the aortic patch with celiac trunk. If the pancreas is also harvested for transplant, then the SMA is divided just above the level where the accessory hepatic artery arises. So, both liver and pancreas are suitable for transplant without jeopardizing its vasculature. After that the attention is directed to the IVC. The anterior wall of the IVC is incised transversely above the level of renal vein. Both entrance of left and right renal vein is checked, and the IVC is transected. The IVC is lifted anteriorly by insertion of a finger from the suprahepatic end, and its posterior side is dissected to reach the suprahepatic end. The posterior side of the IVC is dissected superiorly to the level of division just below the atrium. Care is taken during IVC dissection without jeopardizing the quality of renal vein for kidney transplantation. The right hepatic triangle ligament is dissected, and part of the diaphragm is taken with the liver during the procurement. The liver is now removed freely from the abdomen and immersed in the ice-slush filled basin (**Figure 8**). One technical point is that the liver laceration is easy to occur at the location where the adhesion band is present. Therefore, gentle handling of the liver is emphasized during the dissection and procurement of the liver at all times to avoid the potential injury.

3.2.3. *Procurement of the pancreas*

The pancreas can be retrieved in favor with liver as an en bloc as described in a separate paragraph. Here, we describe a technique for pancreas retrieval as a subsequent procedure following the liver procurement. A 6/0 Prolene suture is placed at the transection of the port vein and splenic artery, respectively, as a mark during the liver procurement if known the pancreas is also procured. A segment of duodenum is routinely procured with the pancreas as exocrine drainage. A GIA stapler is used to divide the duodenum from the stomach distal to the pylorus. Care is taken to ensure that the NGT tube is positioned proximal to the pylorus without being caught in the GIA stapler. A reload GIA is needed to divide the distal part of the duodenum at the level of the fourth part of the duodenum or at the beginning of the jejunum. The distal part of the SMA and SMV is tied, respectively, by pre placed 2/0 Vicryl tie and divided. The transverse mesocolon is divided to free the inferior edge of the pancreas. On the left the dissection is continued to the splenic flexure and on the right to the duodenocolic ligament, which are divided together with the root of mesentery. So, the pancreas with attached duodenum is now free from its attachment. Then, the pancreas is lifted anteriorly

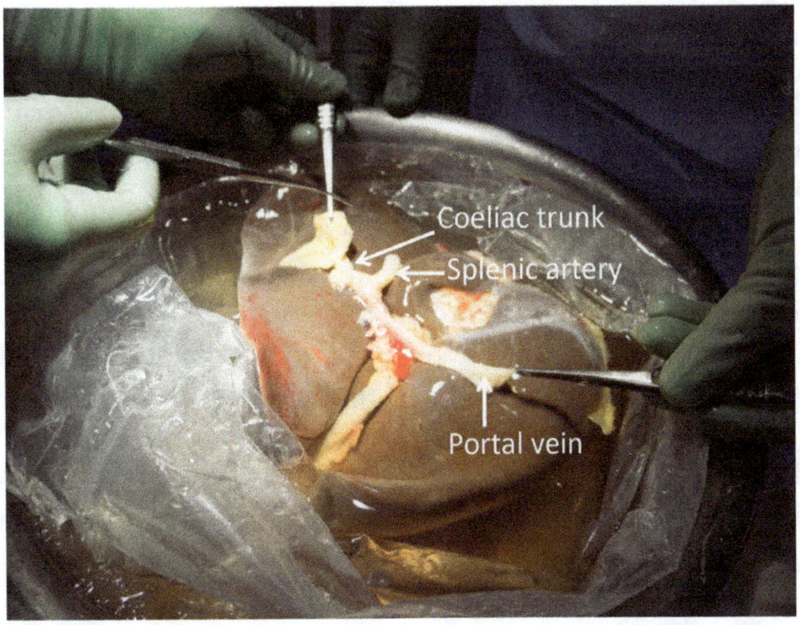

Figure 8. Liver graft harvested and immersed in ice slush.

by holding the spleen, and the dissection to its posterior attachment is performed from the tail toward the body of the pancreas. At this point, the SMA is excised with a small aortic patch, and the pancreas is removed from abdomen and placed in the ice-slush filled basin. Care must be taken during excision of the SMA without jeopardizing the renal artery [2].

3.2.4. Procurement of the liver and pancreas as an en bloc

The liver and pancreas are preferred to have en bloc procurement to minimize warm ischemic injury to these organs. Following cold perfusion, the proximal and distal part of the duodenum is transected by using GIA stapler at the level distal to the pylorus and the fourth part of the duodenum, respectively. The distal part of the SMA and SMV is tied by pre placed 2/0 Vicryl tie and divided. The Transverse mesocolon is divided, and the division is continued on the left to the splenic flexure and on the right to the duodenocolic ligament, which are also divided and the colon retracted inferiorly. The spleen is lifted anteriorly as a handle of the pancreas for dissection posterior to the pancreas. The SMA is excised at the inferior edge with a small aortic patch that is extended superiorly to include the celiac trunk on the same aortic patch. The left gastric artery is divided. The attention is directed to the IVC. The IVC is divided just proximal to the level of the entrance by the renal veins, and the dissection to its posterior is continued superiorly to reach the suprahepatic end of the IVC. At this stage, the liver and pancreas are free to be removed from the abdominal cavity and immersed in an ice basin for separation from each other on the back table [2].

3.2.5. Procurement of the kidneys

The kidneys are the lastly procured abdominal organs. Therefore, care must be taken during cooling and procurement phase to ensure that the kidneys are properly cooled by placing enough ice slush at its surrounding, in particular at its posterior and lateral sides [8].

The right kidney is retrieved first. The bowel is placed superiorly, and the kidneys, the vena cava, and the aorta are left in situ. The perfusion cannula is removed, and the aorta is transected at this level. The superior end of the aorta is also transected at the level where the SMA aortic patch is excised. The left renal vein is excised with a small patch from the vena cava and dissected away from the aorta. The anterior part of the aorta is split open as well as the posterior part of the aorta. Care is taken to keep an equal aortic patch with each side of the renal artery. The renal arteries are inspected at this point and are remained on its patch. The IVC is transected at the level of the confluence of common iliac veins. The right ureter is divided at the level of iliac vessels. The ureter is lifted anteriorly, and its posterior is dissected toward the kidney along the plane anterior to the major psoas muscle. Care is taken to retain plenty of surrounding tissues with the ureter. Then, the kidney is lifted anteriorly within Gerota's fascia together with the ureter, and its posterior side is dissected from the psoas muscle. The dissection is continued posteriorly to the IVC, and the right half of the aortic patch until the kidney is free from the attachment. The right kidney is then removed as a pack from the abdomen and placed in the basin filled with ice slush (**Figure 9**). Care is taken to ensure that the dissection is along the surface of the psoas muscle and spine. So, the injury to the renal artery and renal vein is prevented. The left kidney is procured in the same method as the right kidney.

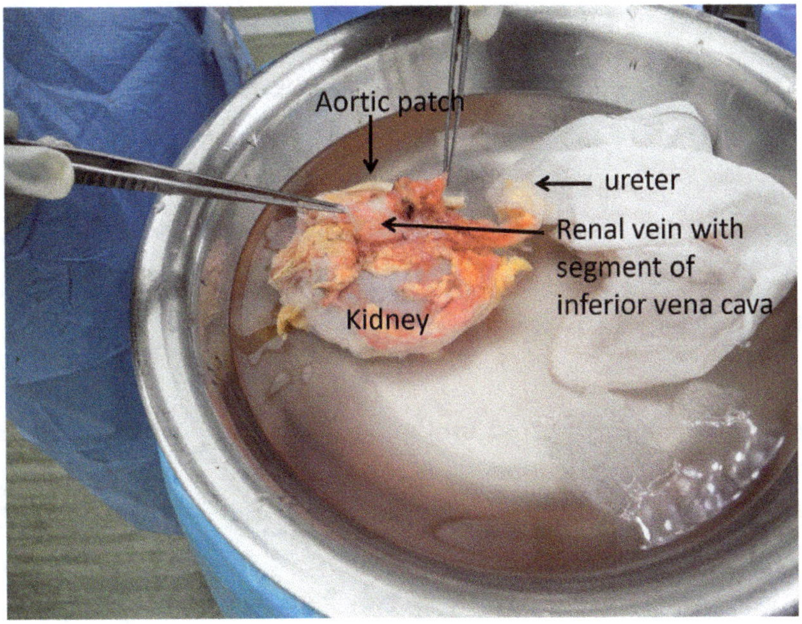

Figure 9. Right kidney harvested and immersed in ice slush.

3.2.6. Procurement of the kidney on en bloc

Alternatively, the kidneys can be procured on en bloc [5] and separated in the ice basin on a back table. The technique is faster to remove the kidney from the abdomen and minimize the risk of warm ischemic injury. In particular, it is preferred for procurement of the kidneys in DCD donors. The bowel is retracted anteriorly and superiorly. The kidneys, the aorta, and the vena cava are left in situ. The aorta and vena cava is transected at the level of its arteriotomy for the cannula. The right ureter is identified and divided at the level crossing over the iliac vessels as well as the left ureter. The ureter is dissected toward the renal hilum with plenty of surrounding tissues to prevent the injury to its blood supply. The dissection is continued superiorly along the plane posterior to Gerota's fascia but anterior to the psoas muscle and spine until reaching the superior end of the aorta and vena cava. Both kidneys are procured and placed in an ice basin on the back table. During the dissection, the assistant holds up both kidneys with ureters anteriorly to facilitate the dissection.

The kidneys are separated on the back table. The left renal vein is excised with a patch at its entrance to the IVC. The anterior side of the aorta is cleaned and incised along its midline allowing the equivalent patch to each side of the renal artery. Similarly, the posterior side of the aorta is incised along the midline. The ostium of the renal artery is inspected as well as the numbers of the renal artery are checked. The kidneys are now separated from each other. The kidney is inspected as described above and packed for transportation.

3.2.7. Procurement of the iliac vessels

A segment of the iliac arteries and veins are harvested as long as possible toward the distal part of the femoral artery and veins. The iliac artery and vein can be taken separately or together as one bundle. Care is taken to avoid injury by over pulling on the vessels. The vessels are stored in a sterile jar with UW solution and parked with two more layers of sterile bags for transportation.

The iliac arteries and veins are routinely retrieved for vascular reconstruction during liver and pancreas transplantation. In pancreas transplantation, the common iliac artery, the external iliac artery, and the internal iliac artery are used as a "Y" graft for reconstruction to the stumps of the splenic artery and SMA and then anastomosed to the recipient common iliac artery at the transplantation. Generally, one set of iliac vessels is sent with the liver, and another set is sent with the pancreas.

4. Organ package and the transportation

All the organs will be further inspected on the back table to ensure its quality and suitability for transplantation. Communication with the transplant surgeon at the recipient end is strongly encouraged to achieve the best outcome for organ transplantation [9].

4.1. Liver

The liver is inspected in the basin. Five hundred milliliter of UW solution (4°C) is perfused to the portal vein system. The common bile duct is flushed with 200 ml of UW solution by using a syringe. The liver is placed into the first sterile bag filled with 700–1000 ml of UW solution, and the bag is tied. The first bag is then placed into the second sterile bag filed with 1 L cold normal saline and tied. The second bag is placed into the third sterile bag and then tied. The liver in the three-layered bag is then placed in the Iskey filled with ice blocks for transportation to the recipient hospital with the document secured in the Iskey (**Figure 10**) [7].

4.2. Pancreas

The pancreas is inspected to ensure its quality for transplantation without injury from the procurement and then is packed by the same method as for the liver. It is placed in the Iskey with retrieved vessels for transportation to the recipient hospital. Often, the pancreas is allocated with the left kidney to the same recipient for simultaneous pancreas-kidney transplantation (SPKT). Care is taken to avoid manipulation over the pancreas. Perfusion to the pancreas on the back table is not recommended to avoid perfusion injury and pancreatitis.

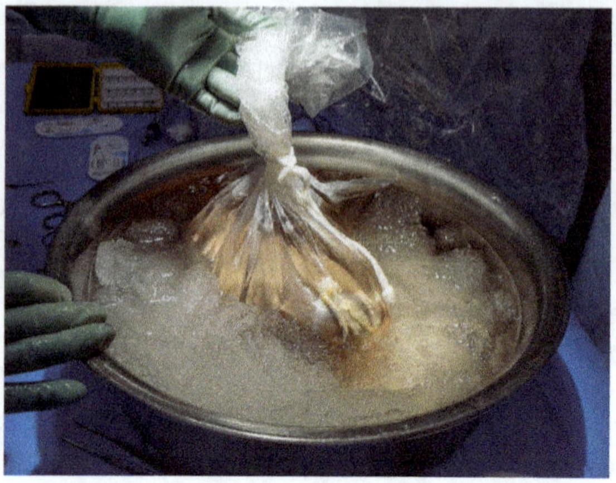

Figure 10. Package of the liver. The first bag filled with UW solution.

4.3. Kidneys

Each kidney is inspected by dissection open the perinephric fat. The quality of perfusion is checked and the mass lesion is excluded. The kidney is placed in the first sterile plastic bag that is filled with 500 ml of UW solution and tied. The first bag is placed into the second bag that is filled with 1 L cold normal saline and tied. The second bag is placed into the third bag and tied. The kidney is placed in the Iskey and buried in the ice blocks for transportation with the document enclosed.

5. Conclusion

Multi-organ procurement is essential for organ transplantation, and proper training is mandatory. It usually involves a few transplant units for organ allocation prior to confirmation of the surgical time. The communication between all parties is very important to minimize the ischemic time and achieve the good outcome for organ transplantation. It should be bore in mind that the anatomical variation may be encountered during the surgery, and care must be taken to avoid any damage to the vessels and organs, which may jeopardize the organ transplantation. Establishment of a surgical protocol is encouraged to achieve a national-wide standard and consistence for organ sharing among the transplant units.

Acknowledgements

We would like to acknowledge DonateLife of Western Australia for their contribution.

Conflict of interest

There is no conflict of interest.

Author details

Bulang He[1*], Xiuwu Han[2] and Michael A. Fink[3]

*Address all correspondence to: bulang.he@health.wa.gov.au

1 Medical School, The University of Western Australia, Sir Charles Gairdner Hospital, Nedlands, Perth, Australia

2 Beijing Chaoyang Hospital (West Campus), Capital Medical University, Beijing, China

3 Department of Surgery/Austin Health, Medicine Dentistry and Health Sciences, The University of Melbourne, Austraila

References

[1] Farinelli PA, Padin JM, Troncoso JC, et al. Short- and long-term outcomes of every graft recovered during a multi-organ procurement procedure including the intestine. Transplantation Proceedings. 2014;**46**:2090-2095

[2] Fridell JA, Powelson JA, Kubal CA, et al. Retrieval of the pancreas allograft for whole-organ transplantation. Clinical Transplantation. 2014;**28**:1313-1330

[3] Merkel FK, Jonasson O, Bergan JJ. Procurement of cadaver donor organs: Evisceration technique. Transplantation Proceedings. 1972;**4**:585-589

[4] Rosenthal JT, Shaw BW Jr, Hardesty RL, Griffith BP, Starzl TE, Hakala TR. Principles of multiple organ procurement from cadaver donors. Annals of Surgery. 1983;**198**:617-621

[5] Starzl TE, Hakala TR, Shaw BW Jr, et al. A flexible procedure for multiple cadaveric organ procurement. Surgery, Gynecology and Obstetrics. 1984;**158**:223-230

[6] Wunderlich H, Brockmann JG, Voigt R, et al. DTG procurement guidelines in heart beating donors. Transplant International: Official Journal of the European Society for Organ Transplantation. 2011;**24**:733-757

[7] Abu-Elmagd K, Fung J, Bueno J, et al. Logistics and technique for procurement of intestinal, pancreatic, and hepatic grafts from the same donor. Annals of Surgery. 2000;**232**: 680-687

[8] Salazar-Banuelos A, Monroy-Cuadros M, Henriquez-Cooper H. Retro-peritoneal cooling for kidney preservation from multi-organ cadaver donors. American Journal of Surgery. May 2018;**215**(5):802-803

[9] https://www.tsanz.com.au/standalonepages/documents/201512thFebruary-OTAVs1ReleaseVersionFinal.pdf. Surgical Technique for Deceased Donor Abdominal Organ Procurement

7

Pancreas Transplantation

Pedro Ventura-Aguiar, Joana Ferrer-Fábrega and
Maria José Ricart

Abstract

Pancreas transplantation is a treatment alternative to patients with type 1 diabetes, particularly to those with associated end-stage renal disease (ESRD). Recently, pancreas transplant centers have widened their criteria for pancreas transplantation to selected type 2 diabetic patients. This chapter reviews the most important topics on pancreas transplantation, including epidemiology and natural history of type I and type II diabetes, indications for pancreas transplantation, different alternatives for pancreas transplant recipients (simultaneous kidney-pancreas transplantation, pancreas after kidney, or pancreas transplant alone—PTA), and their outcomes. This chapter gives a detailed description of the surgical procedure for pancreas procurement and engraftment, as well as the most frequent surgical complications. An approach to the management of the recipient following pancreas transplantation (immunosuppression and infection prophylaxis) is also discussed. Finally, outcomes and complications following the pancreas transplantation are reviewed.

Keywords: pancreas transplantation, surgical complications, acute rejection, diabetes, end-stage renal disease, immunossuppression, kidney transplantation

1. Introduction

Diabetes is a disease characterized by an imbalance in glucose metabolism homeostasis, highly prevalent worldwide, and presents a significant morbidity and mobility due to vascular and neurological complications. It is the single most frequent cause of end-stage renal disease in incident patients on hemodialysis. The clinical presentation and epidemiology of diabetes varies according to the etiology. For selected patients, pancreas transplantation is the best treatment alternative to achieve glycemic control. In this chapter, we describe the most important topics regarding pancreas transplantation, including indication and patient evaluation, surgical techniques, immunosuppression protocols, and outcomes.

2. Epidemiology and pathophysiology of diabetes

Diabetes is a spectrum of diseases characterized by a disorder in glucose metabolism leading to persistent hyperglycemia, with clinical manifestations varying according to disease etiology (**Table 1**).

Type 1 diabetes mellitus (DM) is an autoimmune disorder characterized by the generation of autoantibodies against β cells and the development of a localized inflammatory response with consequent islet destruction. Current models suggest that the disease progresses as a relapsing-remitting disease, with a nonlinear β cell mass loss at each relapse as a result of the imbalance between β cell proliferation and destruction, eventually leading to persistent hyperglycemia. At diagnosis, these patients may present with nearly normal serum concentrations of insulin and C-peptide but with a rapid decrease in the following 8–12 weeks.

Several autoantibodies have been described in patients with type 1 diabetes—antibodies to insulin (IAA), glutamic acid decarboxylase (GAD), Zinc transporter 8 antibodies (ZnT8A), and protein tyrosine phosphatase-like protein IA2 (IA2 or ICA512). The risk for overt diabetes better correlates with the number of autoantibodies present rather than the titter of a single antibody [1].

Type 1 diabetes usually presents at a young age (6 months to 25 years old), and there is a geographical variation, with a tendency toward an increased incidence in developed countries—as

Diabetes	Age presentation	Clinical presentation	Etiology	Prevalence (of total diabetes)	Obesity
Type 1	6 months to young adulthood	Most often acute, rapid	Autoimmune (some genetic associations); β cell mass loss; Insulin deficiency	5–10%	Uncommon
Type 2	Adulthood	Variable; from slow, mild (often insidious) to severe	Insulin resistence; β cell exaustion	80–90%	Common
Monogenic	Often post pubertal except glucokinase and neonatal diabetes	Variable (may be incidental in glucokinase)	Reduced insulin production or secretion; higher glucose sensor threashold	2%	Incidence similar to general population

Table 1. Etiology and clinical presentation of diabetes.

recognized by the World Health Organization (WHO), this may be due to differences in registry data, since few data that exist from sub-Saharian Africa, South America, and Asia [2].

A genetic predisposition has been identified with an increased risk for the disease in siblings and offspring of diabetics. There is an increased incidence in patients with human leukocyte antigen–antigen D related (HLA DR)*03 and DR*04.

Type 2 diabetes is characterized by peripheral cells insulin resistance with a consequent persistent hyperglycemia. Insulin production and secretion is often maintained with normal or high serum insulin and C-peptide. It usually presents in adulthood and is often associated with obesity and a sedentary lifestyle.

According to the WHO, diabetes incidence and prevalence is increasing [3] at a particularly alarming rate among children. This has led to a shift in the paradigm of age of presentation of type 2 diabetes with an ever-increasing incidence in young adults, and consequent presentation of diabetes complications at younger ages [4].

The first line of treatment for type 2 diabetes is lifestyle modification, followed by oral antidiabetic agents. The mechanism of action of oral agents is diverse, from reduction in glucose absorption, to increase in insulin secretion, stimulation of gluconeogenesis, or reduction of tubular reabsorption with an increase in urinary glucose excretion. Despite these alternatives, several patients still need exogenous insulin to achieve glycemic control. Chronic insulin resistance may lead to β cell exhaustion, and insulin and C-peptide levels may decrease below normal range in patients with long-standing type 2 diabetes.

3. Indications for pancreas transplantation

Transplant of β cells is a treatment alternative to insulin-dependent diabetic patients with the objective of reestablishing glucose homeostasis without the need for exogenous insulin.

Both pancreas and islet transplantation are currently used in clinical practice as β cell mass transplant techniques. Islet transplantation is still limited to nearly experimental protocols, though a few centers have introduced them into their clinical practice. According to the Collaborative Islet Transplant Registry (CITR), 1927 procedures have been performed worldwide from 2004 to 2013 [5]. Though conceptually attractive, its high cost of isolation and the sub-optimal insulin-independency results (when compared to whole-organ transplantation) have halted its clinical application.

Pancreas transplantation is indicated in patients with insulin deficiency and end-stage renal disease (ESRD) in those or with brittle diabetes and normal renal function. Indications should take into account disease-related characteristics:

a. Type of DM: pancreas transplantation is indicated in patients with type 1 DM, selected patients with type 2 DM, as well as to those with diabetes secondary other etiologies(acute and chronic pancreatitis, cystic fibrosis, and trauma). According to data obtained from the last US Pancreas Transplant Registry (OPTN/SRTR), pancreas transplantation in type 2 diabetes is increasing worldwide [6], representing up to 8% of all transplants performed in the US [7]. The most recent report demonstrates a 3-year graft survival of 83.3%. Indication in these patients is not consensual. At our center, we indicate in patients <50 years, body mass index (BMI) <30, at least 5 years of insulin therapy, C-Peptide <3.0 ng/mL, and daily insulin at <0.5 U/kg/day. Larger cohorts, standardized inclusion criteria, and long-term results are warranted.

b. Age: an age limit is not established. Though it is usual to accept candidates up to the age of 50 and assessing individually those aged between 50 and 55 years, some groups accept patients who are >60 years old [8].

c. Diabetic complications: the presence and severity of these complications, at the time the patient is studied for transplantation, is another parameter to assess. Successful pancreas transplantation requires suitable vascular permeability for arterial and venous anastomosis. Presence of severe calcifications in the iliac vessels, where the vascular anastomoses of the organs are usually performed, as well as the existence of a severe peripheral vascular disease, can technically allow the implantation of a graft, but it is inadvisable to implant-both organs. In these cases, priority is given to kidney transplantation. Coronary heart disease is also a frequent contraindication for pancreas transplantation. The implantation of two organs requires a major surgery with longer anesthesia time and a greater probability of presenting some type of complication or surgical re-intervention. Other secondary diabetic complications, such as retinopathy and neuropathy, rarely represent by themselves as a contraindication for the transplant, but due consideration should be given to the patient during pre-transplant evaluation.

3.1. Indications according to transplant modality

Pancreas transplantation can be performed individually or simultaneously with kidney transplantation in patients with ESRD. Each type of transplant has certain characteristics that must be highlighted.

3.1.1. Simultaneous transplantation of pancreas and kidney (SPK)

Simultaneous kidney-pancreas transplantation (SPK) is the most common type of pancreas transplant, representing over 98% of all pancreas transplants performed in the US [7]. It is currently the best treatment alternative to patients with ESRD who are candidates to a kidney transplant. In addition to the demographic and clinical parameters previously described, immunological and waiting-list vintage should be considered when proposing a patient to an SPK. The presence of HLA alloantibodies reduces the probability of finding a suitable donor and increases waiting-list vintage. In moderate (cPRA > 50%) and highly sensitized (cPRA > 90%) patients, an individual approach is advised

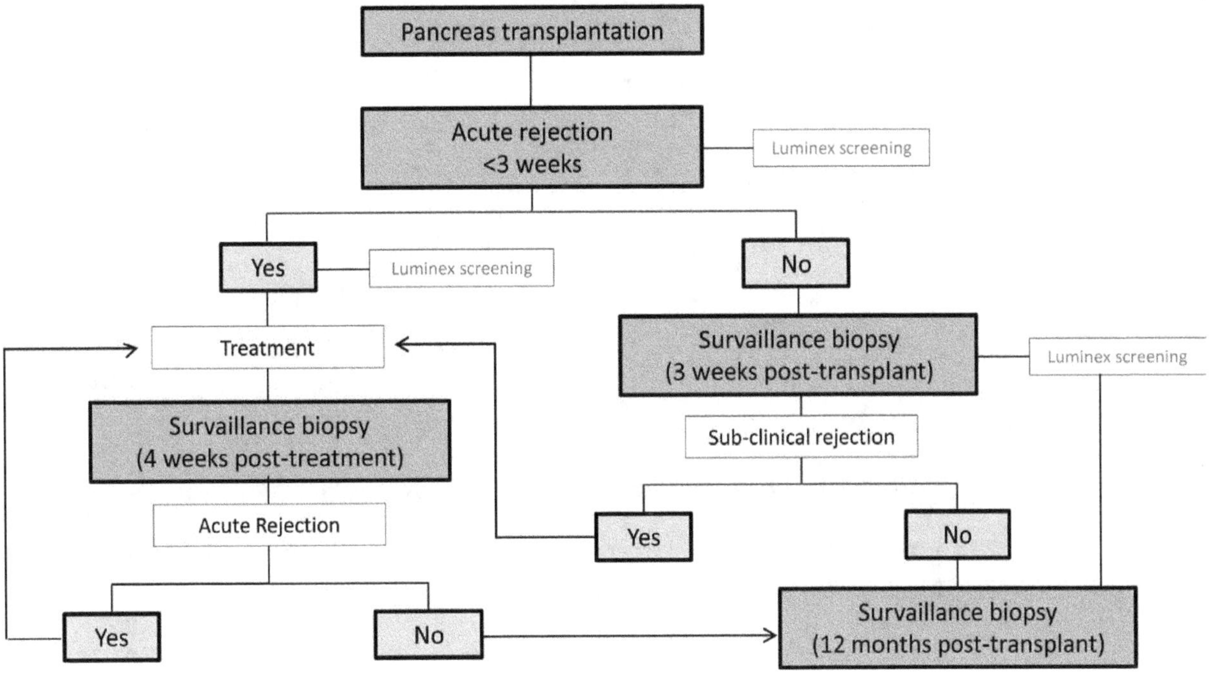

Figure 1. Hospital Clinic's flowchart for performing pancreas graft biopsy. Ultrasound-guided survaillance biopsies are performed at 3 weeks and 12 months post-transplant. Biopsies are also performed if clinicaly indicated, and are followed by a survaillance biopsy 4 weeks after the treatment of rejection.

and a kidney transplant followed by a pancreas transplant alone should be considered. Similarly, centers with long pancreas waiting lists (>2 years) should evaluate the risk of maintaining the patient on dialysis or use a pancrease after kidney transplantation (PAK) approach, since mortality on the waiting list can be up to 42% at 4 years in this population (**Figure 1**) [9].

3.1.2. Pancreas after kidney transplantation (PAK)

This type of transplant is considered for those patients who are candidates for a kidney and pancreas transplant and who have an available living kidney donor or where waiting-list vintage is significantly shorter to kidney when compared to pancreas transplant. The major benefit of PAK is reducing, or avoiding, time on dialysis while waiting for pancreas transplantation. Restoration of kidney function may reduce uremia-induced anticoagulation and possibly reduce bleeding during surgical complications. This approach implies, nonetheless, two different surgical procedures. Moreover, up-to-date results are somewhat poorer for patients who have undergone PAK transplant, with an inferior pancreas graft survival and higher acute rejection incidence [10]. The decision to perform a PAK (live donor kidney) or an SPK will depend fundamentally on the characteristics of the living donor (age, HLA compatibility), the possibility of performing a preventive transplant, the expected time on the waiting list, as well as the patient's expectations (**Table 2**).

	SPK	PAK
Advantages	**a.** Single surgical procedure **b.** Single cycle of induction immunosuppression **c.** Better graft survival	**a.** Minimizes or avoids the need for dialysis (in LDKT) **b.** Shorter surgical procedure **c.** Avoids uremia-asociated complications. **d.** Time to pancreas transplantation usually shorter than for SPK
Disadvantages	**a.** Longer waiting-list time **b.** Lower probability of receiving kidney transplant preemptively	**a.** Two surgical procedures **b.** Two cycles of induction immunosuppression **c.** Higher incidence of acute rejection **d.** Inferior pancreas graft survival

Table 2. Pancreas after kidney transplantation: pros and cons compared to SPK.

This alternative has been gaining increasing interest in recent years due to the current shortage of cadaveric organs from young donors and the consequent increase in waiting-list time for kidney-pancreas transplantation. In some centers, PAK represents up to 50% of pancreas transplants, most of them having received a kidney transplant from a previously living donor.

The indications regarding age, type of DM, and vascular status of the recipient would be the same as in the case of SPK. However, a functioning kidney graft with good and stable renal function (glomerular filtration rate—GFR > 40 ml/min) is recommended prior to inclusion on the waiting list, due to the risk of acute kidney injury following the pancreas transplantation surgery and the increase in doses of immunosuppressors.

One of the issues raised in this type of transplant has been on when to perform pancreas transplantation after the kidney transplantation. There is no established time limit, and it depends on the progression of each patient following the kidney transplant. However, it seems that a better survival of the pancreatic graft has been observed when the interval between both transplants is less than 12 months. For some authors, the optimal interval between both procedures should be less than 4 months.

3.1.3. Pancreas transplant alone

Isolated pancreas transplantation in diabetics without documented kidney disease, and with little or no other secondary complication, would theoretically be the ideal transplant. These would be the ones who could benefit the most from the positive effects of this transplant, by being able to prevent the appearance of secondary complications, thanks to an early metabolic control. However, it is considered that the risk of the intervention, as well as the risk of immunosuppression to which the patient must be subjected for life does not always justify the hypothetical advantages of the transplant.

The results obtained with the PTA are somewhat worse than those of the PAK and SPK. The incidence of technical complications (mainly graft thrombosis) and acute rejection is somewhat higher to the other types of transplant.

It is performed to patients with brittle diabetes and normal renal function, who require repeated hospital admissions due to metabolic decompensation and/or severe hypoglycemic unawareness. These should be confirmed during a hospital stay following treatment optimization using insulin pump and/or continuous glycemic control monitors. It may also be performed to patients with the brittle diabetes and incipient diabetic complications, in order to reduce progression of secondary complications.

The main indications, as well as the absolute and relative contraindications for pancreas transplantation, are presented in **Table 3**.

Indications

SPK: diabetes mellitus and end-stage renal disease (GFR <20 ml/min or dialysis)

PAK: diabetes mellitus and functioning kidney transplant

PTA: Type 1 diabetes with normal renal function (GFR >60 ml/min; proteinuria <1 g/day), and:

- Not aware of severe hypoglycemia (life threatening)
- Frequent hospital admission due to metabolic complications
- Failure to achieve glycemic control using other alternatives—such as insulin pump and/or continuous glycaemic control monitors—during a hospital admission

Absolute contraindications

Severe untreatable coronary heart disease; severe left ventricular disfunction

Chronic liver or pulmonary disease

Active infection

Active or past cancer without adequate remission period (excluded in situ and skin epitheliums)

Severe psycologic or psychiatric disease; drug and alchool abuse

Morbid obesity (BMI >35 kg/m^2)

Active gastrointestinal bleeding

Relative contraindications

Age: <18 and >55 years old

Obesity (BMI < 30 kg/m^2)

Recent acute coronary heart disease

Recent retinal hemorhage

Symptomatic cerebrovascular or peripheral vascular diseases

Severe autonomic neuropathy or diabetic gastropathy

Active smoking

Table 3. Indications and contraindications to pancreas transplantation.

4. Waiting list for pancreas transplantation

4.1. Evaluation of candidates

Evaluation of the candidates for pancreas transplantation should be performed as early as possible, in order to identify those who would benefit the most from the procedure. In patients with chronic kidney disease, we recommend referral to a pancreas transplant center as soon as glomerular filtration rate (GFR) falls below 25–30 ml/min. This early referral offers precious time for patient evaluation and possible inclusion on the waiting-list pre-dialysis. Additionally, and depending on transplant center policies, this allows the study of a possible living kidney donor and a preemptive kidney transplant.

Patient evaluation and clinical workup is similar to that performed for kidney transplantation, such as complete medical history, immunological study, uremic state, liver disease, cancer and infection screening, with some additional particularities related to diabetic disease: hormonal study, β cell autoantibodies, as well as study of the main diabetic complications.

- Hormonal assessment: the main purpose is to determine whether or not the patient has endogenous insulin secretion. For this, it is sufficient to determine the fasting plasma levels of C-Peptide. Its negativity indicates the absence of insulin secretion.
- Autoantibodies: the main objective of pre-transplant quantification of β cell autoantibodies (IAA, GAD, ZnT8A, IA2) is to establish a baseline. These tend to be negative after years of evolution of DM, and therefore negative at the time of transplantation. Their presence does not represent a contraindication for pancreas transplantation. During follow-up, nonetheless, its reappearance is associated with an increased risk for disease relapse.
- Diabetic retinopathy is present in up to 90% of of all transplant candidates, with varying degrees of severity. It is not considered an exclusion criteria for transplantation.
- Diabetic polyneuropathy is also present in majority of patients but rarely contraindicates the transplant. However, it is advisable to take into account the severe dysfunction of the autonomic nervous system, due to post-transplant complications and the negative impact on patient survival. Diabetic neuropathy can often affect the urinary bladder leading to incontinence or incomplete bladder emptying. If urinary exocrine drainage is used, a urinary urethrocystography is recommended to rule out pathology of the bladder and urethra, as well as a cystomanometry to study and evaluate bladder function.
- Cardiovascular evaluation is the most important due to the impact of cardiovascular disease on post-transplant mortality and morbidity. Previous history of myocardial infarction, angioplasty, or coronary bypass should not necessarily be a contraindication to transplantation. Workup should be exhaustive before including the patient on the waiting list. It is advisable to perform an electrocardiogram (EKG) and a pharmacological stress test with MIBI-dipyridamole, as well as an echocardiography to evaluate ventricular ejection fraction and exclude motility disorders. If any of these tests are pathological, coronary angiography should be performed to identify more accurately the existing lesions and

perform the appropriate treatment prior to transplantation (either angioplasty or coronary artery bypass graft—CABG). A recent acute miocardial infarction, untreatable significant coronary angiography lesions, or severe ventricular dysfunction are contraindications to transplantation (**Table 3**).

- Vascular evaluation: an angio-computed tomography (CT) should be performed to rule out vascular lesions, mainly at the level of the iliac vessels and the celiac trunk that could hinder the implantation of the grafts. In pre-dialysis patients, a magnetic resonance imaging (MRI) with no or low dose of low-risk gadolinum contrast can be used.
- Assessment by the transplant team: once the study of potential candidates has been completed, and before being included on the waiting list, it is advisable to carry out a joint assessment by all the members of the transplant team (nephrologist, endocrinologist, anesthesiologist, and surgeons).

4.2. Inclusion on the waiting list

At the time of inclusion on the waiting list, a checklist should be performed to ensure all pre-transplant studies have been completed, and revised by the medical team. It is important to ensure that the patient has received a clear and comprehensible information regarding the advantages, as well as of the possible complications of the transplant, so that he can decide to freely choose this form of treatment.

Logistical issues should also be discussed in advance with the patient, in order to minimize the time from patient contact to the surgical procedure (hence cold ischemia time). The patient and his closest relatives should be aware of the expected duration of the intervention, median hospital stay, and most important post-transplant cares and outpatient visits.

Also, and for as long as they remain on the waiting list, the patient should be made aware of the importance of maintaining regular communication with the transplant center. The high incidence of complications that may occur in these diabetic patients, especially if they are affected by chronic renal failure and are also waiting for a simultaneous kidney transplant, requires strict monitoring and follow-up as long as they are not transplanted. Ideally, they should be visited by a member or collaborating doctor of the transplant team every 3–4 months. Only in this way, it is possible to detect possible events that may represent a temporary contraindication for the intervention.

4.3. Pancreas allocation

Solid organ allocation protocols are the major influence on patients' waiting-list vintage. In the UK, the introduction of a new nationwide allocation system in December 2010 significantly reduced the number of long-lasting patients and increased the number of islet transplants [11]. These protocols must comply with national legislations and logistic constraints. Several factors must be taken into account, such as donor demographics, donor center, geographical proximity to transplant center, and recipient priority indexes. In the UK protocol, weighting factors included expected organ travel time, recipient sensitization, dialysis vintage, waiting-list time,

HLA mismatching, and donor BMI (differential weighting for islet or whole-organ transplantation). Other allocation protocols, such as the US and the Eurotransplant, also include in their weighting factors donor, recipient and center characteristics.

5. Donor selection

Pancreas blood supply is performed under low-flux conditions. This low blood flow rate increases the risk of surgical complications, such as thrombosis and ischemia. In addition, exocrine pancreas produces a large amount of protein cleavage enzymes, making it very susceptible to ischemia-reperfusion injury during transplantation. Pancreas present the highest donor discard rate among abdominal solid organ transplantations, with up to 33% of all pancreas being discarded by surgical teams prior to pancreas extraction, and an additional 50% being discarded following the extraction due to macroscopic appearance.

In an attempt to standardize donor acceptance criteria and predict short-term pancreas graft function, several scoring systems have been developed. P-PASS was one of the first to be described and was used in the Eurotransplant area to increase sensitivity in allocation. It categorized donors in low (<17) or high (≥17) risk donors [12]. The initial enthusiasm was halted by the reports of its inability to predict short- and long-term graft survival [13].

In 2010, Axelrod et al. published a complex scoring system, including donor and recipient variables, which enabled to predict 1-year graft survival [14]. Despite the promising results, it lacked several key factors, which are thought to influence outcomes, such as previous cardiac arrest in donors after brain death and perfusion solution. In 2013, Finger et al. demonstrated that the presence of at least two factors such as BMI ≥30 kg/m^2, donor creatinine ≥2.5 mg/dL, donor age > 50 years, and preservation time > 20 h were associated with technical failure [15].

Donors after brain death (DBD) have been the most widely used deceased donors since late 1980s; donors after cardiocirulatory death (DCD) were the first deceased donors used for organ transplantation in many countries until a brain death diagnosis and its acceptance for organ donation was legislated. Since the mid-2000s, DCDs regained protagonism as a potential source to increase donor pool, with an increasing number of transplanted organs ever since. DCDs should be evaluated carefully, since the definition includes donors with different backgrounds. According to the Maastricht classification, DCD donors can be classified from type I–V (**Table 4**) [16]. For pancreas transplantation, both type II (uncontrolled) and type III (controlled) have been used. Results from single center and registry analysis suggest

Type of donor	Management of cardiac arrest
Type I—brought in dead	Uncontrolled
Type II—unsuccessful resuscitation	Uncontrolled
Type III—awaiting cardiac arrest	Controlled
Type V—cardiac arrest after brain-stem death	Uncontrolled
Type V—cardiac arrest in a hospital inpatient (added in 2000)	Uncontrolled

Table 4. Maastricht classification [16].

that DCD donors are a suitable source of organs for pancreas and islet transplantation in selected donors [17]. Age limit acceptance is usually lower for DBD donors (<45 years), and both warm and cold ischemia times should be strictly respected, at the risk of increased surgical complications.

Table 5 describes the acceptance criteria for both DBD and DCD donors at our center. In summary, all donors under 45 years without other risk factors, with BMI ≤30 kg/m^2, and transaminases and pancreatic enzymes <3× normal values are accepted for transplantation, regardless of being DBD or DCD. Beyond those criteria, individual evaluations are performed.

Characteristic	**DBD donors**	**DCD donors**
Donor age (years)	≤45 (46–55 evaluate individually)	≤45
Donor BMI (kg/m^2)	≤30	≤30
Expected cold ischaemia time (h)	≤12 h (>12 h evaluate individually)	≤8 h (>8 h evaluate individually)
Hepatic transaminases (times above normal value)	<3×s	<3×s
Pancreatic enzymes (times above normal value)	<3×s	<3×s
Warm ischaemia (minutes)	—	• Total (TWIT): <60 • Functional (FWIT): <30 • Hemodynamic instability (SBP <60 mmHg) prior to donation: <60
Clinical risk factors	• Arterial HT • Smoking • Alcoholism • History of pancreatitis	• Arterial HT • Smoking • Alcoholism • History of pancreatitis

Table 5. Hospital clinic pancreas donor acceptance criteria.

6. Surgical techniques

William Kelly and Richard Lillehei performed the first pancreas transplant at the University of Minnesota on December 17, 1966 [18]. In the last decades, the progress in immunosuppressive treatment has been parallel to a decrease in postoperative complications, to an improvement in the surgical technique, and ultimately to a better survival of both the graft and the patient.

The correct evaluation of the viability of the pancreas at the time of extraction in the donor is one of the basic pillars to obtain good results in the recipient. This must invariably be accompanied by a correct surgical technique during the extraction and implantation of the organ.

6.1. Pancreas extraction

Adequate donor selection is crucial in pancreas transplantation, as described in the previous section. The extraction technique is of well-documented importance for a successful outcome [19]. Whether it is advocated for an enteric or bladder drainage, it requires the extraction of the entire pancreas and a segment of the duodenum with its vascularization—perfused by the celiac trunk and superior mesenteric artery—and drained by the portal vein. As this vascularization is shared with the liver, surgical techniques have been developed to allow the simultaneous extraction of both organs. In specific cases of hemodynamic instability, rapid or block extraction must be performed in order to perfuse the preservation solution as quickly as possible.

The surgery begins with a xipho-pubic incision, with sternotomy and opening of the pericardium. The first step is to carry out a thorough examination of all the organs to identify any pathology that contraindicates the donation. It is important to have vascular control to allow rapid cannulation in case of instability, performing the dissection and individualization with ligatures of the aorta above the iliac bifurcation and the infrarenal cava, as well as the inferior mesenteric vein, in the case of portal vein being cannulated through it. The superior mesenteric artery is then dissected, located above and to the left of the confluence of the left renal vein with the cava, and a vessel loop is passed around it.

A first visual evaluation of the organ is performed, after the opening of the smaller sac, sectioning the gastrocolic ligament, to expose the entire anterior surface of the body and tail of the pancreas, together with palpation of the pancreatic head. The next phase comprises the dissection of the hepatic hilum to identify the possible anatomical variants of the hepatic artery. The most frequent are the right hepatic artery from the superior mesenteric artery and the left hepatic artery that derives from the stomatologic coronary artery. The common bile duct is dissected and sectioned at its most distal part. An incision is made in the gallbladder fundus and physiological serum injected into the fundus from the bile duct. The gastroduodenal artery and the hepatic artery are identified and dissected at the celiac trunk. In addition, the left gastric artery and the coronary vein are also identified, as well as all the lymphatic vessels in the upper border of the pancreas. The splenic artery is individualized and referenced with 6/0 prolene suture to prevent its retraction in the pancreas. A silk ligature must be passed through the abdominal aorta above the celiac trunk, following the blunt dissection of the esophageal hiatus. Finally, the dissection of the portal vein is carried out after identifying the stomachatric coronary vein. It is important to perform the Kocher maneuver in order to access the entire duodenum and the posterior aspect of the pancreatic head. The dissection of the pancreas must be done through the "no touch technique." For the release of the pancreatic inferior aspect, mobilization of the entire transverse colon to the splenic angle is required. Subsequently, all the ligaments that fix the spleen to the retroperitoneum are sectioned for its separation from the kidney and the left adrenal gland, as well as the fixation of the body and tail to the retroperitoneum. Likewise, the section of the short gastrosplenic vessels and the dissection of the duodenum below the pylorus and at the level of the fourth portion is completed, for its subsequent sectioning to these two levels by means of a self-suture device.

Once the dissection is completed intrathoracically and abdominally, and prior to cannulation, intravenous sodium heparin (3 mg/kg) is administered. The aorta is then cannulated above the bifurcation, together with the cannulation of the portal system (through the inferior, superior, or portal mesenteric vein) and the supraceliac aorta is clamped to initiate perfusion of the aorta with preservation solution, at which time the vena cava is drained after opening it intrathoracically or through a drainage cannula placed in the inferior vena cava. At this time, crushed ice is placed on the organs to keep them at a suitable temperature. After completing the infusion, pancreas and liver are separated in situ. It is generally accepted that the celiac trunk must go with the liver. The splenic artery divides right after its origin from the celiac trunk. The aorta, at the level of the superior mesenteric artery, is sectioned laterally to visualize the origin of the renal arteries. The superior mesenteric artery must be ligated after the origin of the inferior pancreaticoduodenal artery. In short, the aortic patch is divided into two—the liver with the celiac trunk, and the pancreas—with the superior mesenteric artery. The infrahepatic vena cava is sectioned above the origin of the renal veins. The suprahepatic vena cava is divided along with the diaphragm that surrounds it. Finally, the portal is divided halfway between the liver and the pancreas. Finally, the pancreas is removed once the liver is removed. Some surgeons prefer to perform the extraction of both organs en block and perform their separation on the bench.

The iliac vessels (common iliac arteries/veins together with their bifurcations) are extracted and sent along with pancreas and liver grafts if they are needed for vascular reconstructions during the implant.

The organ is introduced in a sterile bag with preservation solution at 4°C. This bag is protected by inserting it into two other bags and transported to the recipient hospital. Bench surgery can be performed at the extraction site or later at reference hospital.

6.2. Bench surgery

During the bench surgery, the duodenum-pancreatic graft is prepared. This must remain in conditions of hypothermia at 4°C until its implantation.

After ligation of the splenic vessels, splenectomy is performed. If a fatty pancreas is found to be present, it should be removed carefully, making the necessary sutures to minimize the hemorrhage during reperfusion. It is advisable to invaginate the line of staples of the duodenal ends (with continuous 3/0 silk suture, although it is variable depending on the group), to ensure maximum suture tightness and avoid further fistulas.

In case of absence of celiac trunk (usual in simultaneous liver and pancreas extractions), it will be necessary to carry out reconstructions of the arterial vascularization of the pancreas that allow a good anastomosis with the iliac vessels of the recipient.

There are different techniques of vascular reconstruction of the pancreatic graft:

1. Anastomosis of the arteries of the pancreas with a segment of the iliac bifurcation of the donor. It is the most used modality in the USA and Europe.

2. Spleno-mesenteric termino-terminal anastomosis between the splenic artery and the distal end of the superior mesenteric artery of the graft. For some groups, it constitutes the technique of choice for its simplicity.

3. Spleno-mesenteric termino-lateral anastomosis between the splenic artery and the superior mesenteric artery of the graft.

Once the bech surgery is performed, graft is perfused with about 100 cc of preservation solution and is ready to be implanted in the recipient.

6.3. Pancreas implantation

The simultaneous kidney and pancreas transplantation is the most frequent transplant modality performed worldwide. The surgical technique used for the implantation of the renal graft does not differ from that used for kidney transplant alone. For pancreas transplantation, although the surgical technique is not standard among centers, there is unanimous agreement in implanting the complete organ, including the second portion of the duodenum.

Traditionally, the intraperitoneal position has been preferred by most groups. In the last decade, different authors have suggested the implant of the graft in a retroperitoneal location, advocating a more physiological position [20].

The pancreas shloud be implanted prior to the kidney, given its worse tolerance to cold ischemia. The best way to perform the transplant is with a supra-infraumbilical midline laparotomy, from a point midway between the xiphoid and the umbilicus up to 2–3 cm of the pubis. The complete pancreas with a small portion of the donor's duodenum, which contains the Vater's ampulla, is located laterally in the right iliac fossa of the recipient. The cranial or caudal position of the head of the pancreas depends on each group. Placing the pancreas on the left side increases the risk of graft thrombosis.

The intervention begins with the dissection of the ureter and the right iliac vessels. These should be dissected and mobilized widely to facilitate subsequent vascular anastomoses. Hemostasis must be carefully performed, and the major lymphatic vessels must be ligated. To facilitate the venous anastomosis of the portal, it is advisable to mobilize the distal vena cava and the right iliac vein.

Once the iliac vessels are dissected, the venous anastomosis is performed first, between the portal vein of the graft and the most proximal part of the right primitive iliac vein or on the cava before the iliac bifurcation. Before starting the anastomosis, the vena cava is perfused with heparin (1 mg in 100 cc). The termino-terminal venous anastomosis is performed with two continuous sutures of Prolene 5/0.

The arterial anastomosis is then carried out between the right primitive iliac artery of the recipient and the superior mesenteric artery or the segment of the iliac artery of the graft, depending on the bench surgery performed. From the beginning of the anastomosis, the graft should be kept refrigerated by compresses of crushed ice. Once the arterial anastomosis is completed, the vessels are sequentially declamped, first the vein and then the artery. Pancreas should recover a normal coloration immediately.

Systemic venous drainage is most widely used. Some groups advocate the use of portal venous drainage for the hypothetical benefit of maintaining a more physiological insulin level and thus avoiding the hyperinsulinemia attributed to the systemic drainage. However, technically, it is more complex and its potential metabolic advantages are still controversial.

Pancreatic exocrine secretion can be drained to the urinary tract or to the intestinal tract.

The urinary drainage (duodenocistostomy) contributed extraordinarily to consolidate the pancreas transplant, since it allows to monitor the rejection by the determination of pancreatic enzymes in the urine. However, the high incidence of complications associated with it require the conversion to enteric drainage in 15–30% of cases [20].

Therefore, today, enteric drainage is the technique of election. The most common method of enteric drainage is the one in which the anastomosis is performed between the duodenum of the graft and the jejunum of the recipient, with the pancreatic graft positioned intraperitoneally. The enteric anastomosis can be performed to the proximal jejunum or to the distal ileum, in a termino-terminal, termino-lateral, or a latero-lateral anastomosis. The use of direct anastomosis is currently more widely used than Roux-en-Y anastomosis. However, Boggi et al. [21] have shown excellent results with the use of a Roux-shaped "Y" latero-lateral duodenojejunostomy (DY), with the retroperitoneal position of the pancreatic graft, and portal venous drainage. Exocrine drainage techniques to the stomach have also been described [22]. Duodenoduodenostomy (DD) is an interesting option for the drainage of digestive secretions when the pancreas is placed behind the right colon and is oriented in the cranial direction [23]. For the placement of the graft in the retroperitoneal position, the right colon is released medially together with the Kocher maneuver, so that the native duodenum is widely exposed. After the correct mobilization of the duodenum of the recipient, the latero-lateral anastomosis (2.5–3 cm) is performed between the duodenum of the graft and the second and third duodenal portion of the recipient with a doble suture, one internal for the mucosa with resorbable material (Vicryl 3/0) and a seromuscular external one, with nonabsorbable suture (3/0 silk). After this, the right colon is repositioned to its usual position so that the pancreas remains immobile [24].

After the end of the intestinal anastomosis, the peritoneal cavity is washed with povidone-iodine serum. Some groups perform the wash with antibiotic solution to minimize the risk of peripancreatic infection and mycotic aneurysms. The peritoneum is then closed and the surgical field is prepared for the kidney implant on the left side.

6.4. Surgical complications

The absence of complications after pancreas transplantation depends largely on the detailed knowledge of both the donor and the recipient. Therefore, to minimize morbidity, postoperative care begins at the pre-operative and intraoperative periods.

The first 24–48 h is the most crucial for the graft and the recipient due to (a) the surgical trauma to which the patient has been subjected, (b) the ischemia-reperfusion phenomena of the transplanted organ, and (c) immunosuppression. As expected, the combination of these three insults, especially in a diabetic patient with vascular complications, constitutes a challenge for the entire medical and surgical team.

Surgical complications are relevant since they can lead to graft loss. From 1983 to 1987, 25% of the pancreas transplants performed in the world were lost due to technical reasons [25]. However, in the last decade, the percentage of surgical morbidity has decreased drastically [6].

In general, the main complications of pancreas transplantation, in addition to the general complications of solid organ transplants, include those that are more specific as a consequence of certain organ characteristics: low vascular flow and exocrine component.

There are a number of factors that significantly increase the risk of developing surgical complications such as a donor and recipient body mass index >30 kg/m^2, organ preservation time >20 h, cause of death of the non-traumatic donor, and to a lesser extent the intestinal drainage of pancreatic exocrine secretion.

Following are the main surgical complications:

- Vascular complications: arterial or venous thrombosis represents one of the most frequent causes of early graft loss (5–10%). The incidence of thrombosis ranges from 5 to 10% in the simultaneous transplantation of pancreas-kidney and 10–20% in isolated pancreas transplantation. It usually happens to be a venous thrombosis (60%) and appears in the first few days of transplant evolution [26].

  The causes are still not fully understood: technical mistakes when performing vascular anastomoses, prothrombotic disorders and hypercoagulability, microvascular injuries produced during the period of extraction and preservation of the graft, as well as hemodynamic instability that reduce the intrinsic flow. It has also been associated with factors related to the donor, as the age and the cause of death, or a prolonged cold ischemia time.

  Doppler ultrasound in expert hands is the most available image technique to diagnose thrombosis. Computed tomography is used for the evaluation of vascular anastomoses as well as to rule out the presence of other abdominal complications. Arteriography may be used to confirm the diagnosis in cases of partial or total pancreatic vessel thrombosis and even interventional radiology may be necessary.

  In cases of total thrombosis, thrombolysis or thrombectomy should be attempted urgently by performing interventional radiology, and in cases where this is not possible or fails, surgical thrombectomy or transplantectomy should be performed. In partial venous thrombosis, if the thrombus occupies more than two-thrids of the lumen of the vessel, endovascular treatment may be attempted, and in the rest, heparinization. This has made it possible to reduce graft loss due to venous thrombosis to less than 1% [27].

  Other vascular complications of the pancreatic graft include hemorrhage, arteriovenous fistulas, pseudoaneurysms, and stenoses of the anastomoses. **Table 6** summarizes the most important complications observed in pancreas transplant recipients for each period.

- Intestinal complications: they usually present at the anastomosis of the duodenal segment. Its incidence has decreased considerably in recent years, and currently less than 1% of the grafts are lost due to this cause [28]. Its incidence ranges at 5–20% in bladder drainage and between 5 and 8% in the intestinal drainage. Early fistulas are usually attributed to ischemia or technical failure, while later fistulas are usually caused by infections or acute rejection.

They represent the second cause of relaparotomy after hemorrhage. The treatment depends on the type of derivation of the exocrine secretion and the importance of the leak.

- Graft pancreatitis: increase in serum amylase and lypase is common after pancreas transplantation, due to both factors inherent to the donor and lesions that the pancreas can suffer during extraction, preservation, implantation, and reperfusion. They are usually self-limited and do not tend to have an impact on the graft outcome. However, hyperamylasemia may be indicative of true graft pancreatitis, with symptoms that may include fever, abdominal pain, ileus, and abdominal distension. Pancreatitis that appears after the first weeks following transplantation is usually secondary to an acute rejection or infections (such as cytomegalovirus—CMV). In patients with bladder drainage, they can also be attributed to reflux of urine through the pancreatic duct. As a consequence of graft pancreatitis, fistulas, peripancreatic collections or abscesses, and pancreatic pseudocysts may occur.

Post-transplant period	**Complications**
Pre-trasplant	Graft damage during organ procurement: • *Vascular lesions (splenic artery, SMA, portal vein)* • *Duodenal lesion* • *Damage to pancreatic capsule or parenquima*
Peri-transplant	Acute surgical or post-surgical complications: • *Vascular lesion (recipient severe atheromatosis)* • *Hemorrhage* • *Pancreatitis* • *Inadequate graft perfusion* • *Cardiovascular morbidity*
Post-trasplant	Vascular complications • *Graft thrombosis (60% venous, 40% arterial)* • *Late vascular complications (anastomosisstenosis, pseudoaneurisms, arteriovenous fistulas)* • *Vascular complications of kidney graft (in SPK)* Infection of surgical wound Incomplete healing of surgical wound Intra-abdominal infection Fistulas due to duodenal leaks Graft pancreatitis Pancreatic pseudocysts Panreatic leak Hemorrhage (intra-abdominal, bladder, gastrointestinal) Urological complications Infections (bacteria, viral, fungal)

Table 6. Complications according to the time of appearance.

- Infections: they are frequent in this group of transplant recipients (80% throughout the first year), and they play an important role in the patient and graft survival. Diabetes, surgery, and immunosuppression are factors that predispose these patients to suffer infections of all types. Pancreas transplantation presents a risk of infection by CMV of 13–17%, largely due to the use of potent induction immnunosuppression. CMV infection is associated with increases in mortality, the rate of rejection, and the presentation of other types of infections. The incidence of intra-abdominal infections is 10–30%, most of them polymicrobial, with fungi present in less than 10% [29]. The current prophylaxis schemes (against bacterial, viral, and fungal infections), established from the moment of intervention, have managed to reduce its incidence in the short term. However, they still need to be monitored in the longer term.

7. Perioperative management

Recipients of pancreas transplantation are diabetic patients most often with a disease vintage over 10 years and frequently with secondary macro- and microvascular complications. The cardiovascular risk is superior to those of general population or recipients of kidney transplant alone. The perioperative management is of crucial importance not only to avoid the risk of hemodynamic instability and periods of low perfusion of the graft, but is also vital for organs such as brain and heart.

7.1. Volume, acid-base and electrolyte, and hemodynamic stability

Volume and electrolytes should be monitored closely during the first 48 h and fluids administered accordingly to avoid hypovolemia or acid-base and electrolyte inbalances. Although an individualized assessment should be performed in each case, it is considered appropriate to maintain a central venous pressure between 5 and 10 mmHG. The administration of fluids with dextrose should be avoided, as it may prolong the need for insulin.

Since most patients are also recipients of a kidney transplant, close monitoring of urinary output must be performed simultaneously. In the event of polyuria (urinary output >150 ml/h), aggressive volume reposition should be perfomed, usually at a rate of 1:1 during the first 24 h, and thereafter at a rate of 0.7:1 to avoind prolonging the polyuria. Fluid solution should be selected according to acid–base and electrolyte homeostasis, with 0.9% or 0.45% sodium chloride often being the first line of treatment.

In the event of delayed graft function and oliguria (urinary output <50 ml/day), fluids should be restricted to those needed for the minimum daily calories and electrolyte intake to avoid hastening the need for dialysis intended for volume management. When needed, dialysis modality (continuous vs. intermittent) should be discussed with the nephrologist and risk benefits must be weighed—intermittent dialysis may be performed with the need for anticoagulation, and with low ultrafiltration volumes, reducing the risk of surgical complications, while continous dialysis reduces hemodynamic instability and therefore decreases the risk of reducing organ perfusion.

Anemia is frequent among patients with ESRD. It is important to maintain adequate levels of hemoglobin (Hgb >10 mg/dl), especially in the case of postoperative bleeding. Controversy exists regarding the need for immediate anticoagulation (vide Section 8—prophylaxis).

Both hypotension and hypertension should be avoided. A systolic blood pressure < 100 mmHG increases the risk of arterial and venous thrombosis of the graft, especially in the immediate postoperative period. On the other hand, prolonged severe hypertension can lead to a stroke or myocardial infarction and may increase the risk of intra-abdominal hemorrhage. It is advisable to maintain the systolic pressure between 120 and 160 mmHg during the first 24 h post-transplant to ensure adequate perfusion of the graft and minimize the risk of adverse effects.

7.2. Graft function

The immediate evaluation of the graft (both pancreatic and renal, in the case of SPK) can be monitored in various ways. The protocol accepted by most centers combines the use of laboratory parameters together with image tests. The decrease in blood levels of blood urea nitrogen (BUN), creatinine, amylase and lipase is required, together with blood glucose levels within normality, to consider that the grafts function correctly (in case of SPK). Blood levels of amylases and lipases provide additional information regarding pancreatic injury. In the immediate postoperative period, blood levels of pancreatic enzymes may be elevated, with normal blood glucose levels, which translates into an ischemia-reperfusion injury, and usually resolves spontaneously. In cases of exocrine drainage to urinary bladder, the level of amylases in urine can be monitored. A decrease of 50% or more is suggestive of rejection or pancreatitis.

7.3. Image diagnosis

In the post-transplant period, radiological examinations should be perfomed to evaluate graft perfusion and exclude surgical complications, such as collections or thrombosis. Most centers rely on ultrasound as their preferred method, since it is easy to use, nontoxic, and may be pefomed as often as needed. When available, computerized tomography may provide further information, such as contrast-enhanced evaluation of arterial perfusion and venous drainage, as well as exclude possible hemorrhages. Herein, we describe in detail advantages of each option.

7.3.1. Color Doppler Ultrasound

It is the initial imaging technique for control and monitoring of pancreas transplantation. The study with electronic data capture (EDC) allows to assess the size and the structure of the graft, the presence of liquid collections (study in B mode), and the perfusion of the parenchyma (resistance index), as well as the permeability of the vascular anastomoses (Doppler study). An extension of the study can also be done with the ultrasound signal enhancer, if it is considered appropriate by the sonographer who performs the study. It is advisable to make a basal study, between 24 and 48 h post-transplant, and a follow-up study, every 3–4 days until the patient's discharge.

7.3.2. Abdominal CT scan

In some cases, Doppler ultrasound may be technically limited (abdominal distension, obesity) or the study might need to be extended, such as in the patient with abdominal pain, fever, and/or graft dysfunction, intra-abdominal collection not accessible to ultrasound drainage, intra-abdominal collection drained by ultrasound, but without adequate clinical response. If a vascular pathology or bleeding is suspected, a contrast-enhanced CT scan is advised.

7.3.3. Interventional radiology

Interventional radiology may be used for diagnostic confirmation and/or treatment (thrombectomy) of a partial arterial and/or venous thrombosis of the graft.

7.4. Monitoring of vascular thrombosis

Thrombosis is the most common vascular complication in the initial post-transplant (8–10 days post-transplant) period. Therefore, early diagnosis is important to establish adequate treatment.

If a first post-transplant imaging study to confirm the vascular permeability of the graft (splenic and mesenteric artery/vein) is not achieved due to bowel distention, the decision whether or not to extend the radiological procedure will be based on pancreas functionality: (1) in normal functioning graft the study is repeated in 24–48 h, (2) if dysfunctional the study is extended to a non-invasive imaging technique, such as angio-CT. Some groups advocate performing angio-CT as standard monitoring image technique due to its ability to establish a grading score for venous thrombosis [30]. In our experience, in the presence of an experienced radiologist, Doppler ultrasound, with or without contrast-enhanced ultrasound (CEUS), is a reliable screening technique.

During the first 48-h post-transplant, the patient usually stays in the intensive care unit, to be transferred later to the conventional hospital ward if there have been no adverse effects. Progressively, the oral intake is introduced and the abdominal drainage is removed. Before hospital discharge, it is important to to give a detailed description of medication and home care to the patient.

8. Immunosuppression and prophylaxis

8.1. Immunosuppression

Advances in immunosuppression protocols during the last two decades significantely increased short- and long-term pancreas graft survival. The purpose of immunosuppression is control alloimmune response, and protocols often include a combination of different drugs to minimize the damage to the graft and the risks to the patient. They are similar in all solid organ transplants. Nonetheless, it is of particular relevance in pancreas transplant recipients due to the increased risk of acute rejection, especially in recipients of pancreas transplant alone (PTA). The greatest burden of immunosuppression is then usually administered in the recipients of a PTA.

Immunosuppression is usually dived into two major categories—induction and maintenance. The former represents treatments used in the peri-transplant period alone, with the objective of inhibiting both the innate and adaptative immune response when the graft is first exposed to recipient immune system. The drugs used are the same as for other solid organ transplantations and have been described in other chapters. The next section describes how and what drugs are used in pancreas transplantation:

8.1.1. Induction therapy

This consists of the administration of a polyclonal or monoclonal antibodies and is currently assumed as standard treatment for pancreas transplantation. These decrease the incidence of acute rejection or delay its onset, and reduce the number of steroid-resistant rejections. Depleting T-cell antibodies may be polyclonal, most widely used, such as rabbit anti-thymocyte globulin (Thymoglobulin®/ATG-Fresenius®) or monoclonal, such as the anti-CD52 alemtuzumab (Campath®); among non-depleting monoclonal antibodies, anti-IL-2 receptor (anti-CD-25; basiliximab) is the most frequently used.

There is no consensus on which is the best protocol. Depleting antibodies appear to increase graft survival by reducing acute rejection risk [8] and are the most widely used. Nonetheless, due to financial constraints and also due to an increased infection and cancer risk associated with T-cell depleting agents, some groups use monoclonal anti-IL-2 antibodies in low-immunological risk simultaneous pancreas-kidney tranplantation.

8.1.2. Maintenance treatment

As an adjunctive treatment to induction therapy, and as long-term maintenance immunosuppression, a combination of three drugs is most often used: a calcineurin inhibitor (CNI), an anti-prolipherative, and steroids.

The discovery of cyclosporine 35 years ago marked a new era in solid organ transplantation. The incidence of acute rejection was drasticly reduced, and despite an increased risk for renal calcineurin toxicity and subsequent renal failure, the patient and graft survivals observed a spetacular improvement. Tacrolimus (or FK-506), also a CNI, exhibits a better and more potent immunsoppression profile and is currently considered the drug of choice in pancreas transplantation. CNI's act by inhibiting the transduction of the first signal between antigen-presenting cells and T-cells. Several comparative studies have shown a lower incidence of acute rejection, as well as a lower severity of rejection and a better survival of the pancreatic graft in the short and long term, in those patients treated with tacrolimus.

CNI is often associated with an anti-prolipherative agent. Their action focuses on a different pathway of the T- and B-cell activation and prolipheration. Azathioprine, the first to be used, arrests cell cycle in the G2 phase, inhibiting the progress to the M phase and subsequent clonal expansion. On the other hand, antimetabolite agents (mycophenolate-mofetil or mycophenolate sodium) inhibit nucleotide syntisis, removing the substrate to DNA replication, finally achieving the same result as azathioprine—prevents cell prolipheration. Finally, the latest agent to be introduced to solid organ transplantation were mammalian target of rapamycin (mTOR)-inhibitors (sirolimus and everolimus). Both act as anti-proliferative drugs by inactivating the mTOR pathway following the receptor CD25 activation by antigen-presenting cells.

Steroids are perhaps the most widely used immunosuppressive durgs for organ transplantation. Steroids present a pleotropic effect, with an action on both innate and adaptive immune responses. Steroids reduce antigen-presenting cells' cytokine transcription and secretion, reducing the ability of innate immune system to further recruit polynuclear cells. It also inhibits activation of mononuclear cells, such as T- and B-cells. Despite the great immunosuppressive profile, side effects mandate that these are reduced or withdrawn from maintenance treatment.

Triple therapy using one agent from each category has achieved excellent results. The most widely used combination is steroid, tacrolimus, and mycophenolate. An mTOR-inhibitor may be used instead of mycophenolate, but careful management of side effects should be undertaken. Although the results obtained with this association seem to be superimposable, as far as patient and graft survival is concerned [31], the incidence of complications attributable to rapamycin in the immediate post-transplant is greater, so this combination is not as widely used in the initial period of the transplant. However, it is a good option for long-term use.

Several studies have suggested that steroids can be suppressed as maintenance therapy, especially in patients receiving a calcineurin inhibitor associated with an antimetabolite or an mTOR-inhibitor, without affecting the survival of the grafts. However, there is no consensus regarding this topic [32], due to some reported increased risk of rejection following withdrawal. It seems reasonable that the decision to suppress steroids is focused for the moment on those patients with low-immunological risk, and it should be attempted during the first year of transplantation.

8.2. Prophylactic treatments

In pancreas transplantation, prophylactic treatments are usualy wider than those used in kidney transplantation. As previously stated, pancreas low blood flow, complex vascular anastomosis, the duodenal enteric anastomosis, and the increased infection risk due to persistent hyperglycemia prior to transplantation increase the need for thrombotic and infectious prophylaxis.

Antithrombotic prophylaxis: graft thrombosis is one of the most frequent early complications in pancreas transplantation. Therefore, most transplant centers perform prophylaxis. There is no standard protocol among different centers, but the most frequent is the use of heparin and/or aspirin. Some centers use low doses of intravenous heparin, unlike others who use subcutaneous low-molecular-weight heparin. In both cases, it is important to monitor coagulation parameters and adjust dose to renal function due to uremia-induced anticoagulation and/or anticoagulation used during dialysis sessions. Heparin is often associated with low-dose aspirin, which could be continued in the long term to reduce global cardiovascular risk.

Antimicrobial prophylaxis: infection remains one of the main causes of morbidity and mortality after pancreas transplantation. That is why it is usual to use a wider prophylaxis in these patients. At transplantation and during a variable period of time, broad-spectrum antibiotics to cover Gram negative, Gram positive, and anaerobic are recommended. They are used for 3–5 days and several associations are possible, usually cephalosporin + ampicillin or vancomycin or carbapenem + vancomycin depending on local post-transplant epidemiology. Antifungal prophylaxis with fluconazole is also often performed. Currently, some prophylactic guidelines have replaced fluconazole with a new drug, micafungin, with the advantage of avoiding interaction with tacrolimus. Since most patients receive induction treatment with polyclonal antibodies, which is well known to increase the risk of infections, especially viral infections, antiviral prophylaxis with valgancyclovir for CMV is also advisable. Finally, prophylaxis to pneumocystis jirovecii with trimetropin-sulfamethoxazole for 6 months is the treatment method, as used in kidney transplantation.

9. Long-term outcomes and complications

Pancreas transplant outcomes have increased in the last decades, with a median graft survival using current protocols up to 15 years. In order to achieve these outcomes, close ambulatory controls must be perfomed during the first year, with increasing the time between outpatient visits if follow-up is unremarkable. It is usual to perform a weekly control during the first 3 months post-Tx, biweekly until 6 months, and between 6 and 12 months on a monthly basis. They focus primarily on functional graft monitoring, immunosuppression, and complications secondary to diabetes.

To assess pancreatic graft functionalism, baseline glycemia, glycosylated hemoglobin (HbA1c), as well as serum amylases and lipases is determined in each outpatient follow-up. In the post-transplant period, after hospital discharge and again 1 year after transplant, it is convenient to perform an oral glucose tolerance test (OGTT). Subsequently, and as a follow-up guideline, the intervals between these analyses varies according to the teams. It is also advisable to perform a C-peptide determination to monitor insulin secretion throughout the follow-up, as well as the determination of anti-glutamic acid decarboxylase (GAD), in order to detect a possible recurrence of diabetic disease. Both should be checked at least once a year.

During patient follow-up, it is important to control secondary complications of diabetes. Despite having a functioning pancreas graft, recipients should continue to monitor secondary complications present prior to pancreas transplantation, such as diabetic retinopathy or macrovascular complications. Some patients experience an improvement of complications present prior to transplantation, particularly in neuropathic symptoms. As to macro- and microvascular complications, most lesions tend to stabilize [33]. Therefore, it is advisable to perform an annual ophthalmological examination, regularly assess neuropathy of both peripheral and autonomic nervous system, as well as having a special surveillance to the complications related to the vasculopathy, appearance of precordial pain, or peripheral ischemic lesions.

Not least important, patients should be advised to maintain a proper diet to avoid weight gain, promote physical activity, avoid sun exposure, prohibit or limit the consumption of alcohol and smoking, recommend suitable footwear to avoid chafing and periodic podiatric check-up, and, in women of childbearing age, recommend measures of contraception to avoid pregnancy during the first 1–2 years of the transplant.

9.1. Acute and chronic rejection

The incidence of acute rejection is higher in pancreas transplant than those reported in kidney transplantation. The actual incidence must be individualized according to transplant modality, recipient immunological risk, induction and maintenance immunosuppression, and transplant follow-up period.

Overall 1-year rejection incidence varies between 14.7% [34] and 21% [10]. PTA and PAK are associated with significantly higher incidence of acute rejection than SPK recipients [34]. Other risk factors include pancreas re-transplantation [10], absence of induction therapy or basiliximab and induction agent [8], donor age, number of HLA donor-recipient mismatch [10], and the presence of donor-specific antibodies (DSA) [35, 36].

In SPK recipients, monitoring of renal function and/or the performance of a renal biopsy had been advocated as an indirect method to establish the diagnosis and treatment of pancreas' acute rejection, since for many years it has been considered that acute rejection was present in the majority of the cases simultaneously in both grafts. However, it is now well documented that isolated rejection of one of the two organs occurs in up to 36% of cases [37].

To diagnose pancreatic graft rejection, the only biochemical markers available are pancreatic enzymes (amylases and lipases), which are elevated in most of these episodes. Lipase increase is more specific than amylase [10]. On the other hand, in acute rejection, it is possible to observe changes in graft size and eco-structure, with an increase in the resistance index when performing a Doppler ultrasound. Both parameters allow to establish the diagnosis of suspected acute rejection, but they are not specific enough to establish confirmation. This sometimes leads to unnecessary or incomplete empirical treatments, with the consequent repercussion for the patient and the graft. In addition, pancreatic rejection, as recently observed, can also be mediated by antibodies, which requires a different and specific treatment.

Currently, pancreatic biopsy is considered the gold standard for etiologic diagnosis of graft dysfunction. In our center, pancreatic graft biopsy is performed per protocol at 3 weeks and 12months post-transplant, or indicated in the following circumstances (**Figure 1**): (1) patients in whom the existence of an acute rejection of the pancreatic graft is suspected due to biochemical parameters (increase in serum glycemia, amylases, and lipases), and/or ultrasound (increase in size, changes in the graft structure, and involvement of the graft), (2) in whom the existence of a chronic rejection is suspected due to a persistent increase in amylases or serum lipases, progressive increase in glycemia and glycosylated hemoglobin, and/or progressive decrease in C-peptide secretion, and (3) in whom the recurrence of diabetic disease is suspected due to detection or progressive increase of anti-GAD antibodies, and pathologic oral glucose tolerance test. To establish the severity of the histological lesion of acute rejection, the Banff scheme should be taken as reference [38].

Pancreas' acute rejection can be successfully treated using steroids, polyclonal antibodies, and/or plasma exchange and immunoglobulins. Nonetheless, up tp 20% of grafts may be lost during the first year following an acute rejection [10].

9.2. Diabetes relapse

Type 1 diabetes is the most frequent indication for pancreas transplantation. As described in the first section of this chapter, DM1 is an autoimmune disease, characterized by autoantibodies directed to β cells. Disease relapse in pancreas graft is a well-known risk for graft failure. It has been reported in up to 7% of all transplant recipients [39]. Induction and maintenance immunosuppression are likely the reason for such a low incidence. Some factors have been associated with an increased risk for disease relapse, such as donor-recipient sharing of HLA-DR alleles, particularly HLA-DR3 [39], and the increase in autoantibodies, particularly ZnT8A, predicts the risk of disease relapse [40]. As with primary disease, no treatment is established for the management of disease relapse. Increase in baseline immunosuppression maybe attempted. If a pancreas re-transplantation is indicated, recipients must be advised of the risk of relapse in the new graft.

10. Islet transplantation

In addition to pancreas transplantation, β cell mass transfer may be performed through islet transplantation. This procedure consists of islet cell isolation from pancreas as potential donors using both mechanical and enzymatic digestion protocol, following which islets are separated using a Ricordi chamber [41]. Isolated islets are infused into recipient's portal vein, without the need for vascular and/or enteric anastomosis, reducing the surgical risks of the procedure.

The attractiveness of a minimally invasive procedure and the possibility of multiple infusions without the surgical risks associated with whole-organ pancreas transplantation have positioned islet cell transplantation as a promising treatment for patients with diabetes. Despite these advantages, islet transplantation presents two critical drawbacks when compared to whole-organ transplant. Islets obtained from a minimum of 2–3 pancreasas are often needed in order to achieve euglycemia [41], increasing organ demand, and risk of recipients' sensitization. Additionally, islets direct engraftment into a vascularized bed exposes β cells to platelets and lymphocytes. Instant blood-mediated inflammatory reaction (IBMIR) is a well characterized event associated with innate immune reaction and coagulation and complement activation following islet transplantation, leading up to 25% of total islet cell mass loss following vena cava infusion [42]. Moreover, it may increase the risk of rejection and reduces overall graft survival.

In early 2000, the Edmonton group published some promising results using an induction immunosuppression protocol [41]. By the end of 2015, over 15,000 procedures had been performed worldwide [5]. Reported 1- and 5-year insulin independence is up to 80 and 50%, respectively [5].

Novel biocompatible implantation devices and gene editing tools foresee a bright future for islet transplantation. 3D-bioprinting is being used to build an islet-blood interface which enables β cell survival and insulin production, while avoiding immune activation and graft rejection [43]. On the other hand, generation of human-induced pluripotent stem cells (hiP-SCs) has opened the door for personalized medicine and cell-based therapy. iPSCs can proliferate unlimitedly in culture and harbor the potential to generate all cell types in the adult body. Generation of hiIPSC-derived β cells has been published by several groups, using different protocol, with varying degrees of success [44, 45]. The advantage is the possibility to generate tailor-made islet cells, particularly β cells, from recipient-derived hiPSC, evading the risk of alo-rejection. One can envision in the near future hiPSC-derived cells implanted in a biocompatible device for the treatment of type 1 diabetic patient.

For the time being, islet cell transplantation remains at an almost investigation level due to smaller insulin independence when compared to pancreas transplantation. Nonetheless, it is a suitable option for selected type 1 diabetic patients, and to those with a surgical contraindication for whole-organ transplantation. Finally, islet transplantation presents a promising future as the techinique of election for β cell mass transfer.

11. Conclusion

Pancreas transplantation is the best treatment alternative for patients with end-stage renal dis-ease and type 1 diabetes and may be found in the selected group of type 2 diabetic patients. Patient and graft survival have greatly increased in the last decades, particularly due to improve-ments in surgical procedures and immunosuppression protocols, with graft half-life of 15 years. Following transplantation, patients should be carefully monitored due to the risk of acute rejec-tion, disease relapse, or diabetic secondary complications present prior to the transplant.

Author details

Pedro Ventura-Aguiar[1*], Joana Ferrer-Fábrega[2] and Maria José Ricart[1]

*Address all correspondence to: pventura@clinic.ub.es

1 Nephrology and Kidney Transplant Department, Hospital Clinic Barcelona, Spain

2 HepatoBilioPancreatic Surgery and Liver and Pancreas Transplantation Department, ICMDiM, Hospital Clínic Barcelona, Spain

References

[1] Atkinson MA. The pathogenesis and natural history of type 1 diabetes. Cold Spring Harbor Perspectives in Medicine. 2012;**2**(11):a007641

[2] Tuomilehto J. The emerging global epidemic of type 1 diabetes. Current Diabetes Reports. 2013;**13**(6):795-804

[3] www.who.int/mediacentre/factsheets/fs312/en/

[4] Wild S, Roglic G, Green A, Sicree R, King H. Global prevalence of diabetes: Estimates for the year 2000 and projections for 2030. Diabetes Care. 2004;**27**(5):1047-1053

[5] Collaborative Islet Transplant Registry. Eighth Annual Report. CITR www.citregistry.org. 2014

[6] Gruessner AC, Laftavi MR, Pankewycz O, Gruessner RWG. Simultaneous pancreas and kidney transplantation—Is it a treatment option for patients with type 2 diabetes mellitus? An analysis of the international pancreas transplant registry. Current Diabetes Reports. 2017;**17**:44

[7] Kandaswamy R, Stock PG, Gustafson SK, Skeans MA, Curry MA, Prentice MA, Fox A, Israni AK, Snyder JJ, Kasiske BL. OPTN/SRTR 2016 annual data report: Pancreas. American Journal of Transplantation. 2018;**18**(Suppl 1):114-114

[8] Kopp WH, Verhagen MJ, Blok JJ, Huurman VA, de Fijter JW, de Koning EJ, Putter H, Baranski AG, Schaapherder AF, Braat AE, Ringers J. Thirty years of pancreas transplantation at Leiden University Medical Center: Long-term follow-up in a large Eurotransplant Center. Transplantation. 2015;**99**(9):e145-e151

[9] Gruessner RW, Sutherland DE, Gruessner AC. Mortality assessment for pancreas transplants. American Journal of Transplantation. 2004;**4**:2018-2026

[10] Niederhaus SV, Leverson GE, Lorentzen DF, Robillard DJ, Sollinger HW, Pirsch JD, Torrealba JR, Odorico JS. Acute cellular and antibody-mediated rejection of the pancreas allograft: Incidence, risk factors and outcomes. American Journal of Transplantation. 2013;**13**(11):2945-2955

[11] Hudson A, Bradbury L, Johnson R, Fuggle SV, Shaw JA, Casey JJ, Friend PJ, Watson CJ. The UK pancreas allocation scheme for whole organ and islet transplantation. American Journal of Transplantation. 2015;**15**(9):2443-2455

[12] Vinkers MT, Rahmel AO, Slot MC, Smits JM, Schareck WD. How to recognize a suitable pancreas donor: A Eurotransplant study of preprocurement factors. Transplantation Proceedings. 2008;**40**:1275-1278

[13] Blok JJ, Kopp WH, Verhagen MJ, Schaapherder AF, de Fijter JW, Putter H, Ringers J, Braat AE. The value of PDRI and P-PASS as predictors of outcome after pancreas transplantation in a large European pancreas transplantation Center. Pancreas. 2016;**45**(3):331-336

[14] Axelrod DA, Sung RS, Meyer KH, Wolfe RA, Kaufman DB. Systematic evaluation of pancreas allograft quality, outcomes and geographic variation in utilization. American Journal of Transplantation. 2010;**10**:837-845

[15] Finger EB, Radosevich DM, Dunn TB, Chinnakotla S, Sutherland DE, Matas AJ, Pruett TL, Kandaswamy R. A composite risk model for predicting technical failure in pancreas transplantation. American Journal of Transplantation. 2013;**13**(7):1840-1849

[16] Kootstra G, Daemen JH, Oomen AP. Categories of non-heart-beating donors. Transplantation Proceedings. 1995;**27**(5):2893-2894

[17] Rathnasamy Muthusamy AS, Friend PJ, Dor FJ, Crane JS, Papalois V, Herbert P, Sinha S. DCD pancreas transplantation meta-analysis: Ethical and technical considerations. Transplantation. 2017;**101**(2):e57

[18] Kelly WD, Lillehei RC, Merkel FK, Idezuki Y, Goetz FC. Allotransplantation of the pancreas and duodenum along with the kidney in diabetic nephropathy. Surgery. 1967; **61**(6):827-837

[19] Fridell JA, Powelson JA, Kubal CA, Burke GW, Sageshima J, Rogers J, Stratta RJ. Retrieval of the pancreas allograft for whole-organ transplantation. Clinical Transplantation. 2014;**28**(12):1313-1330

[20] Boggi U, Amorese G, Marchetti P. Surgical techniques for pancreas transplantation. Current Opinion in Organ Transplantation. 2010;**15**(1):102-111

[21] Boggi U, Vistoli F, Del Chiaro M, et al. Retroperitoneal pancreas transplantation with portal-enteric drainage. Transplantation Proceedings. 2004;**36**(3):571-574

[22] Linhares MM, Beron RI, Gonzalez AM, et al. Duodenumstomach anastomosis: A new technique for exocrine drainage in pancreas transplantation. Journal of Gastrointestinal Surgery. 2012;**16**:1072

[23] Gunasekaran G, Wee A, Rabets J, Winans C, Krishnamurthi V. Duodenoduodenostomy in pancreas transplantation. Clinical Transplantation. 2012;**26**(4):550-557

[24] Ferrer J, Molina V, Rull R, López-Boado MÁ, Sánchez S, García R, Ricart MJ, Ventura-Aguiar P, García-Criado Á, Esmatjes E, Fuster J, Garcia-Valdecasas JC. Pancreas transplantation: Advantages of a retroperitoneal graft position. Cirugía Española. 2017;**95**(9):513-520

[25] Humar A, Ramcharan T, Kandaswamy R, Gruessner RW, Gruessner AC, Sutherland DE. Technical failures after pancreas transplants: Why grafts fail and the risk factors—A multivariate analysis. Transplantation. 2004;**78**(8):1188-1192

[26] Farney AC, Rogers J, Stratta RJ. Pancreas graft thrombosis: Causes, prevention, diagnosis, and intervention. Current Opinion in Organ Transplantation. 2012;**17**:87-92

[27] Barrufet M, Burrel M, Angeles García-Criado M, Montañà X, Real MI, Ferrer J, Fernández-Cruz L, Gilabert R. Pancreas transplants venous graft thrombosis: Endovascular thrombolysis for graft rescue. Cardiovascular and Interventional Radiology. 2014;**37**(5):1226-1234

[28] Humar A, Kandaswamy R, Granger D, Gruessner RW, Gruessner AC, Sutherland DE. Decreased surgical risks of pancreas transplantation in the modern era. Annals of Surgery. 2000;**231**(2):269-275

[29] Cervera C, Moreno A. Infecciones en el paciente con trasplante renal y pancreático. Enfermedades Infecciosas y Microbiología Clínica. 2007;**25**(5):345-355

[30] Harbell JW, Morgan T, Feldstein VA, Roll GR, Posselt A, Kang SM, Feng S, Hirose R, Freise CE, Stock P. Splenic vein thrombosis following pancreas transplantation: Identification of factors that support conservative management. American Journal of Transplantation. 2017;**17**(11):2955-2962

[31] Gallon LG, Winoto J, Chhabra D, Parker MA, Leventhal JR, Kaufman DB. Long-term renal transplant function in recipient of simultaneous kidney and pancreas transplant maintained with two prednisone-free maintenance immunosuppressive combinations: Tacrolimus/mycophenolate mofetil versus tacrolimus/sirolimus. Transplantation. 2007;**83**(10):1324-1329

[32] Montero N, Webster AC, Royuela A, Zamora J, Crespo Barrio M, Pascual J. Steroid avoidance or withdrawal for pancreas and pancreas with kidney transplant recipients. Cochrane Database of Systematic Reviews. 2014;**9**:CD007669

[33] Boggi U, Rosati CM, Marchetti P. Follow-up of secondary diabetic complications after pancreas transplantation. Current Opinion in Organ Transplantation. 2013;**18**(1):102-110

[34] Dong M, Parsaik AK, Kremers W, Sun A, Dean P, Prieto M, Cosio FG, Gandhi MJ, Zhang L, Smyrk TC, Stegall MD, Kudva YC. Acute pancreas allograft rejection is associated with increased risk of graft failure in pancreas transplantation. American Journal of Transplantation. 2013;**13**(4):1019-1025

[35] Rudolph EN, Dunn TB, Mauer D, Noreen H, Sutherland DER, Kandaswamy R, Finger EB. HLA-A, -B, -C, -DR, and -DQ matching in pancreas transplantation. Effect on Graft Rejection and Survival. American Journal of Transplantation. 2016;**XX**:1-12

[36] Mittal S, Page SL, Friend PJ, Sharples EJ, Fuggle SV. De novo donor-specific HLA antibodies: Biomarkers of pancreas transplant failure. American Journal of Transplantation. 2014;**14**:1664-1671

[37] Parajuli S, Arpali E, Astor BC, Djamali A, Aziz F, Redfield RR, Sollinger HW, Kaufman DB, Odorico J, Mandelbrot DA. Concurrent biopsies of both grafts in recipients of simultaneous pancreas and kidneydemonstrate high rates of discordance for rejection as well as discordance in type of rejection—A retrospective study. Transplant International. 2018;**31**(1):32-37

[38] Drachenberg CB, Torrealba JR, Nankivell BJ, Rangel EB, Bajema IM, Kimf DU, Arend L, et al. Guidelines for the diagnosis of antibody-mediated rejection in pancreas allografts—Updated Banff grading schema. American Journal of Transplantation. 2011;**11**:1792-1180

[39] Vendrame F, Hopfner YY, Diamantopoulos S, Virdi SK, Allende G, Snowhite IV, Reijonen HK, Chen L, Ruiz P, Ciancio G, Hutton JC, Messinger S, Burke GW, Pugliese A. Risk

factors for type 1 diabetes recurrence in immunosuppressed recipients of simultaneous pancreas-kidney transplants. American Journal of Transplantation. 2016;**16**(1):235-245

[40] Occhipinti M, Lampasona V, Vistoli F, Bazzigaluppi E, Scavini M, Boggi U, Marchetti P, Bosi E. Zinc transporter 8 autoantibodies increase the predictive value of islet autoantibodies for function loss of technically successful solitary pancreas transplant. Transplantation. 2011;**92**(6):674-677

[41] Shapiro J, Pokrywczynska M, Ricord C. Clinical pancreatic islet transplantation. Nature Reviews. 2017;**13**:268-277

[42] Eriksson O, Eich T, Sundin A, Tibell A, Tufveson G, Andersson H, Felldin M, Foss A, Kyllönen L, Langstrom B, Nilsson B, Korsgren O, Lundgren T. Positron emission tomography in clinical islet transplantation. American Journal of Transplantation. 2009;**9**(12):2816-2824

[43] Foster GA, García AJ. Bio-synthetic materials for immunomodulation of islet transplants. Advanced Drug Delivery Reviews. 2017;**114**:266-271

[44] Pagliuca FW, Millman JR, Gürtler M, M1 S, Van Dervort A, Ryu JH, Peterson QP, Greiner D, Melton DA. Generation of functional human pancreatic β cells in vitro. Cell. 2014;**159**(2):428-439

[45] Rezania A, Bruin JE, Arora P, Rubin A, Batushansky I, Asadi A, O'Dwyer S, Quiskamp N, Mojibian M, Albrecht T, Yang YH, Johnson JD, Kieffer TJ. Reversal of diabetes with insulin-producing cells derived in vitro from human pluripotent stem cells. Nature Biotechnology. 2014;**32**(11):1121-1133

8

The Process of Organ Donation from Non-Living Donors: A Case-Based Journey from Potential Donor Identification to Organ Procurement

Alyssa Green, Peter G. Thomas, Rebecca Wilde-Onia,
Scott J. Kohler, Joan D. Sweeney,
Deborah M. Stahlnecker and Stanislaw P. Stawicki

Abstract

Each year, thousands of people worldwide succumb to end-organ failure while awaiting life-saving transplantation procedures. The shortage of organs continues with no signs of easing in the foreseeable future. The availability of organs from living donors continues to be constrained. At the same time, the cumulative knowledge of organ preservation is advancing steadily resulting in an enhanced ability to utilize a growing number of previously unsuitable tissue and organ gifts. Our ability to procure and preserve more organs is accompanied by the increasing use of so-called "expanded criteria" donors, or those whose organs may not have been suitable without modern advances in organ preservation science. Within the overall context of organ donation from non-living donors, the importance of physiologic and end-organ optimization cannot be understated. This chapter discusses our current state of understanding of optimized organ procurement approaches derived from practical experiences and "lessons learned" at a high-performing, community-based tertiary referral hospital.

Keywords: clinical optimization, ethical considerations, organ donation, organ procurement, organ procurement organization, transplantation

1. Introduction

The process of organ procurement from non-living donors (OPNLD) is multi-factorial and complex [1]. In the United States, significant progress has been made toward wider availability of organs for transplantation [2, 3]. This includes increased use of organs from donors after cardiac death (DCD) as well as the inclusion of "expanded criteria" donors (ECD) and the introduction of information technology-based tools for better organ allocation [3]. Despite tremendous progress, major challenges remain including the growing number of patients entering transplant waiting lists [4].

It has long been known that more organs may be available than are being currently captured within the existing organ procurement organization (OPO) network [5]. In addition, some organs are lost through suboptimal organ donor resuscitation and/or lack of timely OPO notification [6, 7]. In this chapter, the authors will discuss the modern process of OPNLD, beginning with potential donor identification, then proceeding with physiological optimization, and finally ending with the procurement procedure. To illustrate key points more effectively, a realistic hypothetical case-based scenario will be presented.

2. Case vignette

A 65-year-old male presents via aeromedical flight after a head-on, two-car collision in which he was the restrained passenger. The crash occurred at 7:45 pm–approximately 45 min prior to his arrival at the regional Trauma Center. The patient's wife, the driver, was pronounced dead at the scene. According to the Emergency Medical Services (EMS) report, the patient had Glasgow Coma Scale (GCS) of 9 shortly after the incident and was complaining of left-sided chest pain. It took 30 min to extract the patient from the car.

The patient arrived at the regional Trauma Center at 8:32 pm. On initial assessment, blood pressure was 90/65 mmHg, pulse was 120 beats/min, respiratory rate was 28 breaths/min and the patient had a GCS of 4. Intravenous fluid administration was started and the patient was immediately tracheally intubated. The FAST ultrasound exam was negative. Chest radiograph showed multiple rib fractures and a pneumothorax on the left, for which a chest tube was placed. The secondary trauma survey showed an obvious deformity of the left parietal skull, a left chest wall injury, and a visibly displaced left-sided hip fracture.

Hypertonic saline infusion was begun for treatment of a presumed severe traumatic brain injury (TBI). Detailed timeline of subsequent events now follows:

- 9:00 pm: Once the patient was hemodynamically stabilized, he was taken for computed tomography (CT) of the head, cervical spine, chest, abdomen and pelvis. Immediate review of imaging confirmed left hip fracture-dislocation, multiple left-sided rib fractures and a pneumothorax on the left. Of special concern was the presence of large left epidural and subdural hematomas with evidence of diffuse axonal injury, as well as extensive subarachnoid hemorrhage. The patient was found to have 1.5 cm midline shift with uncal herniation.
- 9:15 pm: Emergent neurosurgery consultation was placed, with immediate arrival of the on-call neurosurgeon. The patient experienced a brief period of hemodynamic instability featuring both bradycardia and tachycardia, followed by the appearance of severe hypertension (systolic blood pressures >200 mmHg), and finally the appearance of bilaterally dilated, unresponsive pupillary exam. The injury was deemed non-survivable.

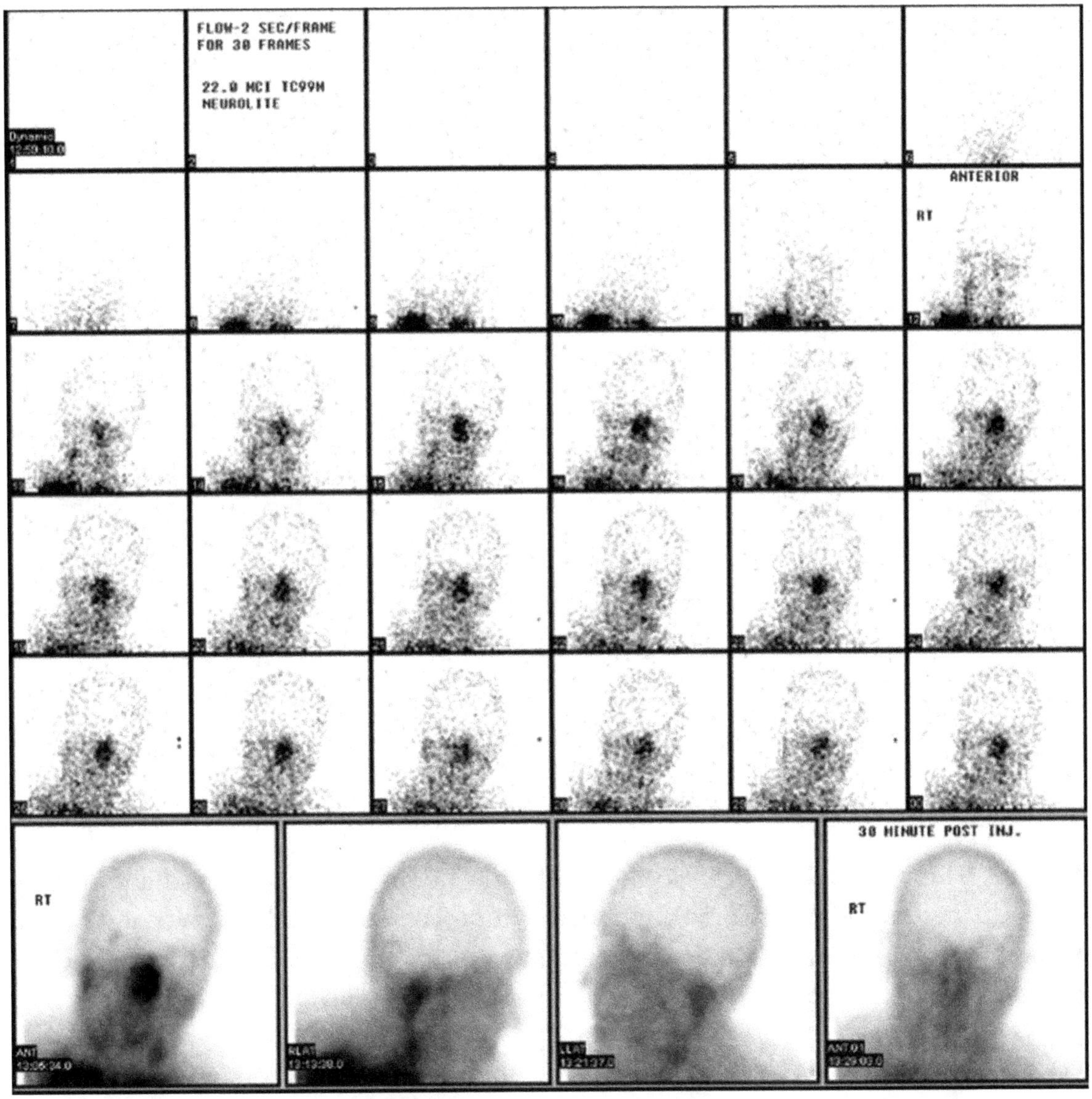

Figure 1. An example of a Tc-99 m radionuclide cerebral blood flow study showing typical appearance of "no flow" within the cranial vault (e.g., the white appearance). At the same time, the facial region is richly perfused with blood (e.g., the "hot-nose" sign), providing a stark comparison to the lack of intracranial flow. **Credit**: Jason Robert Young, M.D. Image used under Creative Commons Attribution-Share Alike 4.0 International license.

- 9:25 pm: The patient's neurological exam was consistent with brain death, as confirmed by two independent physicians credentialed in this clinical area of expertise. Confirmatory testing in the form of cerebral perfusion study was ordered and the patient was taken to the intensive care unit (ICU) in the interim for ongoing medical management. In accordance with applicable State Laws, The Local Organ Procurement Organization (OPO) was contacted for possible organ donation.
- 10:30 pm: The patient's family arrived at the hospital and discussed prognosis and goals of care with the clinical team. At that time, his family members indicated understanding of the diagnosis, and the gravity and irreversibility of his condition. They informed staff that the patient was an organ donor and that they would like to honor his wishes in the event of brain death. Medical management and stabilization continued in anticipation of the cerebral perfusion study.

- 8:30 am: After stabilizing the patient sufficiently for transfer to the radiology department for confirmatory brain flow study, determination was made to proceed with such testing (**Figure 1**). Following the confirmatory study to determine brain death, the patient continued to receive maximum medical management to ensure adequate organ perfusion and maintain tissue oxygenation. Representatives of the local OPO were introduced to the family and the formal process of organ donation was initiated.

- 9:00 am: All required procedures for determining blood type and tissue match were progressing as planned. Organ placement discussions between the local OPO and potential receiving institutions were ongoing. The patient underwent trans-esophageal echocardiography and bronchoscopy to determine his suitability as a heart and lung donor, respectively. Throughout this process, medical optimization of end-organ perfusion continued, including the use of advanced cardiac monitoring, as well as intermittent use of vasopressors and inotropes.
- 11:00 am: After determining that the patient will be able to donate his kidneys, pancreas, and liver. However, due to severe chest trauma his lungs and heart were not suitable for transplantation. At this time, final placement decisions were made.
- 12:00 pm: The patient's family members were allowed to see him prior to the organ procurement operation. The process was to occur within the next several hours, and was predicated on finding a suitable recipient for one of the kidneys. Medical optimization therapy continued.
- 15:30 pm: The patient was taken to the Operating Room for the procurement of bilateral kidneys, pancreas and liver. Three different institutions received kidney, liver and combined kidney-pancreas for transplantation, respectively. Recipients of the above organs underwent uneventful immediate post-transplantation recovery and were able to resume normal lives.

3. Historical background

Organ transplantation and procurement has a rich history, with early accounts of tissue removal and re-implantation involving skin, bone and teeth [8]. During the past several decades, significant progress was made in the area of human transplantation. The evolution of both surgical techniques and immunosuppression resulted in organ transplantation becoming commonplace [9, 10]. Notable medical pioneers of modern transplantation include Dr Christiaan Barnard, Dr Alexis Carrel, Dr Joseph Murray, Dr Thomas Starzl and many others who helped advance the basic scientific and medical understanding required to achieve today's state of knowledge and clinical reliability [11, 12].

From a clinical perspective, the first successful transplants of the modern era involved skin and corneal tissues, and took place in the early 1900s [8]. These experiences, especially involving skin grafting, were plagued by failures well before the concept of tissue compatibility and rejection was fully elucidated [11]. Solid organ transplantation beginning with the kidney was even more challenging. Russian surgeon, Dr Yuri Voronov is credited with the first recorded report of a kidney transplant from a recently deceased donor in the mid-1930s [8, 13, 14]. Although unsuccessful, this procedure foreshadowed the various technical and ethical challenges modern transplantation would face well into the future.

The subsequent years and decades were characterized by a mixture of "trial and error" until the first successful living donor kidney transplant was performed in the mid-1950s by Nobel prize winner, Dr Joseph Murray [8, 11, 13]. The procedure was performed between identical twin brothers, both of whom survived for some time after [15]. Although the understanding of the organ rejection process was still very poor, Murray's successful transplantation strongly implied the need of genetic congruity between donor and recipient. Shortly thereafter, Main and Prehn discovered that chimerism could be induced by using radiation to weaken the immune system of mice, leading to improved acceptance of donor tissue [16, 17]. Several years later, Dr Murray attempted this method in his next successful kidney transplantation, but this was unfortunately preceded by significant mortality among patients who underwent total body irradiation prior to receiving new organs [11, 18]. Of note, this successful non-twin-twin transplant recipient was the first well-documented case to recover from rejection [11, 19]. Subsequent failures associated with total body irradiation, including significant morbidity and mortality, led to increased interest in other potential methods of immunosuppression [13].

As a result of intensive research efforts, immunosuppressive medications were soon introduced to help address the problem of graft rejection [20, 21]. Initially the use of monotherapy was attempted with limited effectiveness. It was Dr Thomas Starzl (whose success rates exceeded most in the field at the time) who proposed a cocktail of immunosuppressive agents capable of reversing rejection [11]. This was yet another critical discovery that over time facilitated the expansion of efforts into transplantation of other solid organs, including the first liver transplant in 1963 by Dr Starzl, the pancreas in 1966 by Dr Lillehei and the heart in 1967 by Dr Barnard [8, 22–24]. Although long-term survival of early transplants and their recipients varied, the 1960s ushered in a new era with transplant centers appearing across the world [8, 11, 24]. Organ preservation science developed out of the necessity to ensure organ viability during transport from donor to recipient [25].

Beginning in the early 1900s, Charles Guthrie proposed that cooling of organs may offer a way to preserve them during transport [11]. It was not until the mid-1960s that the use of cooling agents became standard practice with the introduction of the now widely accepted University of Wisconsin solution [11, 26, 27]. With progress being made in multiple aspects of transplantation, new hope arose for patients suffering from various forms of end-stage organ failure. As organ preservation and technical aspects of transplantation advanced, attention shifted to ensuring adequate organ availability [7]. Along with this challenge came the ethical and legal considerations surrounding death and organ donation, which will be addressed in greater detail later on in this chapter.

4. Ethical considerations

It is the responsibility of physicians to "above all, do no harm" [28]. This concept should permeate each clinical decision made. In theory, this ethical principle is paramount to an equitable and just system of medicine, but oftentimes physicians find themselves in situations where they must weigh the risks and benefits of treatment, and answers are far from apparent [29–32]. The field of transplantation is among the most complex medical settings to navigate from the ethics standpoint. This is even more evident with the emergence of extremity and face transplants [33–35].

As Dr Murray embarked on the first living donor transplant, he faced an ethical dilemma. The concept of retrieving an organ from a perfectly healthy individual for implantation in another patient was, and still is, a gray area considering that by removing an organ from a perfectly healthy donor, you are exposing them to a number of risks. [36]. At the same time, certain organs (e.g., heart and pancreas) can only be procured from deceased donors, which raises a completely different set of ethical issues. These include questions of donor and recipient eligibility, fairness, procurement procedures, the legal definition of death, donor designation versus family permission and compensation [7, 36]. There is also a major concern regarding the potential of inequitable allocation of organs [36, 37]. This dilemma gained international attention with the first successful cardiac transplant in 1967 by Dr Barnard [38]. The concept of taking a still beating heart from someone considered "dead" created a significant conceptual and ethical problem in the eyes of many, with calls for a more concrete definition or list of objective criteria including non-responsiveness and other neurological signs that defined irreversible coma [8, 36]. It would be another 10 years before the Presidential Commission of the Study of the Ethics in Medicine proposed the current legal definition of death which included "irreversible cessation of circulatory and respiratory function" or "irreversible cessation of brain function including brainstem function" [36, 39]. The concepts of brain death and circulatory death will be discussed in greater detail later in this chapter.

Over 33,000 organ transplants were performed in the US in 2016, representing a 20% increase in donations over the past 5 years [40]. Yet about 115,000 individuals are currently on the waitlist for organ donation and 7000 waitlist candidates died in 2016, while awaiting a life-saving transplantation [40]. Although significant strides were made with regard to increasing donations, there continues to be an organ shortage, which has led to some ethically questionable practices [35, 41]. The National Organ Transplant Act of 1984 brought together top content experts and outlined key issues related to the different aspects of the organ procurement process [42–44]. This group established key ethical principles, including the requirement that there would be no payment in exchange for organs and that organs must be voluntarily given [36, 43, 44]. This act also established our current U.S. system of organ allocation [45]. As one can see, there are numerous ethical concerns to take into account from a purely systematic viewpoint. This does not even account for the sensitivity of broaching the topic of organ donation to a grieving family coming to grips with the loss of a loved one. Even with efforts to encourage individuals to make these end-of-life decisions early on through donor registries, it is still common practice in many states to consult the family prior to proceeding with the organ procurement process [7]. Because the primary focus of this chapter is to describe the organ donation process in non-living donors, we will not be discussing numerous other ethical issues that arise when taking into account living donors. The subsequent sections of this chapter will outline OPO's and their critical role in the donation process. We will then proceed to describe the organ donation process in the context of both the above ethical and historical considerations, as well as the vignette presented earlier in the text.

5. Organ procurement organizations

The organ procurement process begins with the identification of a potential organ donor, then proceeds through the stages of notification of next of kin, the decision to donate, the process of physiologic donor optimization, the process of organ procurement and finally the transplantation of donated organs. Throughout this entire sequence of events, the OPO plays a central and an integral role [7]. The evolution of OPOs stems from the increased demand for organ donation, the need to organize and prioritize the process, and the necessity to ensure that organ allocation is performed in a fair and impartial fashion while at the same time efficiently and effectively providing organs to those in need [8, 46].

Prior to the inception of the modern network of OPOs, the organ procurement and allocation process was the responsibility of individual transplant centers [8]. They also shouldered the costs of the procurement and transportation process. As one can imagine this created a fragmented system in which each center would instinctively focus on providing resources to those in need of organs within their own hospital or locality [47, 48]. The evolution of OPO's provided a structured, equitable solution to streamline the process from organ donation to transplantation [7]. The current scope of functions of OPOs is vast and diverse, including interfacing with patient families; providing support to grieving relatives while helping them make critical decisions concerning organ donation; working in conjunction with hospitals and health care practitioners to physiologically optimize donors prior to organ procurement; coordinating with the United Network for Organ Sharing (UNOS) to find proper donor matches; and facilitating professional and public education as well as related research [7, 49].

6. The process of organ procurement

From the time of identification of potential donor to successful procurement and transplant, the process of organ procurement is a complex and intricate undertaking that we will discuss in greater detail in this section. For the purposes of our discussion, we will direct our attention to donation after death since the subject of live donors is outlined in other chapters. A simplified schematic of the overall process is shown in **Figure 2**.

The initial step in donation is centered on the potential organ donor. Although each clinical situation is uniquely different, the first step in the process is the recognition of the irreversible process of brain death, or the circumstances leading to non-heart beating donation [7, 50]. When examining the topic of donation after cardiac or circulatory death, we must go back to the corresponding legal and ethical definitions [23, 51, 52]. How and when does one determine brain death and circulatory death? In the current chapter's vignette, the circumstances of brain death were unequivocal as the patient had suffered a non-survivable injury. We realize that in clinical practice it may not be this straightforward, and repeated exams or confirmatory testing may provide the family with a greater degree of certainty regarding the finality of this devastating diagnosis. More specifically, confirmatory brain death determination with the brain scan showing "no blood flow" to the brain was helpful in the current scenario.

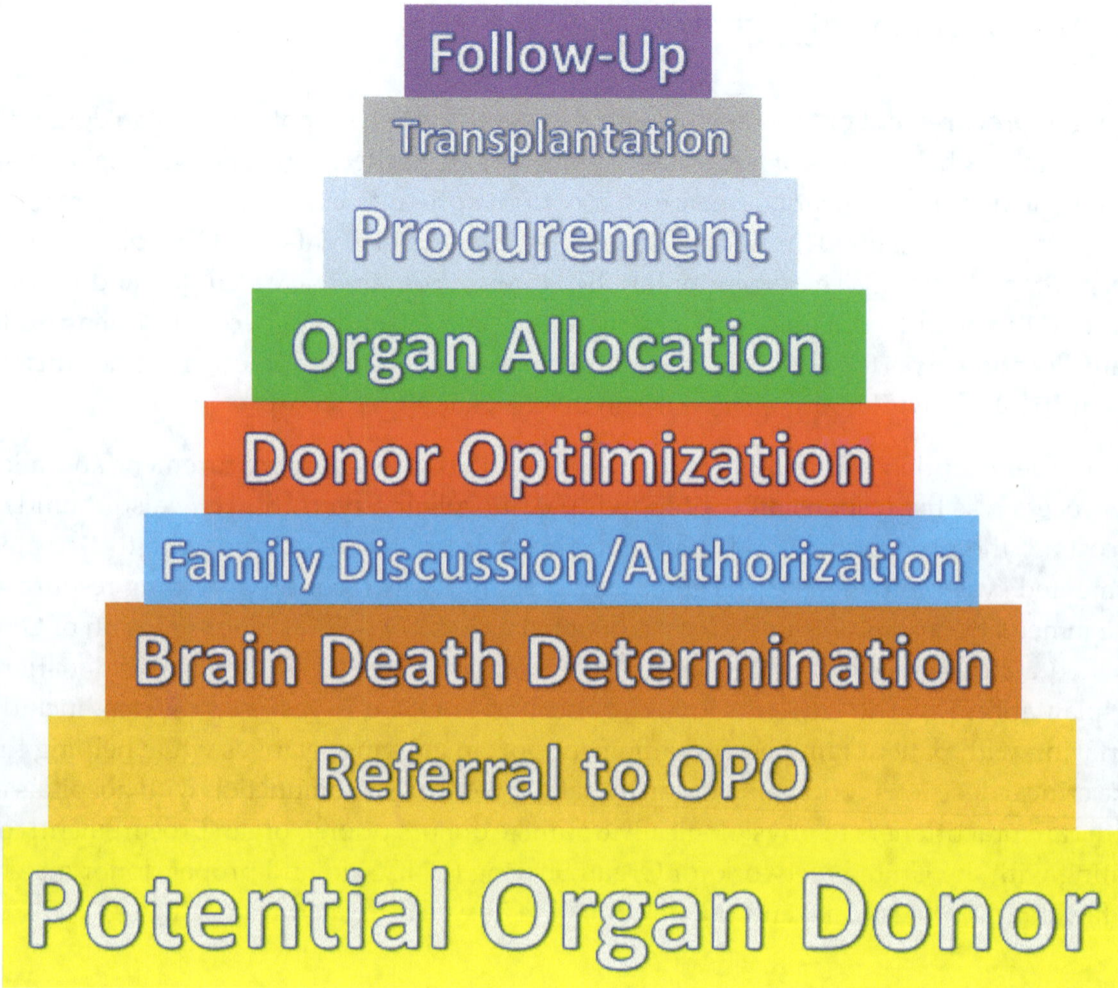

Figure 2. Simplified schematic of the organ donation process. Following the identification of potential organ donor, a cascade of events takes place that ultimately ends with successful organ transplantation. Further details regarding this complex process can be obtained from Wojda et al. [7].

Another critically important consideration is the emotional state of a family coming to grips with the untimely and unexpected loss of a loved one. The grief combined with the immense responsibility of determining what a loved one "may have wanted" can place a significant burden on his or her relatives. This can be especially difficult for families of patients with no advance directive, living will, power of attorney, or prior conversation concerning their organ donation wishes. When dealing with issues related to organ donation, health care providers must be extremely sensitive to family needs and ensure that their local OPO is involved early on in the process in order to prevent any potential conflict of interest [7]. The separation of responsibilities during these proceedings is critical in alleviating any concerns regarding the simultaneous provision of care for the patient along with facilitation of the organ donation process by the same individual and/or team [53, 54].

From the time a potential donor arrives to the hospital and is determined to have non-survivable injury, it is important that they are managed under the assumption that they may donate organs, and that care is both optimal and timely [6, 55, 56]. This includes early notification of the local OPO regarding the presence of a potential donor [7]. A great deal of attention must be paid to prevent hypoxia and systemic hypo-perfusion, both of which could compromise the viability of the donor's organs [56, 57]. As was the case in our hypothetical vignette, the patient should be stable before undergoing any confirmatory testing. In the current example, such stabilization required approximately 10–12 h of continuous effort by the critical care team. Once the decision is made to donate by the family in the case of brain death or circulatory death, the OPO helps coordinate the remainder of the care process, including the distribution of the organs and the provision of highly trained staff to prepare for the actual organ procurement and preservation, as well as highly efficient transport of preserved organs to each recipient's institution [7]. At this time, we will discuss key components of the process of organ donation, including the determination of death and physiologic optimization of the donor.

7. Determination of death

As discussed earlier in the chapter, declaration of death—whether that be circulatory death or brain death—has been a controversial topic over the years. In 2014, an international forum was held in Montreal, Canada with the objective to provide a functional definition of death that encompassed the concepts of brain and circulatory death. They reported that "Death is the permanent loss of capacity for consciousness and all brainstem functions. This may result from permanent cessation of circulation or catastrophic brain injury. In the context of death determination, 'permanent' refers to loss of function that cannot resume spontaneously and will not be restored through intervention" [58]. It is important for health care practitioners of all levels working with potential donor patients to have a good understanding of the definition of death in order to be able to explain to grieving families the reality of the situation and its finality [59]. It is well established that adequate explanation of brain death is one of the critical components of the donation process [60]. The optimal timing of the consent process is also of great importance [61]. Checklists are helpful in maintaining the thoroughness of brain death determination, but do not replace the expertise, knowledge and compassion of physicians in end-of-life discussions with families of the potential donor.

8. Brain death determination

When a patient presents to the hospital with concern for altered consciousness, it is imperative to rule out all reversible causes of coma, first excluding the presence of any substances of abuse, medication side effects, electrolyte, metabolic or acid-base derangements [62]. Once these are ruled out, imaging can often shed some light on potential causes of neurological compromise. In the current case vignette, the CT was utilized in order to give the treating physician an indication of the magnitude of injury and likelihood of recovery. With that being said, official declaration of BD is actually a clinical one [63]. From definitional standpoint, BD is considered to be present when there is irreversible damage to the brain and brainstem [36]. In order to assess brain function, several key components are required, with the most important one being a thorough neurological examination including assessment of brainstem reflexes [62]. Various ancillary tests can also be performed to assess cerebral blood flow and brain electrical activity in cases with equivocal exam findings. The final declaration of BD (including the official time of death) rests with the treating physician.

Determination of brain death (BD) can be a complex issue in the evaluation of catastrophic neurological injury. Clinical diagnosis of BD is relatively uncommon in the acute care setting. Usually acute injury does not progress to the degree of absent brainstem reflexes and apnea. "The small percentage of…cases may be related to many factors including early aggressive care like decompressive craniectomies, change in referral patterns, and early withdrawal of care or decision to proceed with a donation after cardiac death protocol" [64]. There are predefined criteria for the clinical determination of BD which may vary slightly from country to country. The neurological assessment of suspected BD typically requires at least 25 tests and verifications. "The overriding principle is simple: establish cause, exclude confounders, determine futility of interventions, examine brainstem reflexes and test for apnea" [64].

Due to frequent inconsistencies related to the determination of BD, the Quality Standards Subcommittee of the American Academy of Neurology (AAN) met in the 1990s to establish clear definitions of clinical terms and associated testing. The group also determined the validity of ancillary testing versus the clinical exam and its applicability to the organ donation process. Clinical criteria for BD require a formal assessment and are only undertaken once all other potentially reversible cause are excluded. The initial evaluation needs to ensure there are "no lingering effects of prior sedation, or prior use of illegal drugs or alcohol. A reasonable guideline is to calculate 5–7 times the drug's elimination half-life in hours and allow that time to pass before clinical exam is performed" [64]. A core temperature of 36°C is also recommended which can be aided by use of warming blankets if necessary. As in the current chapter's vignette, neuroimaging such as a CT scan of the head should be performed to help determine cause of mental status deterioration. Clinical examination must include a thorough neurological examination including assessment of patient's level consciousness, as well as evaluation for verbal and motor deficits. The above exam must also include the interrogation of brainstem reflexes including pupillary, corneal, pharyngeal, and tracheal responses, as well as oculocephalic reflexes with doll's eye and cold caloric assessments. Apnea testing requires documentation of absence of a respiratory drive after a CO_2 challenge. This methodology also has strict criteria that must be followed to ensure accurate determination of absent respiratory drive [65, 66].

Although ancillary testing, such as electroencephalography (EEG), cerebral angiography, nuclear flow scan, transcranial Doppler, CT angiography and magnetic resonance (MR) angiography, can be utilized in the process of determining BD—due to variability in the interpretation of these studies—it is not a substitute for the clinical examination [67–70]. In aggregate, the above tests can provide additional data on electrical brain function and cerebral blood flow and "…can be used when uncertainty exist about the reliability of parts of the neurological examination or when the apnea test cannot be performed" [71, 72]. Expertise in determining brain death can be inadequate due to multitude of factors, including lack of clinical experience. This is likely one of the reasons why 6 US states require confirmation by a second examiner and some specifically require at least one of these examiners to be either a neurologist, neurosurgeon or intensivist [73].

As one can see, the determination of brain death can be quite complex in and of itself and can be even further complicated when the question of organ donation is raised. This is why we stress the importance of early involvement of a local OPO [73]. After the declaration of BD, assuming the presence of consent for organ and tissue donation, the care of the donor shifts to optimizing organ perfusion and viability [7]. The preservation of organs after determination of BD also requires excellent coordination between the OPO and the medical management team [7, 64]. The key concerns for the medical team are to ensure hemodynamic stability and avoid the development of hyper/hypo-glycemia, acid-base or electrolyte derangements and pulmonary edema [7]. Many diagnostic tests and interventions occur during this phase specifically to ensure viability of key body systems and organs. Accumulated clinical evidence suggests "that a delay in declaration of brain death not only prolongs the time to organ recovery but also may increase the risks to transplantable organs, resulting in more complicated post-operative phases for the recipient" [64]. Finally, there is also evidence suggesting that second BD examination may negatively affect organ donor physiology due to inherent time delays [74], thus lending indirect support for ancillary/confirmatory BD testing.

From historical perspective, transplantation of organs was premised on the so-called "dead donor rule", where donors must be declared dead according to established medical and legal criteria prior to donation [75]. According to Chaten [76], "the dead donor rule (DDR) maintains that it is illicit to procure vital organs from donors until after they have been declared dead". This rule also required adherence to strict BD criteria, directly referencing that the "dead donor rule mandates simultaneous life and death within the same body for organ donation, a biological status that is inherently contradictory" [76]. The best way to decrease variability in BD determination is for all hospitals to implement the established set of AAN brain death guidelines [71, 77]. This would lead to less confusion and fewer inconsistencies among institutions. Due to the many complexities of end-of-life discussions, it is imperative that BD determination protocols become increasingly uniform in both content and application. Wahlster et al. [78] looked at practices and perceptions regarding BD declaration in 91 countries, noting that "countries with an organized transplant network were more likely to have a brain death provision compared with countries without" [78]. Barriers to consensus on universal BD standardization include social, religious and economic factors specific to each country and/or culture. Wahlster et al. [78] further note that "future efforts for uniform policies will need to include physicians with neurologic and critical care expertise, representatives of national and international major medical organizations such as the World Health Organization or World Federation of Neurology, and scientific and medical advisors of government agencies" [76].

9. Circulatory death determination

The shortage of organ donors has prompted resurgence in the utilization of donation after circulatory or cardiac death (DCD) [23, 51, 79]. While the concept of BD has been extensively discussed and there is a reasonable consensus as far as applicable criteria and assessments are concerned, definitive guidelines with respect to DCD continue to pose a challenge. In 1993, the Pittsburg non-beating heart organ donation protocol was proposed in order to provide criterion for organ procurement in the case of circulatory death. This protocol has come under criticism due to its questionable ethical application [80]. Although a definitive consensus is yet to be made from a legal and ethical standpoint, various OPOs are performing organ procurements with their own sets of standards and protocols [80]. Of interest, DCD historically constituted the largest proportion of organ donations prior to the advent of donation after BD. Subsequently, its utilization decreased substantially due to superior graft survival outcomes following donation after BD [81, 82].

10. Physiological optimization of the organ donor

Throughout the process of organ procurement, it is critical to achieve physiologic normalization and maintain systemic homeostasis in order to optimize the number of organs procured from each donor [6, 7, 83]. With this in mind, it is essential that potential donors be attentively managed in order to prevent systemic hypoxia and hypoperfusion to vital organs [7]. As in the current chapter's vignette, the ICU is the ideal location for the resuscitation of organ donors and the associated complex physiological and management needs [56, 84]. Cessation of brain function sets off a myriad of multi-system manifestations (e.g. cardiac arrhythmia, hypotension, profound acid-base and electrolyte imbalances) many of which can result in subsequent end-organ insufficiency and/or failure [56]. Consequently, ICU teams must be cognizant of these considerations and proactively work to counteract deleterious effects of BD through a number of intensive interventions. Adherence to strict protocols for management of the organ donor is of utmost importance to ensure optimal conversion rates and graft survival among recipients [7, 84]. Because such protocols may differ from center to center, it is essential for ICU teams to work with local OPOs to ensure standardization in the approach taken to optimize the organ donor prior to the procurement procedure [7, 84]. This alliance can help standardize the care received by each patient, regardless of the institution, and also provide important feedback on what is working and what may not be working. This then helps facilitate performance improvement from an OPO system standpoint [7].

As previously mentioned, there are multiple adverse physiologic events that may occur when the brain ceases to function (**Figure 3**). These include reflexive hypertension and subsequent hypotension; systemic "endocrine failure" leading to significant hormonal derangements including diabetes insipidus; and finally secondary phenomena such as acute lung injury and neurogenic pulmonary edema [85–88]. When managing patients, who succumbed to BD following TBI and multi-system trauma, special care must be dedicated to preventing any secondary insults

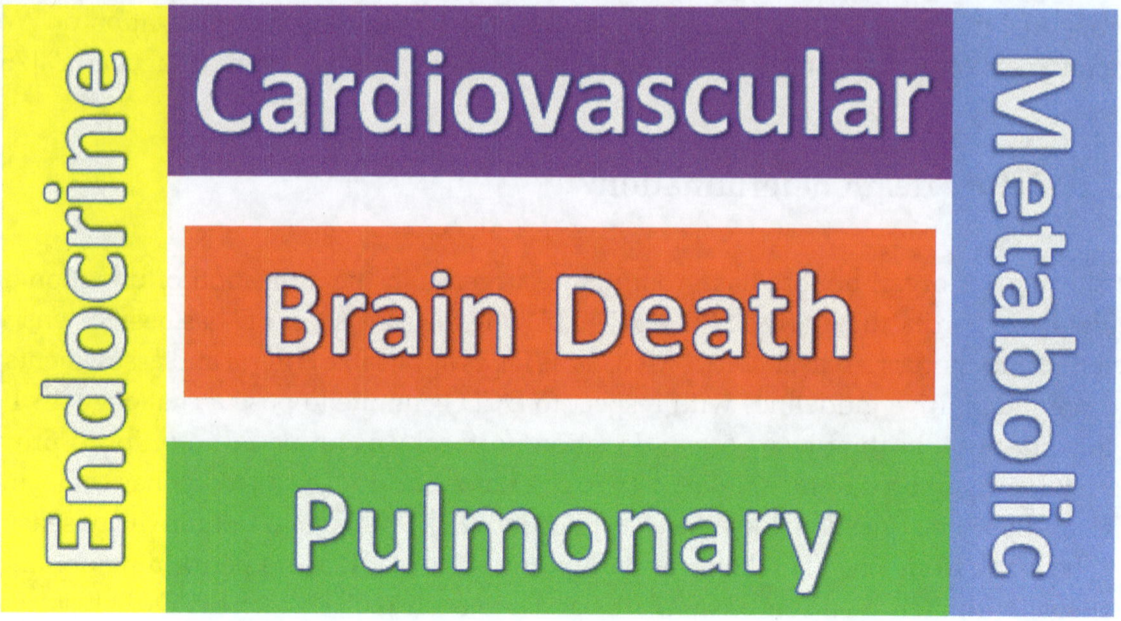

Figure 3. A diagram showing the most important and most commonly reported systemic manifestations following brain death. In the management of an organ donor consideration must be made to all of the above changes, including proactive approaches to normalize any deleterious physiologic disturbances.

from any injury that may pose a potential threat to end-organ viability [87, 89–91]. In order to properly monitor the various changes that may be rapidly occurring within the donor, frequent laboratory assessments and advanced cardiopulmonary monitoring are recommended [7, 57, 62, 92]. Correcting electrolyte and metabolic abnormalities can increase viability of donated organs according to an observational study conducted by UNOS [92]. Another important UNOS report stated that by setting certain parameters or goals for managing donors during the period leading up to organ procurement, care teams were able to augment the number of viable organs from each donor [83]. Among endpoints that increased likelihood of organ viability were maintenance of central venous pressure as well as PaO_2:FiO_2 ratio, optimization of cardiac ejection fraction and normalization of serum sodium and creatinine [83]. Thyroid hormone levels are another important element to closely monitor and correct during organ optimization. Exogenous thyroid hormone is routinely administered along with methylprednisolone and insulin to maximize organ donor viability [62, 83, 92]. Among more progressive developments, the use of extracorporeal membrane oxygenation has been proposed as a method for expanding the donor pool after cardiac death [93]. However, this approach may be prohibitive from a financial standpoint.

11. Conclusion

In summary, the field of transplantation has made significant strides throughout the years. Following its humble beginnings as an experimental science, it evolved into the primary therapeutic option for patients suffering from end-stage-organ failure. Modern transplantation offers hope to those who even a few decades ago would have none. Going hand-in-hand with that hope are the ethical and legal ramifications related to the donor and their families. With the demand for organs far exceeding the current availability, a better framework is needed for both maximizing the procurement of organs from eligible donors and better allocation of these gifts-of-life across patients on transplant waiting lists. Closer examination of all available organ donation avenues is warranted, including the assessment of opportunities offered by the use of expanded criteria donors and greater utilization of donation after cardiac death.

Author details

Alyssa Green[1], Peter G. Thomas[2], Rebecca Wilde-Onia[2], Scott J. Kohler[3], Joan D. Sweeney[3], Deborah M. Stahlnecker[4] and Stanislaw P. Stawicki[1,2]*

*Address all correspondence to: stawicki.ace@gmail.com

1 Department of Research and Innovation, St. Luke's University Health Network, Bethlehem, PA, USA

2 Regional Level I Trauma Center, St. Luke's University Health Network, Bethlehem, PA, USA

3 Center for Neurosciences, St. Luke's University Health Network, Bethlehem, PA, USA

4 Section of Pulmonary and Critical Care, Department of Medicine, St. Luke's University Health Network, Bethlehem, PA, USA

References

[1] Matas A et al. OPTN/SRTR 2012 annual data report: Kidney. American Journal of Transplantation. 2014;**14**(S1):11-44

[2] Hariharan S et al. Improved graft survival after renal transplantation in the United States, 1988 to 1996. New England Journal of Medicine. 2000;**342**(9):605-612

[3] Tuttle-Newhall J et al. Organ donation and utilization in the United States: 1998-2007. American Journal of Transplantation. 2009;**9**(4p2):879-893

[4] Xue JL et al. Forecast of the number of patients with end-stage renal disease in the United States to the year 2010. Journal of the American Society of Nephrology. 2001;**12**(12):2753-2758

[5] Evans RW, Orians CE, Ascher NL. The potential supply of organ donors: An assessment of the efficiency of organ procurement efforts in the United States. JAMA. 1992;**267**(2):239-246

[6] Cipolla J, Stawicki S, Spatz D. Hemodynamic monitoring of organ donors: A novel use of the esophageal echo-Doppler probe. The American Surgeon. 2006;**72**(6):500-504

[7] Wojda TR et al. Keys to successful organ procurement: An experience-based review of clinical practices at a high-performing health-care organization. International Journal of Critical Illness and Injury Science. 2017;**7**(2):91

[8] Howard RJ, Cornell DL, Cochran L. History of deceased organ donation, transplantation, and organ procurement organizations. Progress in Transplantation. 2012;**22**(1):6-17

[9] Doyle AM, Lechler RI, Turka LA. Organ transplantation: Halfway through the first century. Journal of the American Society of Nephrology. 2004;**15**(12):2965-2971

[10] Morris P, Knechtle SJ. Kidney Transplantation-Principles and Practice E-Book. New York, New York: Elsevier Health Sciences; 2013

[11] Barker CF, Markmann JF. Historical overview of transplantation. Cold Spring Harbor Perspectives in Medicine. 2013;**3**(4):a014977

[12] Shumway SJ, Garry DJ. History of cardiac transplantation: Research, discoveries, and pioneers. In: Congestive Heart Failure and Cardiac Transplantation. Cham, Switzerland: Springer; 2017. pp. 417-429

[13] Linden PK. History of solid organ transplantation and organ donation critical care clinics. Critical Care Clinics. 2009;**25**:165-184

[14] Alfonzo JP. Four decades of kidney transplantation in Cuba. MEDICC Review. 2013;**15**(1):23-28

[15] Guild W et al. Successful homotransplantation of the kidney in an identical twin. Transactions of the American Clinical and Climatological Association. 1955;**67**:167-173

[16] Main JM, Prehn RT. Successful skin homografts after the administration of high dosage X radiation and homologous bone marrow. Journal of the National Cancer Institute. 1955;**15**(4):1023-1029

[17] Main JM, Prehn RT. Fate of skin homografts in X-irradiated mice treated with homologous marrow. Journal of the National Cancer Institute. 1957;**19**(6):1053-1064

[18] Murray JE et al. Study on transplantation immunity after total body irradiation: Clinical and experimental investigation. Surgery. 1960;**48**(1):272-284

[19] Hoffart N. The development of kidney transplant nursing. Nephrology Nursing Journal. 2014;**41**(6):575

[20] White D, Calne R. The use of cyclosporin A immunosuppression in organ grafting. Immunological Reviews. 1982;**65**(1):115-131

[21] Murray JE et al. Prolonged survival of human-kidney homografts by immunosuppressive drug therapy. New England Journal of Medicine. 1963;**268**(24):1315-1323

[22] Starzl TE. The saga of liver replacement, with particular reference to the reciprocal influence of liver and kidney transplantation (1955-1967). Journal of the American College of Surgeons. 2002;**195**(5):587-610

[23] Abt PL, Fisher CA, Singhal AK. Donation after cardiac death in the US: History and use. Journal of the American College of Surgeons. 2006;**203**(2):208-225

[24] Groth CG et al. Historic landmarks in clinical transplantation: Conclusions from the consensus conference at the University of California, los Angeles. World Journal of Surgery. 2000;**24**(7):834-843

[25] Petechuk D. Organ Transplantation. Westport, Connecticut: Greenwood Publishing Group; 2006

[26] Faenza A et al. Kidney preservation with university of Wisconsin and Celsior solution: A prospective multicenter randomized study. Transplantation. 2001;**72**(7):1274-1277

[27] D'Alessandro A et al. Current status of organ preservation with University of Wisconsin solution. Archives of Pathology & Laboratory Medicine. 1991;**115**(3):306-310

[28] Smith CM. Origin and uses of primum non nocere—Above all, do no harm! The Journal of Clinical Pharmacology. 2005;**45**(4):371-377

[29] Veatch RM. Models for ethical medicine in a revolutionary age. Hastings Center Report. 1972:5-7

[30] Rothman DJ. Strangers at the Bedside: A History of how Law and Bioethics Transformed Medical Decision Making. New Brunswick, New Jersey: Routledge; 2017

[31] Moulton B, King JS. Aligning ethics with medical decision-making: The quest for informed patient choice. The Journal of Law, Medicine & Ethics. 2010;**38**(1):85-97

[32] Truog RD, Robinson WM. Role of brain death and the dead-donor rule in the ethics of organ transplantation. Critical Care Medicine. 2003;**31**(9):2391-2396

[33] Papachristou C et al. Motivation for living-donor liver transplantation from the donor's perspective: An in-depth qualitative research study. Transplantation. 2004;**78**(10):1506-1514

[34] Clark PA. Face transplantation: A medical perspective. Medical Science Monitor. 2005;**11**(1):RA1-RA6

[35] Chuang TC et al. The main paths of medical tourism: From transplantation to beautification. Tourism Management. 2014;**45**:49-58

[36] Jonsen AR. The ethics of organ transplantation: A brief history. Virtual Mentor. 2012; **14**(3):264-268

[37] Simmons RG, Marine SK, Simmons RL. Gift of Life: The Effect of Organ Transplantation on Individual, Family, and Societal Dynamics. New Brunswick, New Jersey: Transaction Publishers; 1987

[38] Barnard CN. Human cardiac transplantationan evaluation of the first two operations performed at the Groote Schuur hospital, cape town. American Journal of Cardiology. 1968;**22**(4):584-596

[39] Bernat JL. On noncongruence between the concept and determination of death. Hastings Center Report. 2013;**43**(6):25-33

[40] United Network for Organ Sharing. 2016 Annual Report. 2017 [cited 2017 12-20-2017]

[41] Trey T, Caplan AL, Lavee J. Transplant ethics under scrutiny - responsibilities of all medical professionals. Croatian Medical Journal. 2013;**54**(1):71-74

[42] Jones RK. The gift of life and disease of language: Recovering a lost distinction in effectuating the purpose of the National Organ Transplant Act's prohibition on the transfer of human organs for valuable consideration. Temple Law Review. 2007;**80**:1067

[43] Hoffman TJ. Organ donor Laws in the US and the UK: The need for reform and the promise of xenotransplantation. Indiana International & Comparative Law Review. 1999;**10**:339

[44] Weimer DL, Vining AR. Policy Analysis: Concepts and Practice. New York, New York: Taylor & Francis; 2017

[45] Gibbons RD, Meltzer D, Duan N. Waiting for organ transplantation. Science. 2000; **287**(5451):237-238

[46] Koch T. Scarce Goods: Justice, Fairness, and Organ Transplantation. Westport, Connecticut: Praeger ABC-CLIO; 2002

[47] Pritsker AAB. Organ transplantation allocation policy analysis. OR/MS Today. 1998;**25**(4): 1-15

[48] Schwartz HS. Bioethical and legal considerations in increasing the supply of transplantable organs: From UAGA to baby Fae. American Journal of Law & Medicine. 1984;**10**: 397-410

[49] Association of Organ Procurement Organizations. OPO services. 2017 [cited 2017 12-21-17]; Available from: http://www.aopo.org/about-opos/opo-programs/.

[50] Sanchez-Fructuoso A et al. Non-heart beating donors. Nephrology, Dialysis, Transplantation. 2004;**19**(suppl_3):iii26-iii31

[51] Verheijde JL, Rady MY, McGregor J. Recovery of transplantable organs after cardiac or circulatory death: Transforming the paradigm for the ethics of organ donation. Philosophy, Ethics, and Humanities in Medicine. 2007;**2**(1):8

[52] Veatch RM, Ross LF. Transplantation Ethics. Washington, DC: Georgetown University Press; 2014

[53] Steinman TI et al. Guidelines for the referral and management of patients eligible for solid organ transplantation. Transplantation. 2001;**71**(9):1189-1204

[54] Reiner M, Cornell D, Howard RJ. Development of a successful non—Heart-beating organ donation program. Progress in Transplantation. 2003;**13**(3):225-231

[55] Stawicki SP, Hoff WS, Cipolla J. Letters to the editor. Journal of Trauma and Acute Care Surgery. 2005;**59**(2):504-505

[56] Mascia L et al. Management to optimize organ procurement in brain dead donors. Minerva Anestesiologica. 2009;**75**(3):125-133

[57] Stawicki SP et al. Esophageal Doppler monitoring during organ donor resuscitation: New benefits of existing technology. Progress in Transplantation. 2005;**15**(4):320-320

[58] Shemie SD et al. International guideline development for the determination of death. Intensive Care Medicine. 2014;**40**(6):788-797

[59] Evanisko MJ et al. Readiness of critical care physicians and nurses to handle requests for organ donation. American Journal of Critical Care. 1998;**7**(1):4

[60] Franz HG et al. Explaining brain death: A critical feature of the donation process. Journal of Transplant Coordination. 1997;**7**(1):14-21

[61] Niles PA, Mattice BJ. The timing factor in the consent process. Journal of Transplant Coordination. 1996;**6**(2):84-87

[62] Kumar L. Brain death and care of the organ donor. Journal of Anaesthesiology Clinical Pharmacology. 2016;**32**(2):146-152

[63] Bonetti M et al. Diagnosing brain death. In: Emergency Neuroradiology. Berlin, Heidelberg: Springer; 2006. pp. 275-282

[64] Wijdicks EF. Determining brain death. Continuum: Lifelong Learning in Neurology. 2015;**21**(5, Neurocritical Care):1411-1424

[65] Kirkham FJ, Ashwal S. Coma and brain death. In: Handbook of Clinical Neurology. Philadelphia, Pennsylvania: Elsevier; 2013. pp. 43-61

[66] Dulac O, Lassonde M, Sarnat H. Coma and Brain Death. In: Pediatric Neurology, Part I. Philadelphia, Pennsylvania: Elsevier; 2013, pp. 35-40

[67] Shemie SD et al. Brain blood flow in the neurological determination of death: Canadian expert report. Canadian Journal of Neurological Sciences. 2008;**35**(2):140-145

[68] Machado C et al. Brain death diagnosis and apnea test safety. Annals of Indian Academy of Neurology. 2009;**12**(3):197

[69] Hoffmann O, Masuhr F. Use of observational periods or ancillary tests in the determination of brain death in Germany. European Neurology. 2015;**74**(1-2):11-17

[70] Wijdicks EF. The case against confirmatory tests for determining brain death in adults. Neurology. 2010;**75**(1):77-83

[71] Neurology, Q.S.S.o.t.A.A.o. Practice parameters for determining brain death in adults (summary statement). Neurology. 1995;**45**:1012-1014

[72] Rosenberg JH et al. Practice parameters for determining brain death in adults. Neurology. 1995;**45**(5):1012-1014

[73] Wijdicks EF. Brain death guidelines explained. In: Seminars in Neurology. New York, New York: Thieme Medical Publishers; 2015

[74] Lustbader D et al. Second brain death examination may negatively affect organ donation. Neurology. 2011;**76**(2):119-124

[75] Shah SK, Kasper K, Miller FG. A narrative review of the empirical evidence on public attitudes on brain death and vital organ transplantation: The need for better data to inform policy. Journal of Medical Ethics. 2014: medethics-2013-101930

[76] Chaten FC. The dead donor rule: Effect on the virtuous practice of medicine. Journal of Medical Ethics. 2014;**40**(7):496-500

[77] Wijdicks EF et al. Evidence-based guideline update: Determining brain death in adults report of the quality standards Subcommittee of the American Academy of neurology. Neurology. 2010;**74**(23):1911-1918

[78] Wahlster S et al. Brain death declaration practices and perceptions worldwide. Neurology. 2015;**84**(18):1870-1879

[79] Oniscu GC et al. In situ Normothermic regional perfusion for controlled donation after circulatory death—The United Kingdom experience. American Journal of Transplantation. 2014;**14**(12):2846-2854

[80] Spielman B, McCarthy CS. Beyond Pittsburgh: Protocols for controlled non-heart-beating cadaver organ recovery. Kennedy Institute of Ethics Journal. 1995;**5**(4):323-333

[81] Morrissey PE, Monaco AP. Donation after circulatory death: Current practices, Ongoing challenges, and potential improvements. Transplantation. 2014;**97**(3):258-264

[82] Pine JK et al. Liver transplantation following donation after cardiac death: An analysis using matched pairs. Liver Transplantation. 2009;**15**(9):1072-1082

[83] Patel MS et al. The impact of meeting donor management goals on the number of organs transplanted per expanded criteria donor: A prospective study from the unos region 5 donor management goals workgroup. JAMA Surgery. 2014;**149**(9):969-975

[84] Wojda TR, Stawicki S, Yandle KP, Bleil M, Axelband J, WildeOnia R, Thomas PG, Cipolla J, Hoff WS, Shultz J. Keys to successful organ procurement: An experiencebased review of clinical practices at a high performing healthcare organization. International Journal of Critical Illness & Injury Science. 2017;**7**(2):91-100

[85] Hendry R, Crippen D. Brain failure and brain death. ACS Surgery: Principles and Practice Critical Care; 2014: p. 1-10

[86] Edgar P, Bullock R, Bonner S. Management of the potential heart-beating organ donor. Continuing Education in Anaesthesia, Critical Care & Pain. 2004;**4**(3):86-90

[87] Avlonitis VS et al. Pulmonary transplantation: The role of brain death in donor lung injury. Transplantation. 2003;**75**(12):1928-1933

[88] Avlonitis VS et al. The hemodynamic mechanisms of lung injury and systemic inflammatory response following brain death in the transplant donor. American Journal of Transplantation. 2005;**5**(4):684-693

[89] Frontera JA, Kalb T. How I manage the adult potential organ donor: Donation after neurological death (part 1). Neurocritical Care. 2010;**12**(1):103-110

[90] Wisler JR et al. Competing priorities in the brain injured patient: Dealing with the unexpected. In: Brain Injury-Pathogenesis, Monitoring, Recovery and Management. Rijeka: InTech; 2012

[91] Sanchez-Olmedo J et al. Brain death after severe traumatic brain injury: The role of systemic secondary brain insults. In: Transplantation Proceedings. Philadelphia, Pennsylvania: Elsevier; 2005

[92] Kutsogiannis DJ et al. Medical management to optimize donor organ potential: Review of the literature. Canadian Journal of Anaesthesia. 2006;**53**(8):820-830

[93] Magliocca JF et al. Extracorporeal support for organ donation after cardiac death effectively expands the donor pool. Journal of Trauma and Acute Care Surgery. 2005;**58**(6):1095-1102

9

Organ Donation

Young-Nam Roh

Abstract

Organ transplantation is the only way of giving the gift of life to the patients with organ failure; however, the inadequate supply of organs, especially from deceased donors, has created a wide gap between organ supply and organ demand. Many organs from deceased donors are still not being used worldwide because of lack of information, education, and social system. Effective systems such as opt-out, donation after circulatory death, and donor action programs are needed to promote deceased donations. Counseling on organ donations must be an essential step of families of brain-dead patients. Standard practice should include that physicians call an Organ Procurement Organization coordinator before meeting with the families of potential donors. Tight screening for potential organ donor in intensive care unit, decoupling, and professional counseling are key components. The authorities have to consider the establishment of an opt-out system, and social systemic efforts are needed.

Keywords: organ donation, deceased donor, promotion

1. Introduction

Progress in transplantation science and medicine has been impressive in the last decades. Nevertheless, transplantation activity is constrained by the shortage of organs. How can we maximize the utilization of organs that are abandoned from the deceased donors? The process for organ donation is a complex one involving medical, psychological, ethical, and social scientific aspect. Public opinion on organ donation and social maturity is also important factors for a stable and sustainable social system for organ donation. This chapter describes the essential knowledge, principles, and considering factors for the promotion of organ donation.

2. Living and deceased donations

The demand for transplants continues to increase with the increasing aging population and prevalence of renal failure. Thousands of patients on the wait list die annually, and the wait for an organ transplant has significantly increased due to the wide gap between organ supply and demand. Transplantation has become a consolidated therapy to extend or improve quality of life, an activity that constitutes less than 10% of the global transplant needs [1].

Living and deceased donations are two sources for organ transplantation. Each organ donation has its advantages and disadvantages. The advantages and disadvantages for kidney transplantation from living and deceased donations are listed in **Table 1**.

There are also ethical issues associated with each donation. In living donations, it is the safety of the healthy individual undergoing the surgical removal of an organ. This is associated with long-term consequences and affects donors' quality of life. Another important ethical concern is the motivation of the donor. The decision to donate is a psychologically complicated one. Living donors can be impacted by a feeling of moral obligation, not just pure altruism. In addition, there are issues surrounding the commercialization of organ donation and donor rewards. Deceased donations also have important ethical issues. In particular, who should be the one to decide on the donation in the absence of a declared opinion. Does the family have the right to decide? Deceased donations can also result from moral obligation. Financial and non-financial incentives for the families can also affect deceased donations.

Living donor kidney transplantation	
Advantages	Longer graft survival than deceased donation
	Short cold ischemia time
	Planned surgery
	Possible pre-emptive transplantation
	No waiting time
Disadvantages	Requires that the donor undergo major surgery
	Long-term donor safety concerns
Deceased donor kidney transplantation	
Advantages	No harm to the donor
	Possible options for patients without a living donor.
Disadvantages	Shorter graft survival than living donation
	Long cold ischemia time
	Long waiting time on list
	Requires an unplanned surgery

Table 1. Living versus deceased kidney donation.

The medical safety associated with living kidney donations is an ongoing issue. The premise of living donations of the kidneys is that the removal of one does not impair survival or long-term kidney function of the donors. Data have shown that live kidney donations are safe in northern European populations who underwent nephrectomy [2–5]. Nevertheless, Ellison et al. [6] identified 56 live kidney donors in the OPTN database who were subsequently listed for a kidney transplant. The rate of ESRD in donors (0.04%) is comparable to the rate in the general US population (0.03%). In a meta-analysis evaluating reduced renal mass in humans, Kasiske et al. [7] demonstrated that living donations were free of progressive renal dysfunction or an increased incidence of proteinuria. The data indicated little long-term medical risks in healthy donors after unilateral nephrectomy. However, it is recommended that before the donation, the donor receives a complete medical and psychosocial evaluation, provides informed consent, and is capable of understanding the information presented to ensure a voluntary decision.

Although living and deceased donations are important sources of organs for transplantation, a proportion of organs from deceased donors worldwide are not being used due to a lack of information, education, and social system. The use of organs from deceased donors could be significantly increased with the implementation of public education and social systems. Unlike the practical problems observed in living donors, the ethical issues associated with deceased organ donations occur post mortem and can be solved by social agreement and systemic supplementation. In addition to the efforts to increase living donation, a social infrastructure, including education and the creation of laws, should be established to promote deceased donations.

Most of the progresses made in modern transplantation were to overcome the organ shortage (**Figure 1**). Medical and surgical progresses include ABO-incompatible transplantation, en bloc transplantation, and using expanded criteria for donors. On a social level, progress includes the legalization of donations after circulatory death, an opt-out system, and donor action program. The establishment of these systems is needed to promote deceased

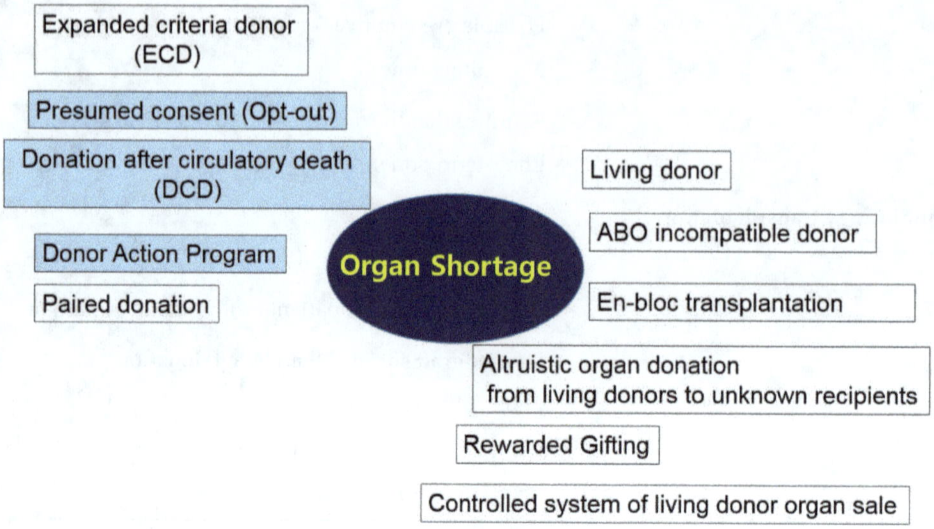

Figure 1. Measures used to overcome organ shortage.

donations. However, organ donation also needs to be socially accepted, and public opinion should change before the change of social system.

3. Deceased donation: Donations after brain death versus Donations after cardiac death

Organ donation has traditionally been possible only after brain death. It now includes donations after cardiac death (DCD), which is increasing in European countries, North America, and Australia. However, the majority of deceased donor organs continue to be from donations after brain death (DBD). DCD are from donors who do not meet the criterion for brain death, and whose cardiac function stopped before the organs were procured. The cessation of cardiac function could have occurred spontaneously or initiated deliberately. There are two types of DCDs, controlled and uncontrolled. In controlled DCD, the donor is withdrawn from life support and his or her family has given written consent for organ donation in a controlled environment. The clinical steps for controlled DCD are shown in **Figure 2**. In uncontrolled DCD, the donor died in the emergency department or elsewhere in the hospital before consent for organ donation was obtained. Catheters are placed in the femoral vessels to cool organs and infuse perfusate until consent can be obtained.

DCD now accounts for 17% of the 31,812 donors reported to the Global Observatory on Organ Donation and Transplantation in 2015 [1]. DCD is used in a limited number of countries, because of legislative and ethical obstacles, lack of technical expertise, and/or insufficient organizational capabilities [2, 8]. There are also differences in DCD practices, including differences in legislative and ethical frameworks, patterns of end-of-life care, and approaches for the treatment of patients with cardiovascular arrest outside of the hospital [9]. Although transplant outcomes from organs obtained from DCD donors are appropriate overall, they need improvement [9]. It is generally accepted that DCD can substantially increase the availability of deceased donor organs with optimal results.

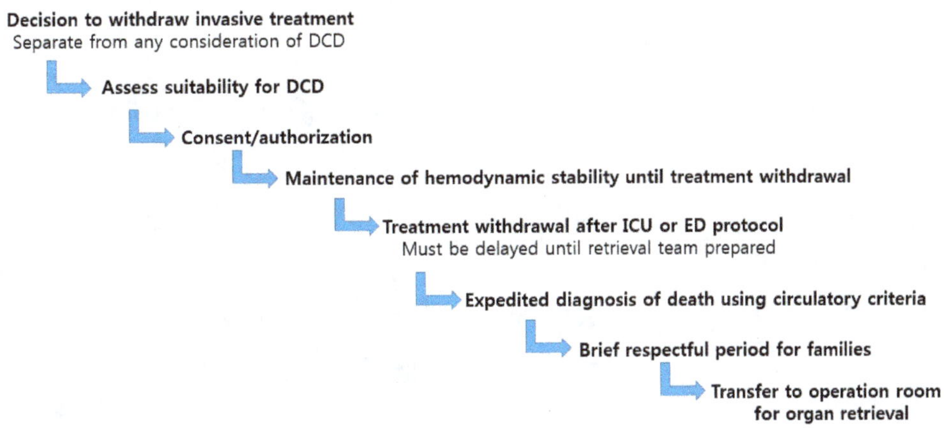

Figure 2. Clinical steps for controlled DCD.

4. Practical issues with organ donation after brain death

The clinical course of patients with severe brain injury varies depending on the degree of injury and the clinical decisions made by the primary physician. The latter are impacted by legislative and ethical frameworks, as well as patterns of end-of-life care. Organ donation is one of the options in end-of-life decision, which must be considered in every patient who may become brain dead (**Figure 3**). Organ donation counseling is an essential step that should be incorporated in end-of-life decisions.

Although the consent rate for organ donation in Europe is 50–80% with approximately 85% of families being requested to donate, only 50% provide consent. Other studies have confirmed these findings [10–14]. It is important to identify potential cases of brain deaths and obtain informed consent for organ donation from the families of the patients. Because most countries have an opt-in system, voluntary consent is considered an essential factor in organ donation. Only a small portion of these brain-dead donors are being used for solid-organ transplantation, primarily because of the low percentage of families who consent to donation [15]. Several studies have evaluated the factors associated with these types [1–4, 12, 14–16], which are listed in **Table 2**.

How to ask for an organ donation correctly is another important practical issue. The physician should call an Organ Procurement Organization (OPO) coordinator before meeting with the family of a potential donor and it must be a standard practice. Including an OPO coordinator in conversation is critical to successfully counsel families. Studies have shown that the time spent with an OPO coordinator is strongly associated with a family's decision to donate organs [15]. Incomplete or inaccurate information about the donation process may limit consent. Furthermore, the early involvement of an OPO coordinator is the best way to deliver complete and accurate information to families. Discussion of common fears and misinformation about organ donation should be part of the organ donation request process during counseling. Important questions families typically have regarding organ donation focus on the process, physical impairment during organ recovery, and the way the organs are used.

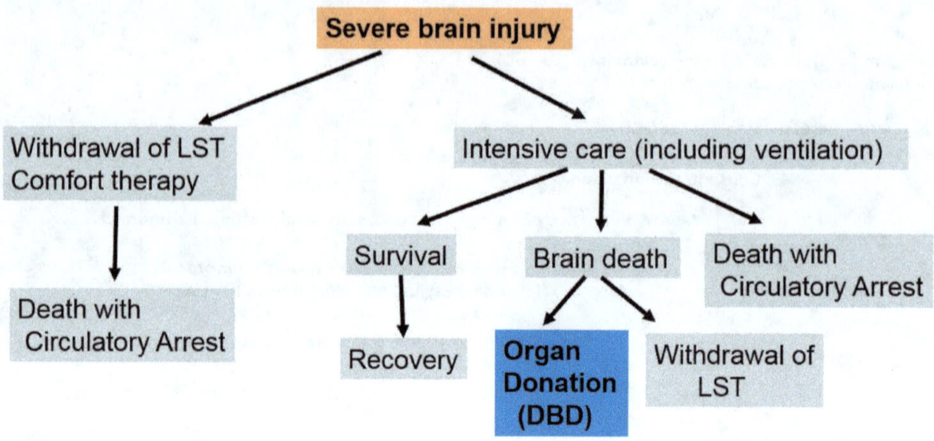

Figure 3. Clinical pathways of potential brain-dead donor. LST, Life-Supporting Treatment; DBD, Donation after Brain Death.

Factors
Patient factors
Age
Religion
Cause of death
Wish to terminate life support
Wish for organ donation
Health-care factors
Request factors
Timing and preparation for decision
Decoupling
Time to decide
Accurate information before decision
Behavior of care professionals
Care for patient and relatives
Supportive communication
Critical events before request
Respect for patients
Care professional's attitude toward organ donation
Family factors
Prior knowledge and opinion
Family culture
Religion
Education
Information about brain death
Information about organ donation
Opinion about who has to decide
Decision making
Emotional stress and grief
Family relationship
Agreement among relatives
Economic status
Financial incentives

Table 2. Factors affecting deceased donation.

In addition, incentives for organ donations are a topic of interest. Most physicians cannot deliver enough information about these topics to the families. The early involvement of OPO coordinators is easy, and a definite solution for this problem has been recommended in many studies. A physician must be accompanied by an OPO coordinator before beginning family counseling, and precise information with supportive care must be given if the families need more information (**Figure 4**). Common reasons families refuse organ donation include the following:

1. Protecting and respecting the body
2. Fear that the surgery will disfigure the body
3. Belief that their loved ones have already experienced enough trauma
4. Concerns about the wholeness and integrity of the dead body
5. Wish to keep the body intact
6. Observation of a lack of respect for the deceased by the hospital staff
7. Gift of life is frequently considered by the relatives to be a sacrifice
8. Financial incentives do not influence the decision

OPO coordinators can counsel families on these specific topics. Families are often concerned about the physical impairment and pain sensation associated with preserving the donor's body or thinking that the donor will feel the pain. In addition, a significant portion of families believes that the surgery causes excessive physical damage. These are significant concerns associated with decision making in families. Therefore, it is important that the medical staff or a transplantation coordinator offers specialized information about this subject during counseling. Efforts to address families' concerns are an important step toward gaining consent to donate. OPO coordinators can provide the right information to families and address negative perspectives on organ donation (**Figure 5**).

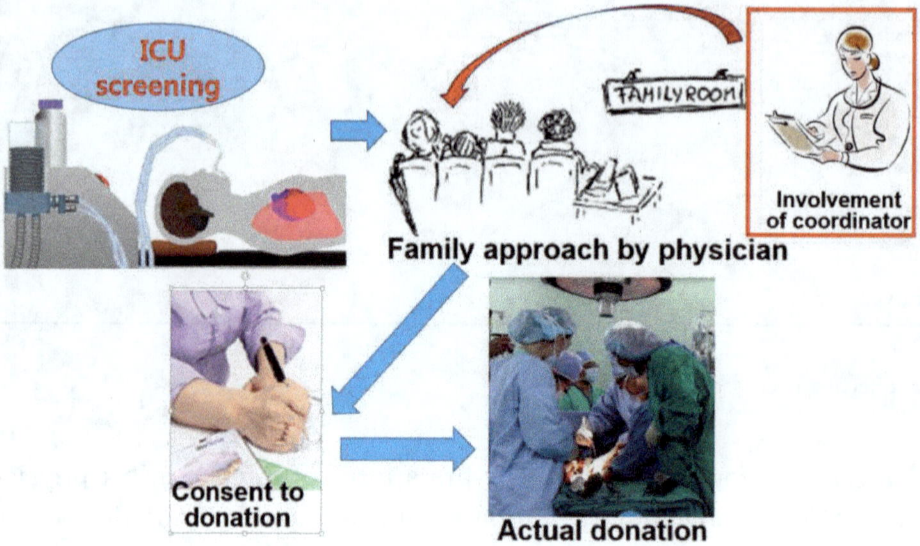

Figure 4. Early involvement of OPO counseling.

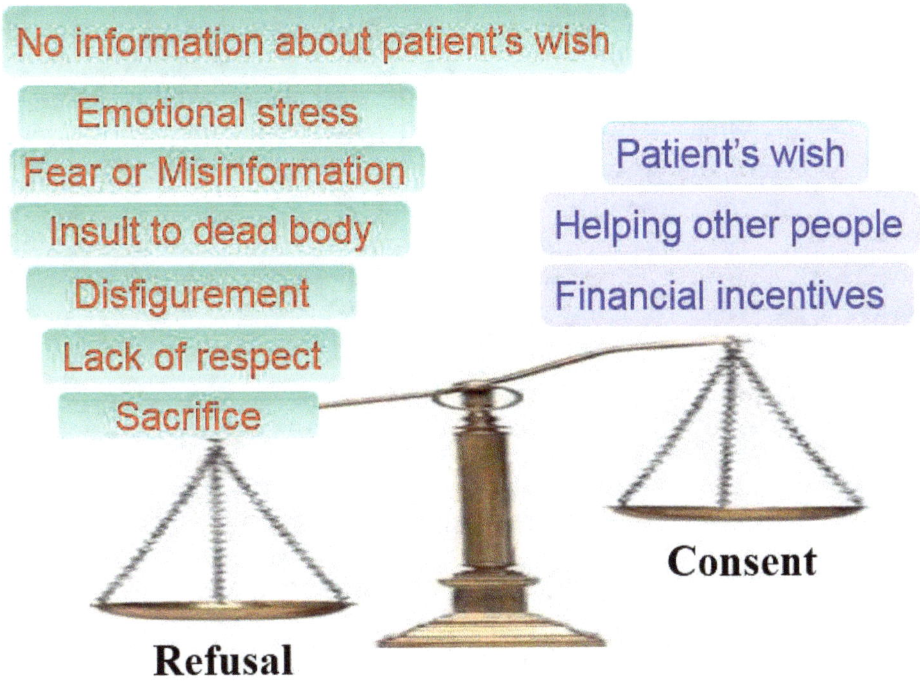

Figure 5. Key negative perspectives on organ donation.

The decision to donate is often forced on families during complex clinical situations, at a time when they may be shocked and stunned, and ill-equipped to make a decision [16–19]. It can be difficult to accept the death of a loved one, and many family members are not prepared to understand the medical concept of brain death because of emotional stress. In addition, one of the most stressful situations is when a family member has to make this type of decision without his or her previously specified opinion about organ donation. Even when counseling is done correctly, nearly half families refuse to donate. However, some of the families refuse to donate to avoid the request as a nonresponse. Frutos et al. suggest discussing organ donation as an option more than once with relatives who initially refuse or are unsure [20]. Relatives should also have the opportunity to spend time with the donor and say their final farewell. More than one-third of relatives regret declining to donate soon after the funeral [18].

Emotional upheaval in acutely bereaved families and lack of clarity on brain death cause dissonance and distress that adversely affect decision making in families and grieving over time [21–23]. Several factors have been shown to affect decision making in family members [12, 14, 15]. The complex situation and emotional stress make it difficult for families to understand the nature of brain death and accept the actual death of their loved one. This ultimately impacts the decision-making process regarding organ donation. Multiple factors negatively affect the decision to donate and lead to time delay for the final decision. A final decision may require several hours to days. This time delay, though justifiable, can be associated with the refusal to donate or failure of a successful donation. In one study, researchers reported that a delay in decision making does not reflect a negative attitude about organ donation, but a reasonable and necessary amount of time for deliberation [24]. Therefore, the medical attendant and OPO coordinator should continue their efforts to maintain organ viability and consider extended repetitive counseling to encourage donation.

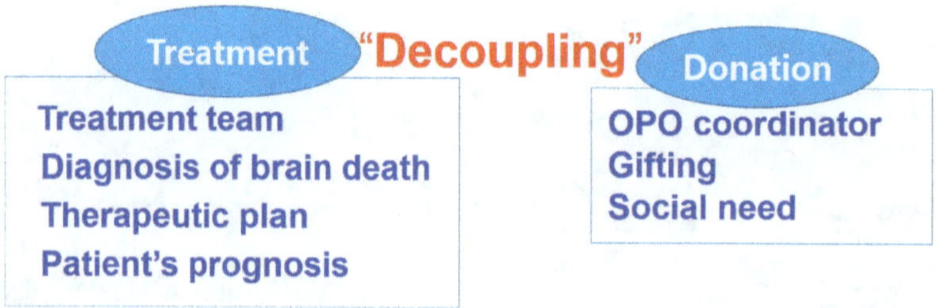

Figure 6. Principle of decoupling.

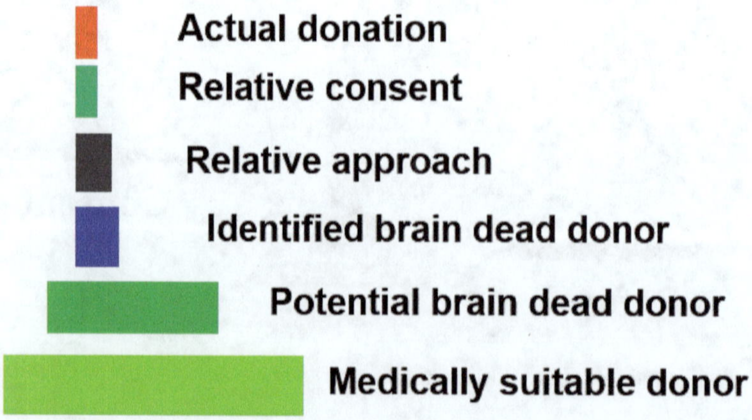

Figure 7. Multiple steps for organ donation after brain death in intensive care unit.

Decoupling is one of the best principles in which making a donation request is delayed until the family understands that brain death is the same as death and has the opportunity to realize that their loved one is dead (**Figure 6**). This principle of waiting to discuss organ donation until the family is ready to make end-of-life decisions is important to correctly timed request. The principle of decoupling is a well-known way to increase the consent rate for organ donations [25]. In a study by the Kentucky Organ Donor Affiliates in 1989–1990, researchers reported that the consent rate increased from 18 to 60% if there was a separation between when death is pronounced and the approach for organ donation [25]. However, decoupling frequently becomes impossible when the hemodynamics of a potential donor worsens. The patient's attending physician may feel an ethical conflict about providing active or invasive life-support care that seems to have no therapeutic benefit on the patient's recovery and appears to have significance solely for maintaining organ quality, especially when the family's opinion about organ donation is not specified yet. This frequently occurs in the emergency department or the intensive care unit [26]. In addition, decoupling is sometimes not consistent with the current recommendation of early referral to the OPO coordinator [26]. If we profoundly believe that there is value in organ donation, a more flexible high-dimensional strategy is needed when a potential donor is progressing to circulatory death.

Identifying a potential brain-dead donor is the fundamental step for a successful donor action program. The typical steps of actual organ donation in the intensive care unit are illustrated in **Figure 7**. OPO coordinators or transplantation teams typically identify only a small portion of potential brain-dead donors. If the OPO coordinator approached the families and appropriate counseling was performed, the families consent is an invincible one. A tight screening system must be established to increase the rate of identification of potential donors in the intensive care unit. The generally accepted criteria for potential deceased donors are shown in **Table 3**.

Every ventilated patient with
Glasgow coma scale of <5
Brain death test being considered
Do-not-resuscitate or comfort care being considered
Withdrawal of life support being considered
Family initiates conversation about donation
Within 1 h of every cardiovascular death

Table 3. Criteria for referral of a potential donor.

5. Social system for organ donation

Strategic efforts by the government and local authorities, as well as individual efforts by medical personnel, are necessary to promote organ donation. These include the revision of laws, simplifying the required procedures for receiving consent, expansion of the donor card system, adoption of a presumed consent concept known as an opt-out system, and the establishment of a DCD system. The strategic processes put in place in Europe and the United States have resulted in a progressive and gradual increase of organ donation [27–30].

Despite the effectiveness of these strategies, public acceptance of organ donation is essential before these measures can be implemented in other countries. The establishment of social systems for organ donation depends on public consensus. There are currently two moral values on organ donation: deontologism versus consequentialism. This means where we put our maximum value of some behavior, as it were, the legitimacy of process or the benefit of consequence (**Table 4**). Many procedural details in organ donation and recovery have points of conflict, which can be solved with social agreement.

Asking families for organ donations to families is generally regarded as a stressful task by primary physicians. Only a small portion of potential donors are being asked about organ donation as an option of end-of-life decision, and it is decided according to the primary physician's point of view or belief. Despite the important role of the medical staff in recommending organ donation to families, imposing this burden on physicians alone may not be adequate. If we, including local authorities and the general population, agree on the importance of organ donation, its promotion would not be the sole responsibility of individual medical staffs. The authorities have to consider establishing an advanced system that links potential donors to organ donations, known as an "opt-out" system. Many valuable lessons can be learned from the efforts of European countries to adopt it [28].

Religious beliefs were found to be important. Officially, nearly all religious groups support organ transplantation as long as it does not impede the life or hasten the death of the donor [31]. However, only a small portion of the public knows about the stance of their religion on organ donation. More active involvement of religious bodies is needed to raise the public's awareness and encourage organ donation.

Deontologism	Consequentialism
Moral principle	*Moral principle*
Duty or obligation-based ethics	Outcome-based ethics
Action or process is more important than the consequences.	A morally right act is one that will produce a good outcome.
A moral obligation may arise from rules	The end justifies the means
Donation system	*Donation system*
Donor's will	Social need
"Opt-in" system	"Opt-out" system
Informed consent	Presumed consent
Explicit consent	Implicit consent
No donor incentives	Donor incentives
Individual decision	Social campaign
Donor management after consent	Donor management before consent
Volunteering	ICU screening and family approach
Resuscitation for organs forbidden	Resuscitation for organs allowed
Femoral cannulation after consent	Femoral cannulation before consent

Table 4. Moral dilemma surrounding organ donation.

Asian countries have delayed the creation and adoption of social systems for organ donation. Despite the socioeconomic development of several Asian countries, the number of organ donations per million is extremely low, compared with western countries. In addition, most of the data on organ donation consent after brain death are largely based on findings from Western populations. The current opinion on organ donation after brain death is unclear in Asian countries. Traditionally, the body of a loved one should not be tampered with after death in Asian cultures, especially in Korean, Japanese, and Chinese. This belief originates from the Confucian tradition, and it is believed that this tradition may be the main reason for the low consent rate of organ donation in Asian countries. In addition to cultural differences, it is thought that widely differing opinions, perceptions, and concerns may be related to low frequency of organ donation in Asia. However, these factors are not well studied. The general opinion on brain death and organ donation appears to be quite positive in Asia [24, 32]. The perception of brain death as death is widely accepted [32]. However, there were several perceptional barriers against organ donation in Asia [32]. Evidence-based strategies focused on these barriers should be established to increase the rate of organ donation effectively.

6. Summary

- Living and deceased donations are two sources of organs for transplantation. Each type of donation has its advantages and disadvantages.
- Many organs from deceased donors are still not being used worldwide because of lack of information, education, and social system.

- Effective systems such as opt-out, donation after circulatory death, and donor action programs are needed to promote deceased donations.
- DCD is developed in a limited number of countries, because of legislative and ethical obstacles, lack of technical expertise, and/or insufficient organizational capabilities. It is generally accepted that DCD can substantially increase the availability of deceased donor organs with optimal results.
- Counseling on organ donations is an essential step for stable end-of-life decision of families. Standard practice should include that physicians call an Organ Procurement Organization (OPO) coordinator before meeting with the families of potential donors.
- Delays in deciding on organ donation do not reflect a negative attitude, but a reasonable and necessary time for families to deliberate.
- Decoupling is important to properly timed organ donation requests. However, a more flexible high-dimensional strategy is required when the potential donor is progressing toward circulatory death.
- A tight screening system must be established to increase the rate of identification of potential donors in the intensive care unit.
- The authorities have to consider the establishment of an opt-out system.
- More active involvement of religions is needed to encourage organ donation. The participation of religious societies in public campaigns would also be helpful.

Author details

Young-Nam Roh

Address all correspondence to: ironman0913@hanmail.net

Keimyung University, Dongsan Medical Center, Daegu, South Korea

References

[1] Transplantation. Gooda. Available from: http://www.transplant-observatory.org/ [Accessed: October 25, 2017]

[2] Fehrman-Ekholm I, Elinder CG, Stenbeck M, Tyden G, Groth CG. Kidney donors live longer. Transplantation. 1997;**64**:976-978

[3] Najarian JS, Chavers BM, McHugh LE, Matas AJ. 20 years or more of follow-up of living kidney donors. Lancet. 1992;**340**:807-810

[4] Narkun-Burgess DM, Nolan CR, Norman JE, Page WF, Miller PL, Meyer TW. Forty-five year follow-up after uninephrectomy. Kidney International. 1993;**43**(5):1110

[5] Ramcharan T, Matas AJ. Long-term (20-37 years) follow-up of living kidney donors. American Journal of Transplantation. 2002;**2**:959-964

[6] Ellison MD, McBride MA, Taranto SE, Delmonico FL, Kauffman HM. Living kidney donors in need of kidney transplants: A report from the organ procurement and transplantation network. Transplantation. 2002;**74**:1349-1351

[7] Kasiske BL, Ma JZ, Louis TA, Swan SK. Long-term effects of reduced renal mass in humans. Kidney International. 1995;**48**:814-819

[8] Dominguez-Gil B, Haase-Kromwijk B, Van Leiden H, Neuberger J, Coene L, Morel P, Corinne A, Muehlbacher F, Brezovsky P, Costa AN, Rozental R, Matesanz R, European Committee on Organ Transplantation. Council of E. Current situation of donation after circulatory death in European countries. Transplant International. 2011;**24**:676-686

[9] Minambres E, Rubio JJ, Coll E, Dominguez-Gil B. Donation after circulatory death and its expansion in Spain. Current Opinion in Organ Transplantation. 2018;**23**:120-129

[10] Beasley CL, Capossela CL, Brigham LE, Gunderson S, Weber P, Gortmaker SL. The impact of a comprehensive, hospital-focused intervention to increase organ donation. Journal of Transplant Coordination. 1997;**7**:6-13

[11] Gortmaker SL, Beasley CL, Sheehy E, Lucas BA, Brigham LE, Grenvik A, Patterson RH, Garrison N, McNamara P, Evanisko MJ. Improving the request process to increase family consent for organ donation. Journal of Transplant Coordination. 1998;**8**:210-217

[12] Hulme W, Allen J, Manara AR, Murphy PG, Gardiner D, Poppitt E. Factors influencing the family consent rate for organ donation in the UK. Anaesthesia. 2016;**71**:1053-1063

[13] Siminoff LA, Arnold RM, Caplan AL, Virnig BA, Seltzer DL. Public policy governing organ and tissue procurement in the United States. Results from the National Organ and Tissue Procurement Study. Annals of Internal Medicine. 1995;**123**:10-17

[14] Simpkin AL, Robertson LC, Barber VS, Young JD. Modifiable factors influencing relatives' decision to offer organ donation: Systematic review. BMJ. 2009;**338**:b991

[15] Siminoff LA, Gordon N, Hewlett J, Arnold RM. Factors influencing families' consent for donation of solid organs for transplantation. Journal of the American Medical Association. 2001;**286**:71-77

[16] Jacoby L, Jaccard J. Perceived support among families deciding about organ donation for their loved ones: Donor vs nondonor next of kin. American Journal of Critical Care. 2010;**19**:e52-e61

[17] Burroughs TE, Hong BA, Kappel DF, Freedman BK. The stability of family decisions to consent or refuse organ donation: Would you do it again? Psychosomatic Medicine. 1998;**60**:156-162

[18] DeJong W, Franz HG, Wolfe SM, Nathan H, Payne D, Reitsma W, Beasley C. Requesting organ donation: An interview study of donor and nondonor families. American Journal of Critical Care. 1998;**7**:13-23

[19] Rodrigue JR, Cornell DL, Howard RJ. The instability of organ donation decisions by next-of-kin and factors that predict it. American Journal of Transplantation. 2008;**8**:2661-2667

[20] Frutos MA, Ruiz P, Requena MV, Daga D. Family refusal in organ donation: Analysis of three patterns. Transplantation Proceedings. 2002;**34**:2513-2514

[21] Long T, Sque M, Addington-Hall J. Conflict rationalisation: How family members cope with a diagnosis of brain stem death. Social Science & Medicine. 2008;**67**:253-261

[22] Long T, Sque M, Payne S. Information sharing: Its impact on donor and nondonor families' experiences in the hospital. Progress in Transplantation. 2006;**16**:144-149

[23] Sque M, Long T, Payne S. Organ donation: Key factors influencing families' decision-making. Transplantation Proceedings. 2005;**37**:543-546

[24] Han SY, Kim JI, Lee EW, Jang HY, Han KH, Oh SW, Roh YN. Factors Associated with a family's delay of decision for organ donation after brain death. Annals of Transplantation. 2017;**22**:17-23

[25] Garrison RN, Bentley FR, Raque GH, Polk HC Jr, Sladek LC, Evanisko MJ, Lucas BA. There is an answer to the shortage of organ donors. Surgery, Gynecology & Obstetrics. 1991;**173**:391-396

[26] Venkat A, Baker EF, Schears RM. Ethical controversies surrounding the management of potential organ donors in the emergency department. The Journal of Emergency Medicine. 2014;**47**:232-236

[27] Evenson AR. Utilization of kidneys from donation after circulatory determination of death. Current Opinion in Organ Transplantation. 2011;**16**:385-389

[28] Rieu R. The potential impact of an opt-out system for organ donation in the UK. Journal of Medical Ethics. 2010;**36**:534-538

[29] Rithalia A, McDaid C, Suekarran S, Myers L, Sowden A. Impact of presumed consent for organ donation on donation rates: A systematic review. BMJ. 2009;**338**:a3162

[30] Summers DM, Watson CJ, Pettigrew GJ, Johnson RJ, Collett D, Neuberger JM, Bradley JA. Kidney donation after circulatory death (DCD): State of the art. Kidney International. 2015;**88**:241-249

[31] Donation. RVoO. Available from: http://donatelifecalifornia.org/education/faqs/religious-views-on-organ-donation [Accessed: June 11, 2017]

[32] Lee HJ, Jin MJ, Han SY, Han KH, Oh SW, Jang HY, Park UJ, Kim HT, Roh YN. Survey regarding attitude of family about organ donation after brain death in Korea. Annals of Transplantation. 2017;**22**:646-655

10

Xenotransplantation

Sean Stevens

Abstract

Xenotransplantation, defined as the transfer of cells, tissues or organs between species, has been a subject of significant interest for decades as a response to the increasing demand for biological materials to treat patients. In this review, the history and recent progress in xenotransplantation research will be discussed, including the immunological challenges that need to be overcome and the molecular biological methods which are required to allow the complex genome engineering to meet the critical need for organs.

Keywords: xenotransplantation, immune rejection, swine, transgene, gene editing, gene knockout, tolerance

1. Introduction

Over the course of the past 100 years, the rapid progress in drug development and surgical techniques has created a paradox for the area of transplantation medicine. Surgical protocols have become more successful and medicines have overcome many mechanisms of chronic rejection and allowed increased survival of transplant patients. However, the number of organs available for transplant has remained essentially constant. In addition, not all organs available through donation are viable for transplant. Organs such as lung, which are more prone to damage due to trauma, disease or deterioration, are available in drastically reduced numbers compared with heart or kidneys. Therefore, while there is an increasing number of patients who would survive and thrive long-term after organ transplantation, the limited number of organs available means a smaller percentage of eligible patients can actually undergo transplant surgery.

A hard truth about human organ donation is that even with exponential increases in donor numbers, it is unlikely that the organ shortage would be relieved. The diversity of the human species, paired with the efficiency of the immune system, significantly reduces the chances that a given organ will be compatible with the patients in greatest need. Although immunosuppressive drugs can enhance length of survival, chronic rejection remains a risk the greater the mismatch between organ and patient. Furthermore, the donor geographic proximity, organ size and timing of availability of a compatible organ with a matching patient may be limiting. Thus, even as human organ donation continues to be optimized, there remains an immense need for additional organs above and beyond the availability of human donors.

In order to address the above concerns and provide sufficient numbers of compatible organs, a number of approaches, both biological and mechanical, are being actively explored. Use of animal organs provides solutions to the challenges of availability and function. Multiple mammalian species possess organs which may substitute effectively for their human analogs and, in the case of agricultural species, can be rapidly bred in sufficient numbers to overcome organ shortages. Through use of controlled facilities, production of animals can be regulated and disease exposure eliminated. Additionally, careful breeding schedules can provide organs of appropriate size for any given patient on a predictable schedule for optimal timing of surgery. Finally, recent advancements in DNA sequencing and assembly and genome engineering technologies, paired with the advanced understanding of the cellular and molecular immunology responses in transplant rejection, allow the creation of animals which could provide an unlimited supply of rejection-free organs.

2. Early beginnings

Examples of xenotransplantation can be found recorded as early as the seventeenth century, in which the transfusion of blood from animals into human patients was described [1]. In the eighteenth century, more complex tissues such as skin were tested as grafts in human patients [2]. In 1905, Princeteau transferred rabbit kidney sections into a child with immediate positive results, however, after 16 days the child died of pulmonary complications [3]. Soon thereafter, two kidney xenotransplants were attempted, with one patient receiving an organ from goat, the other from pig. Unlike Princeteau's experiment, neither organs functioned and both apparently failed due to thrombosis [4]. Similarly, an attempt by Unger in 1910 to transplant kidneys from a chimpanzee into humans led to failure due to thrombosis in about a day [5]. In 1923, Neuhof transplanted a kidney from a lamb into a human patient, allowing the patient to survive 9 days [6].

In the early twentieth century, an odd offshoot of xenotransplantation was created due to interest in "rejuvenation" via transplant of animal testis in human males, as demonstrated by Voronoff in Russia [7] and Brinkley in the US [8] using chimpanzee or goat testis, respectively. So popular was the use of goat testis in the US, an entire radio empire was built around advertising the services, with many patients claiming enhanced fertility and sexual function [8].

The field of immunology developed in parallel with surgical approaches to xenotransplantation. As the mechanisms of immune rejection were better defined, the enormity of the challenges facing transplant of organs between members of the same species were recognized.

During and after WWII, pharmaceutical companies created a series of increasingly effective immunosuppressive drugs which could inhibit some rejection responses, renewing interest in xenotransplantation.

3. First attempts at human xenotransplantation with primate organs

During 1963–1964, Reemstma carried out a series of transplants into 13 human patients using chimpanzee kidneys, with one patient surviving 9 months after transplant surgery [9]. The need for these experiments was driven in part by the desperate human organ shortage and lack of alternatives. Cadaveric organs often proved insufficient in quality, and volunteer human kidney donation, high risk at the time, was untenable for ethical and legal reasons. Although chronic dialysis had been demonstrated by the early 1960s, it was not widely available for patient treatment [10]. Therefore, despite the risks, xenotransplantation was considered a potentially viable solution.

Reemstma was not alone in exploring xenotransplantation as a means to overcome critical organ shortages. Hume attempted transplanting a chimpanzee kidney into a human, but the organ failed to show renal function [11]. Hardy and team focused on heart, observing survival for only 2 hours after transplanting a chimpanzee heart into a human patient [12]. Starzl carried out a series of transplants in human patients with baboon kidney [13] and livers, with variable results [14]. These seminal attempts at xenotransplantation showed that although surgical techniques and immunosuppressive drug treatments had greatly improved, they were insufficient to address the multitude of challenges in overcoming the xenorejection response. Indeed, it was nearly a generation later before Bailey used a baboon heart for transplantation into an infant, who survived several weeks after receiving the organ [15].

4. A shift in species

Although the close evolutionary relationship between non-human primates and humans would suggest an advantage in using chimpanzee or baboon organs for xenotransplantation, clinical, practical and ethical considerations prevent them from being a viable option. Non-human primate organs do indeed function almost identically to human organs, but are subject to a variety of diseases which are readily transmissible to humans [16]. Given the relatively fragile state of patients receiving multiple immunosuppressive drugs, the risk of primate zoonoses is too great. In addition, chimpanzees, baboons and many other non-human primates are impractical for large scale breeding. The low numbers of progeny of non-human primates limits the production of large numbers of animals by natural breeding or *in vitro* fertilization compared with agricultural species. Finally, use of non-human primates as organ donors faces insurmountable ethical barriers.

A much more viable approach is the use of pig organs for xenotransplantation. Porcine organs are structurally and physiologically close to humans, and therefore can functionally substitute for analogous human organ functions. Unlike non-human primates, pigs are more evolutionarily distant from humans and thus have a greatly reduced risk of transmission of diseases to human patients, which can be essentially eliminated through genetic manipulation [17].

Husbandry techniques for pigs are extremely well-understood, with large litter sizes and rapid cycle times, allowing production of populations that could overcome organ shortages in a much shorter timeframe than possible with non-human primates. Furthermore, a suite of genome engineering technologies is available for use in pigs to make critical changes to enhance survival and function of the pig organ, while avoiding the human immune rejection response. In fact, the complex engineering approaches now available may actually provide organs with advantages over even closely-matched human organs.

5. Current status and challenges for xenotransplantation

A variety of academic, clinical and industrial institutions have made substantial progress in recent years in the understanding of the molecular mechanisms of the xenorejection response and the genetic modification of pigs to overcome these mechanisms [18]. Professional organizations are working with the FDA to develop guidelines for clinical use [19], with several groups indicating their intention to initiate clinical trials in the near term with porcine organs [20].

For xenotransplantation to become a viable routine human therapeutic option, there are a number of challenges that still need to be overcome. These challenges fall into two broad categories; the biology of the xenorejection responses and the engineering technologies needed to restructure the porcine genome to overcome these responses.

6. The immune system and rejection

The immune system is an evolutionarily ancient collection of structures, mechanisms and cells that detect and eliminate harmful organisms from the host. In older texts, the immune system is often described as distinguishing "self" from "non-self," but more recent research demonstrates that there are a variety of roles for the microbiome ("non-self" micro-organisms resident within, on or around the host) in maintaining the health of the host organism. Thus, the host immune system must be able to not only identify and eliminate harmful pathogens, it must also tolerate the presence of a variety of beneficial bacteria, fungi and yeast [21]. Because transplantation of cells, tissues and organs is an unnatural situation created through deliberate medical intervention, the human immune response uses incredible precision to identify even closely related human cells as "non-self" and efficiently removing them, a process referred to as "immune rejection." In general, the strength of the response is proportional to the degree of difference between the host and donor materials, therefore, when exposed to materials from an animal, the rejection response is much faster and stronger, increasing the challenge in controlling the immune response.

7. Xenotransplant rejection

Xenorejection is a much more exaggerated and rapid form of the allorejection response. Four overlapping and inter-related reactions occur temporally; hyperacute rejection (HAR), acute vascular rejection/acute humoral xenograft rejection (AVR/AHXR), acute cellular rejection (ACR) and chronic rejection (CR) (**Figure 1**) [22]. Although these processes can be characterized as distinct stages based on histological and clinical data, each is due to highly interconnected pathways and mechanisms that are challenging to separate. In fact, these responses were defined as pathologic observations prior to development of more detailed analyses of the molecular immunology mechanisms.

HAR is primarily due to immediate binding of pre-existing host natural antibodies specific for xenoantigens expressed by the donor tissues. Antibody binding can activate the endothelial cells, causing the release of immune activators, as well as inducing the complement-mediated destruction of the endothelial layer, reducing the barrier function and allowing host cells to infiltrate the organ. Cell debris released by the damage to the endothelium and products of the complement cascade also stimulate coagulation and the innate inflammatory response. These pathways synergize during rejection to create stronger responses that are more pathogenic and can be less amenable to control.

AVR/AHXR, like HAR, is also mediated by host antibodies. However, instead of pre-existing natural antibodies, AVR/AHXR is often the result of humoral responses which lead to production of antigen-specific antibodies. The AVR/AHXR is delayed due to the time it takes to induce

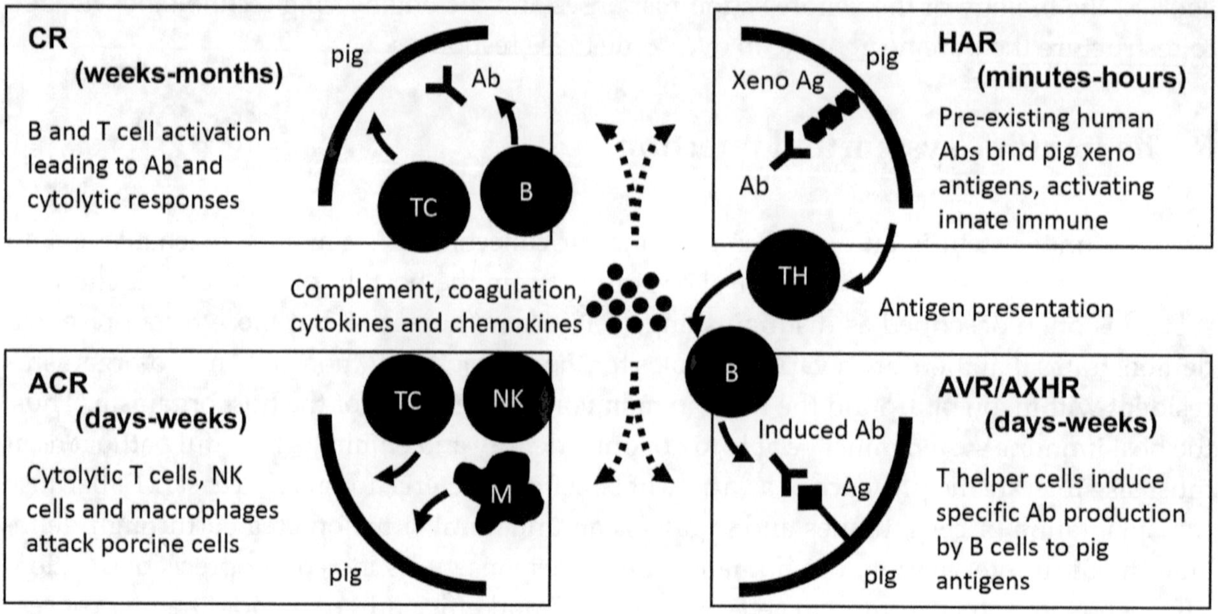

Figure 1. Overview of the xeno-rejection response. The human immune response to xeno-organs initiates within minutes to hours with hyperacute rejection (HAR, upper right), in which pre-existing antibodies (Ab) in human serum bind to xenoantigens (xeno Ag) on the surface of the pig cells. This results in cell destruction and presentation of porcine antigens to human helper (TH) and cytolytic (TC) T cells, as well as groups of pro-inflammatory and pro-immunity cytokines and other soluble mediators. Activation of human helper T cells (TH) stimulates human B cells (B) over the course of days to weeks, resulting in production of induced antibodies (induced Ab) as part of the acute vascular rejection/acute humoral xenograft rejection (AVR/AHXR, lower right) response. These secondary antibodies are often more specific and higher affinity than the pre-existing human serum antibodies, and also cause cellular destruction of the xenograft. in parallel with AVR/AHXR, the acute cellular rejection response (ACR, lower left) is carried out by human NK cells (NK), macrophages (M) and the xenograft-specific cytolytic T cells (TC) recruited to the xeno-organ within days to weeks. The activated cells express a variety of molecules to attack the porcine cells, as well as secrete additional cytokines to recruit more human immune cells. After weeks to months, the human immune response may be again induced to react to the xeno-organ during chronic rejection (CR, upper left), leading to specific antibody (Ab) responses from B cells (B) or cytolytic T cell (TC) destruction. A large collection of cytokines, chemokines, complement and coagulation factors (center) play a key role in regulating the complex set of reactions occurring in every aspect of rejection.

an adaptive immune response via germinal center reactions, typically days to weeks. Much like natural antibodies, the induced antibodies recognize components of the xeno-organ and, similar to HAR cause activation of the endothelial cells and their destruction via the complement system. The specific antibody binding also attracts multiple elements of the cellular immune system, such as NK cells and phagocytes, creating further damage of the target tissues and secreting soluble factors, such as cytokines and chemokines, which further enhance immune responses.

ACR includes predominantly cellular responses to the graft, such as T cell activation, which occur within days to weeks of organ transplant. Although ACR is well-established in allotransplant, the importance of ACR in the xenorejection response is not entirely clear. This may be due to either the more rapid activation of hematopoietic populations in HAR and AVR/AHXR compared with allotransplantation. However, some groups have proposed that reduction of the HAR and AVR/AHXR in earlier stages of xenorejection would unmask ACR which would otherwise be unnoticed amidst the earlier more pathogenic responses. In either case, ACR is expected to be substantially similar between allo- and xenotransplantation and thus more readily controlled by immunosuppressive drugs already in use for allotransplant.

CR is longer term, occurring within months or even years after transplantation. CR can be due to complications due to other immune activity, such as infection, or escape of humoral or cellular responses from immunosuppressive drug control. CR is well-understood in allotransplant and effective treatments are available for control and reversal of CR.

HAR and AVR/AHXR are the most unique and most critical to address in xenotransplantation. These earlier reactions can greatly enhance later reactions, with some of the mechanistic elements of the xenorejection response initiated even before the transplant surgery itself occurs. Therefore, it is essential to control the initiating events as early as possible in order to reduce the course of later responses. Much like the layers of an onion, removing one layer reveals the next, but as each layer is removed the overall size may be diminished.

The latter two responses, ACR and CR, are mechanistically similar between xeno- and allorejection responses [23]. Use of currently-available immunosuppressive drugs are believed to be able to control both responses as evidenced by the extensive data from allotransplants in humans. However, the speed and violence of the HAR and AVR reactions against xeno-organs can greatly accelerate and strengthen ACR and CR. Thus, even well-established treatments for allorejection may need to be reviewed as xenotransplantation proceeds toward clinical trials.

8. Innate and adaptive immunity in xenotransplantation

The immune system has two inter-related arms; the innate and the adaptive immune systems, both of which contribute to the rejection of xenotransplanted cells, tissues and organs. Although often described as separate, the systems have a large network of connections which are interdependent, and thus are not completely distinct. Both systems utilize multiple mechanisms to protect the host, creating a series of defense layers of increasing specificity. When functioning properly, a given layer may not be 100% efficient, but in aggregate will capture the overwhelming majority of pathogens. In addition, the ability to detect subtle differences between highly related cells has the potential benefit of identifying and eliminating cells with oncogenic mutations, preventing tumors before they have a chance to establish themselves [21].

8.1. The innate immune system and xenorejection

The innate immune system is evolutionarily ancient, with related mechanisms found in both plants and animals. The innate immune system consists of relatively invariant mechanisms for the identification of pathogens, and, although less specific, is extremely rapid and strong in response. The rapidity of the innate immune system provides an immediate barrier to pathogen infiltration and infection of the host, limiting the pathogen burden and giving the adaptive immune system time to develop more specific responses [24].

The use of physical barriers is one of the most critical elements of innate immunity. Although organ transplant bypasses the skin as a protective layer, the endothelium of the blood vessels, which connect the organ to the host circulatory system, remains as the main interface between the human hematopoietic system and xeno-organ tissues. As such, many of the immediate mechanisms of the innate response are greatly influenced by the interactions between the human immune cells and the porcine endothelial cells. Once the human innate immune system attacks the porcine endothelium, the barrier function is quickly lost, followed by rapid influx of human immune cells, pro-inflammatory infiltrates and edema, and then necrosis and destruction of the xeno-organ. It is important to note that the endothelium is an extremely active part of the immune response, which responds to soluble factor and cellular interactions to induce a variety of immune and inflammatory responses. Therefore, any efforts to improve the engraftment of xeno-organs must take into account the functional role of the endothelium in regulating the rejection response [25].

8.2. Inflammation

Inflammation is one of the earliest innate responses, driven by pattern recognition receptors found on human immune cells which recognize damage-associated molecular patterns (DAMPs). The binding and signaling of DAMPs causes the immediate secretion of proinflammatory mediators, such as cytokines and chemokines, which attract additional innate immune cells and induce a variety of local responses which would be highly beneficial during an infection but destructive to xeno-organs. For example, vasodilation and increased vascular permeability, which would normally allow host immune cells greater access to tissue to rapidly eliminate pathogens, instead causes the xeno-tissue to be more quickly infiltrated by human innate immune cells, which in turn leads to more inflammation and destruction. Similarly, there are blood-borne proteinaceous biochemical cascades activated by inflammation, such as the coagulation and the complement systems, which further degrade xeno-organ function and survival [26].

8.3. Xenoantigens

The genes encoded by the porcine genome can encode proteins that are substantially different from their human counterparts or may carry post-translational modifications which are not present in humans. Interestingly, some of these molecules, referred to as "xenoantigens", are recognized by pre-existing natural antibodies found in human serum. One subset of these antigens is the swine leukocyte antigens (SLA), which are the physical and functional equivalent of the human leukocyte antigens (HLA). Much like the case for human allotransplant, the SLA genes are highly diverse and individual patients will have a variable level of cross-reactive antibodies in their serum for a given set of SLA genes [27]. A separate group of xeno-antigens are glycan molecules, such as Gal alpha (1,3) Gal and Neu5Gc, which are expressed in porcine, but not human, cells [28].

Although specific induced antibodies are produced by B cells as part of the adaptive response, the presence of pre-existing antibodies in human serum contributes to the innate response. The specific reasons for the existence of these human natural antibodies are not entirely clear. In the case of glycan structures, one hypothesis is that the molecules are related to those found in pathogens, and that the natural antibodies are cross-reactive to each. Alternately, consumption of porcine materials in the human diet may induce antibody formation. Regardless of the specific source in human serum, xenotransplantion of porcine cells and tissues in humans leads to binding of these pre-existing natural antibodies, activation of complement and eventual destruction of target cells carrying the xenoantigens.

Several approaches have been taken to address xenoantigens, including cross-matching donors and recipients for reduced immunoreactivity, removal or modification of the xenoantigen from the donor pig, or the reduction of the ability of the antibodies to induce the complement cascade. In the first case, typing of patients and porcine donors to find the best matches would be very similar to the current system used for determining allotranplant cross-reactivity [29]. Use of gene targeting or editing technologies can eliminate the genes encoding SLA or the enzymes required for expression of the relevant glycan. This has been proven to be highly effective for ablating the genes GGTA1 (the gene encoding alpha 1,3-galactosyltransferase essential for Gal alpha (1,3) Gal), CMAH (cytidine monophosphate-N-acetylneuraminic acid hydroxylase critical for Neu5Gc biosynthesis) and B4GALNT2 (beta 1,4 N-acetylgalactosam inyltransferase). In each case, the elimination of the glycan leads to greatly reduced recognition of porcine cells by natural antibodies in human serum, and reduction in complement-mediated destruction [28]. Unfortunately, as the number of antibody targets increases there is a risk that one or more of the xenoantigens alone or in combination may have essential functions which cannot be eliminated without damaging the development or function of the pig. Therefore, efforts to introduce more subtle mutation in SLA which remove immunogenic epitopes while leaving critical antigen-presentation functions intact, or even replacement of SLA with HLA, may be more effective.

The second approach, which is often used in combination with the first, is to reset the threshold at which the complement cascade is activated, making it more difficult for the binding of human natural antibodies to targets on porcine cells to induce the complement cascade. There are a series of "complement regulatory proteins" (CRPs), such as CD46, CD55 and CD59, expressed on the cell surface which prevent complement activation by the inadvertent non-specific binding of human antibody to human cells [30]. By overexpressing one or more of the CRP molecules on the porcine endothelium, the amount of antibody binding required for complement activation is increased, which reduces the amount of antibody-mediated cell destruction due to human natural antibodies [31].

8.4. Coagulation

Inflammation and vascular leakage, due to loss of endothelial barrier function, both induce coagulation, which normally is required to repair localized endothelial damage. In the case of xenotransplantion, the attack of the endothelium is rapidly occurring at multiple sites, therefore, coagulation spreads throughout the blood vessels in the xeno-organ and can overcome the normal control mechanism. The thrombosis produced by the procoagulant environment leads to occlusion of the vessels within the graft, known as thrombotic microangiopathy (TM). The lack of blood flow results in hypoxia and tissue damage and necrosis, further complicating transplant function. The relatively greater amount of endothelial injury and coagulation in xenotransplant therefore creates more frequent and extensive TM and contributes to the more rapid destruction of the graft [32].

In addition to physiological pathways induced by human innate immune responses, there are non-physiological activities caused by mismatches between porcine and human constituents of the coagulation cascade [33]. For example, porcine von Willebrand factor (vWF) has been shown to bind more avidly to the human GP1b receptor and activate human platelets, leading to coagulation and rapid loss of platelets from the circulation [34]. Ongoing efforts seek to engineer porcine vWF to eliminate the inappropriate interactions with GP1b, while maintaining normal coagulative phenotypes. In addition, porcine proteins which provide positive and negative feedback to control the coagulation cascade do not function as efficiently upon the human coagulation targets, leading to dysregulation of the cascade. The targeting the porcine genome to express human regulatory proteins in porcine cells has been shown to help control human coagulation in response to exposure to the modified porcine materials [35].

8.5. Innate immune cells

Macrophages and neutrophils are two of the earliest host cell types to infiltrate xeno-organs. Both cell types are instrumental in the phagocytosis and destruction of pathogens during infection. During a xenorejection response, the damaged porcine cells release a variety of DAMPs which are recognized by the human innate cells, inducing phagocytic functions which further damage the xeno-organ and increasing production of additional proinflammatory and other immune mediators which attract more innate immune cells [36, 37].

Similar to the molecular mismatch described above for vWF and coagulation, macrophages express the SIRPA receptor, which must interact with the surface receptor CD47 to prevent the target cell destruction by the macrophage. Thus, the CD47 receptor expressed on the cell surface binds to SIRPA to instruct the macrophage not to consume the target cell. In the case of porcine CD47, the interaction with human SIRPA appears to be unproductive and cannot inhibit the macrophage activity. Expression of the human form of CD47 in porcine cells has been shown to greatly reduce human macrophage activity directed against the porcine cells [38].

NK cells are functionally analogous to cytolytic T cells, and even share some mechanistic pathways for targeted cell destruction. NK cells express a collection of stimulatory and inhibitory receptors on the cell surface, which engage conserved targets on the surface of target cells. The balance of activation and inhibition via combinatorial signaling determines whether the NK cells are stimulated to kill or ignore the target cell. The target cell receptors, such as HLA-E, may be perturbed by pathogens or tumorigenesis, which is detected by the NK cells and the target cells eliminated [39].

In the case of xenotransplantation, the porcine cell receptors, although expressed normally, are not sufficiently well-conserved with their human counterparts and thus cannot inhibit NK cell attack. By expressing on porcine cells the human versions of receptors which stimulate the inhibitory receptors on NK cells, the damage may be averted. With careful genetic modification, the normal mechanisms for detection of infection or other dysfunction may be maintained, allowing normal NK functions while eliminating the xeno-specific destruction [40, 41].

8.6. Resolution of innate immune responses

There are a variety of mechanisms used to resolve innate immune reactions. Many of the soluble mediators of innate immunity have extremely short half-lives which allows them to dissipate quickly. In addition, immune receptors become increasingly desensitized to further stimulation during the course of the innate response, reducing reactions. A variety of negative regulators are also produced to further inhibit the innate effectors. All of these mechanisms are in place to prevent over-reaction of the immune system and the destruction that it can cause once the pathogenic threat has been eliminated [42]. In the case of a xenorejection response, however, the "threat" that is recognized comes from every porcine cell and thus the innate response is never fully resolved without intervention. It may be possible to take advantage of these resolution mechanisms to create porcine cells with an enhanced ability to curtail or end a human inflammatory response through careful genetic modification.

8.7. The adaptive immune system and xenorejection

The adaptive immune system is comprised of cellular and antibody components which recognize pathogens and develop highly specific responses, which can increase in specificity and effectiveness over time and exposure. The adaptive immune response also creates immunological "memory" to allow more rapid reactions should similar pathogens be encountered in the future. Because of the time required to develop specific responses, the adaptive immune system generally becomes more critical after the initial innate immune response [21].

8.8. Antigen presentation and T cells

Antigen presentation is a crucial mechanistic part of the adaptive immune response and plays a major role in the decision between immunity and tolerance for a given target. There are two main routes for antigen presentation to the immune system, reflective of the different classes of pathogen antigens, intracellular or extracellular.

Intracellular antigens, either natural cellular proteins or those derived from viral or bacterial infection of cells, are enzymatically cleaved into peptides which bind to the ubiquitously expressed class I human lymphocyte antigens (HLA). The peptide-HLA class I complex is displayed on the cell surface where it can be surveyed by the binding of cytolytic T cells expressing T cell receptors (TCR) and CD8 co-receptors on the T cell surface. Similar to antibodies, TCRs are assembled combinatorially, creating a diversity of specificities for HLA-peptide complexes, with only a small subset of TCRs binding to a given complex. Should a given CD8 T cell be activated by the HLA-peptide complex, it will express a series of cytolytic molecules which kill the target cell. This system works due to the efficient T cell selection mechanisms applied during T cell development. After initial production of a rearranged TCR, the nascent T cell is tested in the thymus for inappropriate reactivity against cellular antigens. If the T cell survives the selection process, it exits to the body and theoretically will only be activated when it encounters and antigen that does not naturally exist in body, such as a peptide from a pathogenic organism, or a mutant peptide from an oncogenic cell [43].

Extracellular antigens can be any molecule taken up by a cell from its environment and degraded in lysosomes intracellularly. The resulting peptides are then loaded onto HLA class II molecules which, unlike HLA class I, are expressed on only a subset of immune-related cells. The class II HLA-peptide complex is recognized by a different T cell subset expressing TCRs with the co-receptor CD4. The CD4 T cell subset also undergoes thymic selection as observed with CD8 T cells, to eliminate recognition of self-antigens [44]. However, CD4 T cells can be induced to create different phenotypes once they specifically recognize class II HLA-peptide complexes. A large variety of T cell subsets have been described, including production of helper T cells, which participate in the activation of B cells for the production of antigen-specific antibodies, or regulatory T cells, which act to inhibit the immune response [45]. The choice of outcomes is driven by the soluble mediators, such as cytokines, found in the local environment, and the collection of co-receptors expressed on the antigen presenting cells.

HLA itself is a significant direct contributor to rejection responses outside of its role in antigen presentation. As described above, T cells are selected for lack of recognition of self-antigens. This not only includes the recognition of self-peptides bound to HLA molecules, but of the HLA molecules themselves. Normally, T cells bearing TCRs with inappropriately high affinity for binding HLA molecules, even in the absence of peptide, are eliminated early in T cell development. Because the human T cells have not been exposed to, or selected by, the class I or II swine lymphocyte antigens (SLA), a subset of human TCRs will bind to SLA and induce strong T cell activation, regardless of the peptide presented in the SLA [46]. As porcine cells are attacked by the human immune system, donor peptides are efficiently presented by human cells via HLA to human T cells as part of the normal human adaptive response. Conversely, depending upon the organ transplanted, there can also be donor T cells and antigen presenting cells transferred which result in donor immune responses against the host tissues, referred to as graft versus host disease (GvHD) [47]. In all cases, the immune cells are responding normally, but in the setting of xenotransplantation can be extremely pathogenic due to the artificially high concentration of immunogenic targets present.

Because HLA matching is part of organ selection in allotransplantation, a frequent question is whether introduction of human HLA in place of porcine SLA would help overcome rejection. Although SLA ablation may be helpful in averting antibody-dependent damage, this approach does not resolve some of the challenges related to antigen presentation in xenorejection responses [29]. It is true that the human T cell binding directly to pig SLA could be eliminated by substitution of SLA with HLA, however, the HLA genes are highly polymorphic, hence the need to HLA match human patients. This means that for a given patient, a donor pig would need to be engineered to specifically express the HLA homologous to that patient, which would be limiting given the timelines necessary for production and validation of genetically-modified pigs. In addition, in the normal situation human cells display human peptides in the HLA, the overwhelming majority of which will be conserved between a human donor and recipient, and thus much less likely to induce a response. If pigs were engineered to express human HLA which is perfectly matched to the patient, the donor porcine cells could now be significantly more efficient at displaying porcine peptides to the human immune system and more rapidly induce T cell activation. Therefore, introduction of human HLA in place of porcine SLA may not provide a benefit without additional engineering.

Humans possess a number of pre-existing antibodies specific for porcine antigens which can contribute to the xeno-organ damage during HAR. As the donor tissue is damaged, the antigens are released and presented to T cells as described above, causing the activation of helper T cells. These T cells interact with B cells in lymphoid organs, inducing the activation of any B cells which express antibodies specific for the xeno-antigens. This initiates the germinal center reaction, in which antigen-specific B cells rapidly proliferate and mutate their antibody sequences and are then progressively selected for improved antibody function. The resulting B cells expressing the affinity-matured antibodies exit the germinal center and can differentiate further to plasma cells, which act as factories that can produce extraordinarily high levels of serum antibody [48]. These induced antibodies, like natural antibodies, further amplify AVR/AHXR and contribute to the destruction of the xeno-organ.

The *de novo* production of antibodies can be quite rapid and are a risk for the lifetime of the transplant whether for allo- or xenotransplantation. There are a number of drugs available for the control of B cell reactions. One of the most effective approaches is the depletion of B cells using antibody therapeutics such as Rituxan, specific for the CD20 surface molecule [49]. However, the constitutive ablation of host B cells will create long term immunosuppression and could be prohibitively expensive. Although highly related to CR in allotransplant, the B cell responses in xenotransplant are stronger and more challenging and likely to require more stringent therapeutic control.

9. Immune suppression and tolerance in xenotransplantation

Advancements in understanding of immune mechanisms in immune rejection have elucidated a number of targets and pathways for intervention, and discovered a variety of small molecule and protein therapeutics for the suppression and manipulation of the immune system. However, the restraint of the immune system required to prevent xeno-organ rejection places the patient at significant risk of infections, tumors and other diseases which are preventable by an intact immune system. Therefore, there is a growing interest in the application of immune tolerance mechanisms in the transplant setting.

Immune tolerance is the natural unresponsiveness of the immune system to targets which may otherwise create an immune response. As mentioned previously, there are many mechanisms used by the immune system to identify non-self-antigens to prevent autoimmune diseases. As the body of literature regarding the molecular basis of immune tolerance has grown, interest in testing tolerance mechanisms in xenotransplantation has also increased [50].

Mixed chimerism is one route that has shown significant promise in both allo- and xeno-transplant settings. This approach combines the transfer to the recipient of both the organ and hematopoietic cells from the donor. Typically, the patient is pre-treated with radiation or drugs to allow hematopoietic cell engraftment prior to the organ transplant. The combination of hematopoietic cells from host and donor allows cross-tolerance of host immune cells to donor tissue as well as donor immune cells to host tissue. Therefore, the resulting immune system is a combination of the donor and host, or a "mixed chimera," which recognizes the donor organ and host tissue as "self" despite the differences in genetic origin [51].

A further refinement of mixed chimerism includes transplant of donor thymus into the recipient, allowing selection of host T cells via donor antigen presentation [52], suggesting that tolerance is T cell dependent. A large body of evidence points to the role of regulatory T cells (Treg) as a driver of immune tolerance. Treg cells are antigen-specific but upon binding of the specific HLA-peptide complex on antigen-presenting cells will produce a variety of immune inhibiting and tolerogenic factors. The Treg cells may be derived from either thymus selection (central tolerance) or selection in tissues (peripheral tolerance), with central tolerance believed to be more durable, and the conceptual basis for donor thymus transplantation in mixed chimerism [53].

A critical factor in the maintenance of tolerance is the balance between Treg and effector T cells over time. Any imbalance that increases the number of effector T cells can rapidly lead to immune rejection. If indeed the Treg population is the main active component of immune tolerance, then it may be desirable to specifically bolster the numbers of Treg cells transferred to the recipient to more greatly ensure that the balance is biased firmly toward tolerance. A number of groups have established protocols for the generation of Treg cells that are specific for xeno-organs and tissues through *in vitro* selections and expansions [54]. While this has been shown to have positive effects in allograft tolerance, the durability is variable and, worse, some studies have described conversion of Treg to effector T cells which then contribute to rejection [55]. Despite these concerns, mixed chimerism, with or without Treg supplementation, remains a potentially valuable approach to immune tolerance.

10. Genome engineering to improve xenotransplantation

The progress of xenotransplantation research in recent times has closely paralleled the advancement in genome engineering technologies. As the complexity of the engineering toolsets has increased, so too has the complexity of porcine genomic manipulations increased to address the immunological challenges described in previous sections.

Complex mammalian genome engineering has advanced much more rapidly in mice than in virtually any other species, including pigs. The reason for the rapid progress in mice is the availability of embryonic stem (ES) cells which can be maintained in culture for extended periods time and undergo extensive transfection/transduction protocols and drug selection without losing the ability to produce large numbers of fertile progeny via blastocyst injection [56]. Although several labs have made strides in this area, similarly manipulable and viable ES cells are not currently available for routine use in the generation of cloned pigs [57].

The most common approach for production of genetically-modified pigs is very similar to the protocol described in the creation of "Dolly the sheep." Briefly, the nucleus from a pig cell carrying the desired genome changes is extracted and introduced into a pig oocyte, which has previously had its own nucleus removed, and then induced to initiate embryogenesis using electrical and chemical induction, a process referred to as somatic cell nuclear transfer (SCNT). The newly-created cells are implanted into surrogate female pigs and allowed to develop to birth. Compared to genetically-modified mouse production, this process is significantly less efficient and more costly, limiting the number of facilities capable of effectively carrying out this complex process [58].

A key factor in the success of SCNT is the source of the donor nucleus. These cells are typically primary cells derived from fetal sources. Extended culture, transfection, or drug selection of these donor cells can all cause a significant loss of viability for subsequent productive SCNT. Therefore, the approaches commonly used for mouse ES cell manipulation such as multigenic targeting and selections with various drugs over long periods in culture would not allow for production of modified pigs using SCNT. Similarly, any genome manipulations of pig cells must also maintain the viability of the cells for SCNT, which alters the approaches available compared with mice.

10.1. Gene knockouts

One of the earliest genome engineering approaches applied to pigs was introduction of gene knockouts (KO). For any given gene, mutations which remove or disrupt the coding sequence can eliminate the expression of the gene and, provided that the KO is not lethal, create an organism which is entirely missing the gene product. The introduction of gene KO technology has been a key factor in the rapid advancement of the field of xenotransplantation [59].

As discussed above, there are several glycan molecules present in pigs which are absent in humans. These glycans are recognized by antibodies present in human serum which leads to rapid and extensive antibody-mediated damage to the porcine cells. Therefore, the elimination of the specific carbohydrate structures should help prevent human antibody recognition of the pig tissues. Unlike protein antigens which are directly coded by the DNA, glycosylation is due to the action of enzymes which create post-translational modifications of a variety of proteins produced by the cell. Therefore, glycosylation pathways must be examined to identify the key enzyme that creates the immunogenic glycan while otherwise leaving cellular metabolism intact.

The GGTA1 gene is responsible for creating the Gal alpha (1,3) Gal epitope in pigs. Although the specific reasons for this are unclear, human patients can express high levels of antibody specific for the Gal alpha (1,3) Gal epitope, presenting a major challenge to xenotransplantation [60]. The KO of the GGTA1 gene is one of the earliest genetic modifications of pigs for application in xenotransplantation, and results in greatly reduced human antibody recognition of porcine cells [61]. However, elimination of the GGTA1 gene alone has been shown to be insufficient due to a variety of other xenoantigens present in pig cells which are recognized by antibodies present in human serum. Generation of KO of CMAH [62], B4GALNT2 [28] and other xenoantigen genes have further decreased the reactivity of porcine cells to human serum. However, it is important to keep in mind that the greater the number of gene KO, especially when made in combination, may lead to detrimental effects on pig health.

10.2. Gene insertions

The use of gene KO approaches is highly useful for eliminating xenoantigens but does not address the need for expression of human or synthetic versions of genes necessary for control or proper function of dysregulated pathways. This requires the ability to permanently introduce heterologous DNA into the genome in a manner which maintains gene function.

The initial approach to gene insertions was simply random integration of DNA into the target genome. These genes are introduced from elsewhere and thus termed "transgenes" (TG). Once the ability to introduce DNA into mammalian cells was established using a variety of technological approaches, it became clear that over long-term culture a subset of cells could be isolated which have permanently incorporated the heterologous DNA. Because many transgenes do not provide a straightforward means to identify cells which have incorporated foreign DNA from the population that have not, TGs often include genes encoding drug resistance markers. In order for cells to survive drug treatment they must incorporate the resistance gene, greatly reducing the population to be screened, and increasing the chance of identifying cells which incorporate the TG of interest along with the drug resistance gene [63].

The integration of transgenes is rapid but relatively uncontrolled. Although there may be some preferences for integration site based upon chromatin accessibility, these are hard to predict and may be related to DNA breakage sites at which repair mechanisms fortuitously insert the transgene DNA [64]. The random nature of the insertions can create risks. For example, the same transgene inserted at different sites can yield highly variable results in expression. Furthermore, some insertions may be deleterious to cell function, causing them to grow more slowly or die off, or, if these cells are used for generation of animals *in vivo*, there is a possibility of insertions creating mutations, instability or even lethality.

Due to the risks of random integration, significant effort has focused on protocols to create targeted integration, or gene knock-in (KI), of heterologous DNA into the genome. This is accomplished in mice by taking advantage of ES cells which undergo homologous recombination. In this approach, the transgene of interest is flanked by DNA sequences that are identical to regions of the genome to be targeted. After introduction of the heterologous DNA, the regions of DNA sequence identity are aligned with the target sequence and the homologous recombination machinery creates crossover events to switch the endogenous sequence with the heterologous sequence. This approach is much less efficient than random integration of TG, therefore drug selection schemes often need to be employed to identify the relatively rare targeting events [64].

Homologous recombination is well-established for targeting in mice but requires ES cells which express the enzymes necessary for the targeting event. Unfortunately, porcine ES cells are not available that both possess homologous recombination function and can reliably generate cloned animals. For reasons that are not entirely clear, generation of ES cells competent for homologous recombination and cloning seems to be challenging for most species other than mice [57]. Therefore, alternate approaches are required for targeted integration in the pig genome [65].

10.3. Tools for genome engineering

A number of novel enzymatic molecules have been created which help resolve the dilemma of targeted integration in porcine cells. Zinc Finger Nucleases (ZFN), Transcription Activator-Like Effector Nuclease (TALEN) and Clustered Regularly Interspaced Short Palindromic Repeats (CRISPR) are all synthetic molecules based on genuine proteins which allow the precise targeting of genomic DNA based upon sequence [66–68]. In each case there are two functional components, a targeting module which recognizes a specific genomic sequence, and an enzymatic module which introduces a double-stranded DNA break at the target site. In the case of ZFN and TALEN, the targeting module is a complex array of protein sequences which have previously been shown to recognize specific DNA sequences and can be mixed in a modular way to bind to any desired sequence. Although both technologies have shown great success, the effort and cost required to identify a single functional molecule can be significant. In contrast, the relatively more recently recognized CRISPR, and related prokaryotic systems, is much more easily applied in mammalian cells. The DNA binding module in this case is RNA base-pairing to provide sequence specificity. The enzymatic module cleaves DNA, creating a double strand break similar to ZFN and TALEN. When heterologous DNA is present, the cellular repair machinery may use the synthetic DNA to repair the break, inserting the TG at the desired genomic site. It is important to note that all of these systems, ZFN, TALEN or CRISPR, are essentially the same in that they introduce double strand DNA breaks at a selected site in the genome and do not directly affect the rate of DNA insertion. Therefore, it is often necessary to include selection schemes for identification of the modified cells. The greater efficiency and ease of use of these systems, CRISPR in particular, has allowed targeted insertion of DNA into genomes that were not previously able to be modified [69].

Due to the challenges of creating genomic modifications in porcine primary cells while maintaining their viability for SCNT, more efficient engineering methods are desirable. One approach to enhance efficiency is to target a specific region of DNA, called a landing pad, with multiple genes at once. By inserting a DNA vector bearing multiple therapeutic genes at once, a large amount of breeding and testing can be circumvented using a single event. This approach has the added advantage of avoiding inefficient crossbreeding necessary to bring loci from distinct chromosomes together in one lineage. When combined with the use of tools such as ZFN, TALEN and CRISPR more rapid progress in the genetic modification of animals has been greatly facilitated [70].

11. Conclusions and future prospects

The increasing sophistication and accessibility of genome engineering toolsets and deeper understanding of immunological rejection mechanisms has allowed greater advancement in xenotransplantation than ever before. A key question is just how many genetic changes are required in order to make a pig organ suitable for transplantation? While the critical experimental data needed for such an assessment is still accumulating, it is clear that the number of alterations required for one organ may be different from another. For example, xeno-hearts with relatively minimal genetic modifications have demonstrated months to years survival in transplantation studies with non-human primates, whereas xeno-lungs with more extensive modifications have yet to survive more than a few weeks. This is due to the relative differences in structure and function of organs, the resilience to trauma, and susceptibility to rejection responses. Furthermore, tolerance mechanisms may be able to supplant the need for some genetic modifications, and thus the specific protocols and treatments will govern the ultimate complement of alterations.

The immediate need in xenotransplantation is to define the specific genetics required for xeno-organ survival, however, it is possible to project further enhancements such that porcine organs may be superior to human organs for human transplant. Synthetic biology approaches have created novel genetic circuits which can react in real time to human immune responses, inducing counter-reactions in the porcine cells to circumvent and tolerize the xeno-organ against human rejection. Furthermore, xeno-organs may be engineered to express protein therapeutics to further control human immunity while saving hundreds of thousands of dollars in expensive biotherapeutic treatments. Thus, the first version of pigs appropriate for xenotransplantation are likely to be further refined and improved to create increasingly useful rejection-free organs.

Author details

Sean Stevens

Address all correspondence to: sean_m_stevens@yahoo.com

Synthetic Genomics, Inc., La Jolla, CA, USA

References

[1] Roux FA, Sai P, Deschamps JY. Xenotransfusions, past and present. Xenotransplantation. 2007;**14**(3):208-216

[2] Gibson T. Zoografting: The early, early years. British Journal of Plastic Surgery. 1955;**8**(3):234-242

[3] Princeteau M. Greffe renale. Journal de Medicine de Bordeaux. 1905;**26**:549

[4] Jaboulay M. Greffe de reins au pli coude par soudres artielles et veincuses. Lyon Médical. 1906;**107**:575

[5] Unger E. Nierentransplantation. Klinische Wochenschrift. 1910;**47**:573

[6] Neuhof H. The Transplantation of Tissues. New York: Appleton and Co.; 1923. p. 260

[7] Hamilton D. The Monkey Gland Affair. London: Chatto and Windus; 1986

[8] Lee RA. The Bizarre Careers of John R. Brinkley. Lexington, KY: University Press of Kentucky; 2002

[9] Reemstma K, McCracken BH, Schlegel JU, Pearl MA, Pearce CW, DeWitt CW, Smith PE, Hewitt RL, Flinner RL, Creech O. Renal transplantation in man. Annals of Surgery. 1964;**160**:384

[10] Blagg CR. The early history of dialysis for chronic renal failure in the United States: A view from Seattle. American Journal of Kidney Diseases. 2007;**49**(3):482-496

[11] Hume D. Discussion of paper by Reemtsma and others. Annals of Surgery. 1964;**160**:384

[12] Hardy JD, Chavez CM, Kurrus FD, Neely WA, Erasian S, Turner MD, Fabian LW, Labecki TD. Heart transplantation in man. Journal of the American Medical Association. 1964;**188**:1132

[13] Starzl TE, Marchioro TL, Peters GN, Kirkpatrick CH, Wilson WE, Porter KA, Rifkind D, Ogden DA, Hitchcock CR, Waddell WR. Renal heterotransplantation from baboon to man: Experience with 6 cases. Transplantation. 1964;**2**:752-776

[14] Starzl TE, Fung J, Tzakis A, Todo S, Demetris AJ, Marino IR, Doyle H, Zeevi A, Warty V, Michaels M. Baboon-to-liver transplantation. Lancet. 1993;**341**(8837):65-71

[15] Bailey LL, Nehlsen-Cannarella SL, Concepcion W, Jolly WB. Baboon-to-human cardiac xenotransplantation in a neonate. Journal of the American Medical Association. 1985;**254**(23):3321-3329

[16] Editorial. US guidelines on xenotransplantation. Nature Medicine. 1999;**5**:465

[17] Fishman JA, Patience C. Xenotransplantation: Infectious risk revisited. American Journal of Transplantation. 2004;**4**:1383-1390

[18] Yung GLP, Rieben R, Buhler L, Schuurman HJ, Seebach JD. Xenotransplantation: Where do we stand in 2016? Swiss Medical Weekly. 2017;**147**:w14403

[19] Cooper DKC, Pierson RN, Hering BJ, Mohiuddin MM, Fishman JA, Denner J, Ahn C, Azimzadeh AM, Buhler LH, Cowan PJ, Hawthorne WJ, Kobayashi T, Sachs DH. Regulation of clinical xenotransplantation-time for a reappraisal. Transplantation. 2017;**101**(8): 1766-1769

[20] Pullen LC. Xenotransplantation: Time to get excited? American Journal of Transplantation. 2017;**17**(12):2995-2996

[21] Delves PJ, Martin SJ, Burton DR, Roitt IM, editors. Roitt's Essential Immunology. United Kingdom: Wiley-Blackwell; 2017

[22] Samstein B, Platt JL. Physiologic and immunologic hurdles to xenotransplantation. Journal of the American Society of Nephrology. 2001;**12**:182-193

[23] Cooper DKC, Ayares D. The immense potential of xenotransplantation in surgery. International Journal of Surgery. 2011;**9**:122-129

[24] Medzhitov R, Janeway CA. Innate immunity: The virtues of a nonclonal system of recognition. Cell. 1997;**91**:295-298

[25] Bach FH, Robson SC, Ferran C, Winkler H, Millan MT, Stuhlmeier KM, Vanhove B, Blakely ML, van der Werf WJ, Hofer E. Endothelial cell activation and thromboregulation during xenograft rejection. Immunological Reviews. 1994;**141**:5-30

[26] Ezzelarab MB, DKC C. Systemic inflammation in xenograft recipients (SIXR): A new paradigm in pig-to-primate xenotransplantation? International Journal of Surgery. 2015;**23**(Pt B):301-305

[27] Barreau N, Godfrin Y, Bouhours JF, Bignon JD, Karam G, Leteissier E, Moreau A, Dantal J, Menoret S, Anegon I, Imbert BM, Brouard S, Soulillou JP, Blancho G. Interaction of anti-HLA antibodies with pig xenoantigens. Transplantation. 2000;**69**(1):148-156

[28] Estrada JL, Martens G, Li P, Adams A, Newell KA, Ford ML, Butler JR, Sidner R, Tector M, Tector J. Evaluation of human and non-human primate antibody binding to pig cells lacking GGTA1/CMAH/β4GalNT2 genes. Xenotransplantation. 2015;**22**(3):194-202

[29] Martens GR, Reyes LM, Butler JR, Ladowski JM, Estrada JL, Sidner RA, Eckhoff DE, Tector M, Tector AJ. Humoral reactivity of renal transplant-waitlisted patients to cells from GGTA1/CMAH/B4GalNT2, and SLA class I knockout pigs. Transplantation. 2017;**101**(4):e86-e92

[30] Kim DD, Song WC. Membrane complement regulatory proteins. Clinical Immunology. 2006;**118**(2-3):127-136

[31] McCurry KR, Kooyman DL, Alvarado CG, Cotterell AH, Martin MJ, Logan JS, Platt JL. Nature Medicine. 1995;**1**(5):423-427

[32] Houser SL, Kuwaki K, Knosalla C, Dor FJ, Gollackner B, Cheng J, Shimizu A, Schuurman HJ, Cooper DK. Thrombotic microangiopathy and graft arteriopathy in pig hearts following transplantation into baboons. Xenotransplantation. 2004;**11**(5):416-425

[33] Robson SC, Cooper DK, d'Apice AJ. Disordered regulation of coagulation and platelet activation in xenotransplantation. Xenotransplantation. 2000;**7**(3):166-176

[34] Lau CL, Cantu E 3rd, Gonzalez-Stawinski GV, Holzknecht ZE, Nichols TC, Posther KE, Rayborn CA, Platt JL, Parker W, Davis RD. The role of antibodies and von Willebrand factor in discordant pulmonary xenotransplantation. American Journal of Transplantation. 2003;**3**(9):1065-1075

[35] Cowan PJ, Robson SC, d'Apice AJ. Controlling coagulation dysregulation in xenotransplantation. Current Opinion in Organ Transplantation. 2011;**16**(2):214-221

[36] Korsgren O. Acute cellular xenograft rejection. Xenotransplantation. 1997;**4**(1):11-19

[37] Wang H, Yang YG. Innate cellular immunity and xenotransplantation. Current Opinion in Organ Transplantation. 2012;**17**(2):162-167

[38] Yang YG. CD47 in xenograft rejection and tolerance induction. Xenotransplantation. 2010;**17**(4):267-273

[39] Stringaris K, Barrett AJ. The importance of natural killer cell killer immunoglobulin-like receptor-mismatch in transplant outcomes. Current Opinion in Hematology. 2017;**24**(6):489-495

[40] Seebach JD, Waneck GL. Natural killer cells in xenotransplantation. 1997;**4**(4):201-211

[41] Weiss EH, Lilienfeld BG, Müller S, Müller E, Herbach N, Kessler B, Wanke R, Schwinzer R, Seebach JD, Wolf E, Brem G. HLA-E/human beta2-microglobulin transgenic pigs: Protection against xenogeneic human anti-pig natural killer cell cytotoxicity. Transplantation. 2009;**87**(1):35-43

[42] Serhan CN, Savill J. Resolution of inflammation: The beginning programs the end. Nature Immunology. 2005;**6**(12):1191-1197

[43] Neefjes J, Jongsma ML, Paul P, Bakke O. Towards a systems understanding of MHC class I and MHC class II antigen presentation. Nature Reviews. Immunology. 2011;**11**(12):823-836

[44] Pieters J. MHC class II-restricted antigen processing and presentation. Advances in Immunology. 2000;**75**:159-208

[45] Zhu J, Yamane H, Paul WE. Differentiation of effector CD4 T cell populations. Annual Review of Immunology. 2010;**28**:445-489

[46] Davila E, Byrne GW, LaBreche PT, McGregor HC, Schwab AK, Davies WR, Rao VP, Oi K, Tazelaar HD, Logan JS, McGregor CG. T-cell responses during pig-to-primate xenotransplantation. Xenotransplantation. 2006;**13**(1):31-40

[47] Ferrara JLM, Deeg HJ. Graft-versus-host disease. The New England Journal of Medicine. 1991;**324**:667-674

[48] Shlomchik MJ, Weisel F. Germinal center selection and the development of memory B and plasma cells. Immunological Reviews. 2012;**247**(1):52-63

[49] Feugier P. A review of rituximab, the first anti-CD20 monoclonal antibody used in the treatment of B non-Hodgkin's lymphomas. Future Oncology. 2015;**11**(9):1327-1342

[50] Vagefi PA, Shah JA, Sachs DH. Progress towards inducing tolerance of pig-to-primate xenografts. International Journal of Surgery. 2015;**23**(Pt B):291-295

[51] Griesemer A, Yamada K, Sykes M. Xenotransplantation: Immunological hurdles and progress toward tolerance. Immunological Reviews. 2014;**258**(1):241-258

[52] Barth RN, Yamamoto S, LaMattina JC, Kumagai N, Kitamura H, Vagefi PA, Awwad M, Colvin RB, Cooper DK, Sykes M, Sachs DH, Yamada K. Xenogeneic thymokidney and thymic tissue transplantation in a pig-to-baboon model: I. Evidence for pig-specific T-cell unresponsiveness. Transplantation. 2003;**75**(10):1615-1624

[53] Sakaguchi S, Miyara M, Costantino CM, Hafler DA. FOXP3+ regulatory T cells in the human immune system. Nature Reviews. Immunology. 2010;**10**(7):490-500

[54] Muller YD, Golshayan D, Ehirchiou D, Wekerle T, Seebach JD, Bühler LH. T regulatory cells in xenotransplantation. Xenotransplantation. 2009;**16**(3):121-128

[55] Tang Q, Vincenti F. Transplant trials with Tregs: Perils and promises. The Journal of Clinical Investigation. 2017;**127**(7):2505-2512

[56] Capecchi MR. Gene targeting in mice: Functional analysis of the mammalian genome for the twenty-first century. Nature Reviews. Genetics. 2005;**6**(6):507-512

[57] Wheeler MB. Development and validation of swine embryonic stem cells: A review. Reproduction, Fertility, and Development. 1994;**6**(5):563-568

[58] Wilmut I, Beaujean N, de Sousa PA, Dinnyes A, King TJ, Paterson LA, Wells DN, Young LE. Somatic cell nuclear transfer. Nature. 2002;**419**(6907):583-586

[59] Tai HC, Ezzelarab M, Hara H, Ayares D, Cooper DK. Progress in xenotransplantation following the introduction of gene-knockout technology. Transplant International. 2007;**20**(2):107-117

[60] Galili U. The α-Gal epitope (Galα1-3Galβ1-4GlcNAc-R) in xenotransplantation. Biochimie. 2001;**83**(7):557-563

[61] Phelps CJ, Koike C, Vaught TD, Boone J, Wells KD, Chen SH, Ball S, Specht SM, Polejaeva IA, Monahan JA, Jobst PM, Sharma SB, Lamborn AE, Garst AS, Moore M, Demetris AJ, Rudert WA, Bottino R, Bertera S, Trucco M, Starzl TE, Dai Y, Ayares DL. Production of alpha 1,3-galactosyltransferase-deficient pigs. Science. 2003;**299**(5605):411-414

[62] Cimeno A, Hassanein W, French BM, Powell JM, Burdorf L, Goloubeva O, Cheng X, Parsell DM, Ramsoondar J, Kuravi K, Vaught T, Uluer MC, Redding E, O'Neill N, Laird C, Hershfeld A, Tatarov I, Thomas K, Ayares D, Azimzadeh AM, Pierson RN 3rd, Barth RN, LaMattina JC. N-glycolylneuraminic acid knockout reduces erythrocyte sequestration and thromboxane elaboration in an ex vivo pig-to-human xenoperfusion model. Xenotransplantation. 2017;**24**(6):e12339

[63] Clarke AR, editor. Transgenesis Techniques. Totowa, NJ: Humana Press; 2002

[64] Smith K. Theoretical mechanisms in targeted and random integration of transgene DNA. Reproduction, Nutrition, Development. 2001;**41**(6):465-485

[65] Wells KD, Prather RS. Genome-editing technologies to improve research, reproduction, and production in pigs. Molecular Reproduction and Development. 2017;**84**(9):1012-1017

[66] Urnov FD, Rebar EJ, Holmes MC, Zhang HS, Gregory PD. Genome editing with engineered zinc finger nucleases. Nature Reviews. Genetics. 2010;**11**(9):636-646

[67] Mahfouz MM, Li L, Shamimuzzaman M, Wibowo A, Fang X, Zhu JK. De novo-engineered transcription activator-like effector (TALE) hybrid nuclease with novel DNA binding specificity creates double-strand breaks. Proceedings of the National Academy of Sciences of the United States of America. 2011;**108**(6):2623-2628

[68] Eid A, Mahfouz MM. Genome editing: The road of CRISPR/Cas9 from bench to clinic. Experimental & Molecular Medicine. 2016;**48**(10):e265

[69] Kim JS. Genome editing comes of age. Nature Protocols. 2016;**11**(9):1573-1578

[70] Fischer K, Kraner-Scheiber S, Petersen B, Rieblinger B, Buermann A, Flisikowska T, Flisikowski K, Christan S, Edlinger M, Baars W, Kurome M, Zakhartchenko V, Kessler B, Plotzki E, Szczerbal I, Switonski M, Denner J, Wolf E, Schwinzer R, Niemann H, Kind A, Schnieke A. Efficient production of multi-modified pigs for xenotransplantation by 'combineering', gene stacking and gene editing. Scientific Reports. 2016;**6**:29081

11

Experimental Brain Death Models in Liver Transplantation

Maria Eugenia Cornide-Petronio,
Araní Casillas-Ramírez,
Mónica B. Jiménez-Castro and Carmen Peralta

Abstract

Most organs for transplantation are currently procured from brain-dead donors; however, brain death is an important risk factor in liver transplantation. In addition, to counteract the shortage of liver grafts, transplant centers accept the use of sub-optimal livers, which may show higher risk of primary non-function or initial poor function. Very few literatures exist regarding liver transplantation using brain-dead donors, or about brain death and its effects on sub-optimal grafts in such surgical situation. This chapter aims to describe the pathophysiological changes occurring in liver grafts during brain death and focuses on the strengths and limitations of experimental models used to study the effect of brain death on optimal and sub-optimal (specially steatotic) liver grafts. Depending on the use of experimental models that simulate as much as possible the surgical conditions present in clinical practice, therapeutic strategies designed in animal models could be more successfully translated to the bedside.

Keywords: liver transplantation, ischemia-reperfusion injury, brain death, experimental models

1. Introduction

Liver transplantation (LT) has evolved to become a standard therapy for certain end-stage liver diseases [1]. Nowadays, 80% of organs come from donors who have suffered brain trauma (brain-dead donors) [1–4]. Brain death (BD) has been defined as the irreversible loss of brain and brain stem function, usually caused by major hemorrhage, hypoxia or metabolic dysregulation [5, 6]. Hemodynamic events, hormonal changes and inflammation and immune activation occur consequently to BD [6–9]. It has been described that BD markedly reduces the tolerance of liver grafts to preservation and reperfusion injury and reduces graft survival [2–4, 10]. The detrimental consequences of BD have been clinically described; however the underlying mechanisms and their relevance in LT remain poorly understood. Indeed, few studies have evaluated the effect of BD on LT, and most of the experimental studies focused in establishing surgical or pharmacological strategies to reduce liver graft damage associated with transplantation have been performed in the absence of BD [6].

Shortage of donor organs remains a major obstacle to the widespread application of LT in patients with end-stage liver disease [11–14]. To overcome this problem, transplant centers developed strategies to expand the organ donor pool [15]. This shortage could be alleviated by routine use of sub-optimal donor livers including elderly donors, steatotic donors, split livers and donor with viral infections or with malignancy. These sub-optimal livers exhibit a greater risk of organ dysfunction and primary non-function compared with optimal livers, when used as grafts in transplantation [1, 4, 9]. Multiple methods are currently being investigated to minimize the effects of ischemia-reperfusion (I/R) injury to allow the use of sub-optimal liver grafts, including anti-inflammatory approaches to attenuate cytokines, blockade of adhesion molecules, antiapoptotic strategies, among others. However, these studies are performed in non-BD surgical conditions. Only a recent study describes, for the first time, a potential treatment in steatotic liver grafts undergoing LT from cadaveric donors [1].

Since consequences of BD are linked to an inferior graft function and a more potent immune response, studies in animal models could be critical in uncovering its basic mechanisms and to provide a rationale for the development of novel targets that may prevent the deteriorating consequences of BD in clinical practice [16]. Virtually, all experimental organ transplantation studies generally utilize young, healthy living animals as donors; in clinical practice; however, a relatively low percentage of organs are acquired from living sources. Among other variables, the difference between living and brain-dead donors includes the effect of profound physiological and structural derangements [17]. Although a wide variety of animal BD models have been used to study the effect of BD on donor organ quality (without transplantation) [18–26], the lack of standardization of BD models makes difficult to compare results from different research groups. Undoubtedly, there is a need for a more controlled and standardized BD model allowing studies of organs in a situation closely resembling the reality in the intensive care unit [27].

In the first part of this chapter, we highlight the actual knowledge and new insights into the pathophysiology in BD focusing on liver graft undergoing transplantation. Following, the different experimental models reported in literature used to study the effect of BD on quality of optimal and sub-optimal liver grafts are presented, focusing on the strengths and limitations. Since recognize the underlying mechanisms of detrimental effects of BD is a critical question to design therapeutic strategies to protect liver grafts undergoing transplantation, we discuss if the existing BD animal models mimic the clinical findings in transplants with BD donors, and highlight which BD model could be more appropriated.

2. Effects of brain death on liver graft undergoing transplantation

Liver I/R injury is a local proinflammatory response mediated by the immune system. The central nervous system plays a fundamental role in the regulation of molecular markers triggering inflammation and tissue damage, and BD results in a breakdown of these mechanisms, hence initiating the cascade of I/R injury liver transplants and exacerbating the hepatic damage caused by I/R [9]. However, although the detrimental consequences of BD have been clinically described, the underlying mechanisms and their relevance in LT remain poorly understood [6]. Following, systemic events that happen after BD and the specific effects of BD on hepatic graft undergoing transplantation are presented.

BD is followed immediately by an acute and transient rise in blood pressure (Cushing reflex), that is immediately followed by a transient bradycardia communicated through parasympathetic activation [16, 24, 28–31]. Later after BD, deteriorating hemodynamics and a compromised perfusion of abdominal organs is becoming evident. Accordingly, a shift from aerobic to anaerobic metabolism and acidosis is registered, clinically reflected by elevated serum levels of lactate and free fatty acids and promoted by decreasing insulin secretion and hyperglycemia [21, 32, 33]. Alterations of specific mitochondrial functions may lead to an impaired production of ATP and a reduced uptake of substrates for mitochondrial metabolism and eventually limit resistance and survival of cells and organs to damaging insults [34]. It is well known that ATP degradation during hepatic ischemia leads to an acceleration of glycolysis [35]. Although glycolysis is essential for cell survival, it may also be detrimental because of the accumulation of glycolytic products such as lactate [35]. In the liver, the increase in cAMP levels due to ischemia triggers the activation of glycolysis. This causes the accumulation of hexose 6-phosphates, which proceed down the glycolytic pathway to form lactate [35–38]. Some authors [39] have shown that normotensive BD had no influence on the general viability of the liver, as measured by ATP content. In this research work, no differences were found in ATP content in livers from BD-induced rats and control rats, implicating that the phase of BD up to 6 h does not reduce general liver viability. However, it has also been described that the ATP content after 3 h of reoxygenation after graft harvesting was significantly increased in liver biopsies from brain-dead rats, may be because of a stress response, caused by increased catecholamine levels induced by BD and exaggerated reoxygenation times of liver tissues, exacerbating the I/R injury [39].

Hemodynamic instability, hormonal alterations, blood coagulation factor consumption, lung tissue changes, hypothermia, and electrolyte disturbance generated by BD invariably influence hepatic functions. Increased AST and ALT concentrations indicated liver dysfunction in brain-dead pigs and hepatocyte edema, hepatic sinusoid compression, and other microscopic observations in such animals demonstrated damage to liver cells [40, 41]. Also, BD causes time-dependent general dysfunction in rats, as indicated by elevated LDH and creatinine, AST and α-GST levels [42]. The disruption of liver function seems to be due to circulatory collapse and hemodynamic instability [41]. Morphological changes in the liver following BD are even less well defined. Recent experimental findings show that hepatocytes in livers from brain-dead donors show an altered cell membrane permeability and integrity [17, 43]. It has also been reported increased caspase-3 activity indicating that apoptosis occurs in liver tissue of brain-dead donors [3].

A systemic inflammatory response is present in most patients at the diagnosis of BD [44]. The intense cellular and molecular activation that quickly follows the acute onset of BD involves acute transcriptional upregulation of inflammatory cytokines, both on a systemic and intra-organ level [16]. In liver, aside from microcirculatory changes, early effects of I/R injury and BD are mediated via Kupffer cells. When I/R injury occurs, Kupffer cells and neutrophils are activated, together with an increased expression of adhesion molecules and infiltration of monocytes and lymphocytes [9, 45]. Cell death by necrosis and apoptosis is initiated. In addition to mitochondrial damage, synthesis of oxygen-free radicals is boosted and accompanied by a decreasing activity of antioxidant enzymes. All of this results in immediate organ damage, contributing to hepatic failure after transplantation. In BD models many of these events have been also documented, exacerbating the hepatic damage that already occurs by I/R. In this sense, expression of adhesion molecules in endothelial and epithelial cells, initiating the release of proinflammatory cytokines and the infiltration of immune competent cells is induced by BD [16, 46–50]. VCAM-1 expression was found after 6 hours of BD in both hypotensive and normotensive donors. The pattern of VCAM-1 expression was similar to that described by others during periods of inflammation or rejection of the liver. Also, the ICAM-1 expression observed in all brain-dead rats was similar to expression patterns during episodes of inflammation [42, 51–55]. Leukocyte recruitment to the underlying parenchyma was facilitated, as expected, with upregulated VCAM-1 and ICAM-1 expression, with a significant increase in infiltrating leukocytes in the liver tissue of brain-dead rats. Also, naive as well as activated macrophages (i.e., ED1- and ED2-positive cells) were significantly increased in brain-dead donors versus controls [42]. The detrimental changes observed during experimental BD were confirmed in more limited clinical studies. Inflammatory changes were found in cadaveric donor livers that showed increased proportion of CD3+ lymphocytes, CD68+ monocytes, and macrophages relative to livers from living donors [33, 56, 57]. Clinical events after BD included more frequent acute rejection episodes and increased lymphocytic infiltrates [33, 56]. In human liver transplants, donor BD triggered upregulation of inflammatory cytokines IL-6, IL-10, TNF-α, TGFβ, IFN-γ, and MIP-1α. Those findings correlated with more pronounced cellular infiltrates, a higher incidence of primary graft dysfunction, and frequent acute rejection episodes [16, 58]. Findings in small animal models of BD parallel clinical observations [16], for instance upregulation of IL-10 and iNOS mRNA in liver has been demonstrated after 6 h of BD [39]. On the contrary, another study has not found iNOS induction in brain-dead animals. This contradictory result may be explained by the fact that the phase of BD in this later study was maintained for only 2–3 h [39].

3. Experimental models used to study the effect of brain death on liver graft quality

Future research in experimental models of LT using BD donors is required to understand the pathophysiology of BD and elucidate the consequences of BD on graft function and survival [6]. The knowledge of the underlying mechanisms on the detrimental effects of BD is a critical question to promote better preservation of the organ and to improve outcome after LT [1].

A wide variety of BD models have been described in the literature, and in most of them an increase in intracranial pressure is generated by an expanding intracranial balloon, finally leading to BD [26]. This section will discuss about experimental animal models used to evaluate the effects of BD on optimal and steatotic liver grafts.

3.1. Experimental BD in small animals

Irreversible pontine ischemia is the essential hallmark of experimental BD. As hemodynamic instabilities related to cardiovascular collapse may bias experimental results, invasive monitoring is important for accurate determination of volume and maintenance of physiological blood pressure. The initial spike in blood pressure during brain stem herniation, apnea, and transient spontaneous reflexes with subsequent absence of spinal reflexes are characteristic criteria of the central catastrophe in experimental models of BD [16, 24, 28, 29, 31, 59]. To produce BD in small laboratory animals, a Fogarty balloon catheter (2–4 French) is inserted through a parietal bore hole into the subdural space and inflated. Reported inflation volumes for induction of the condition range from 200 to 500 μL in rats and 80–103 μL in mice. The inflated balloon catheter is left in place during the entire period of observation to avoid intracerebral hemorrhage and hemodynamic collapse. Computerized axial tomography or magnetic resonance imaging in brain-dead animals can document that the catheter inflation causes the hindbrain to herniate through the foramen magnum [16, 21, 28, 29, 60, 61]. Two types have been described: the so-called 'sudden onset' BD model and the 'gradual onset' model. In the gradual onset model described by [26], induction of BD was started by gradually increasing the intracranial pressure by inflating the balloon with 16 μL saline per minute. During balloon inflation, a hypotensive period occurred followed by a short peak and a subsequent drop in blood pressure. When the blood pressure returned to its basal level during an increasing peak, inflation of the balloon was stopped and anesthesia was withdrawn. The state of BD was confirmed 30 min after the onset of BD, by the absence of corneal reflexes and a positive apnea test, and such condition was maintained during 1 h or for 4 h [26]. In contrast to the sudden onset model, the gradual onset model simulates cerebral hemorrhage by slowly increasing the intracranial pressure, resulting in less hemodynamic instability and maintenance of normotension during BD for several hours. So far, only a few studies in abdominal organs have described BD induction using a gradual expansion of an intracranial balloon [24, 26].

Authors using a sudden onset model of BD [60] have demonstrated upregulations of proinflammatory markers in different organs, including the liver. BD was produced by rapid balloon inflation of a Fogarty arterial embolectomy catheter introduced into the subdural space through an occipital burr hole; this maneuver suddenly increases intracranial pressure and causes herniation of the brain stem within 20 min in all animals. The rats were tracheostomized and mechanically respirated for periods up to 6 h. [60]. Authors conclude that the experimental system described provides a potentially clinically relevant model in which to study the systemic effects of BD in detail and suggests means to prevent changes in peripheral organs [60]. Thus, it has been postulated that sudden onset BD reflects the situation of the hemodynamically instable donors [23]. In a sudden onset' BD model described by [23], through a frontolateral trepanation a balloon catheter was introduced in the subdural space with the tip pointing caudally. Inflating the balloon for 1 min increased the intracranial pressure thereby inducing rapid progressive brain injury leading to BD, which was based on the sharp rise and subsequent drop of blood pressure and heart rate. The state of BD was confirmed 30 min after induction by the absence of corneal reflexes and an apnea test and the effect of BD was studied at 1 h and 6 h after BD induction [23]. Hemodynamic changes in this model, mimicking acute isolated cerebral trauma, included first a sudden increase and subsequently a gradual drop of both heart rate and mean arterial pressure [23]. This BD model appears to be a reliable tool to mimic the type of fast occurring brain injury due to isolated cerebral trauma in man. In this BD model that reflects the situation of the hemodynamically instable donor, expression of immediate early genes was found in tissues of liver and kidney coinciding with progressive dysfunction of these organs and suggest a progressive detrimental effect of BD on donor organ quality, especially in livers from hemodynamically instable donors [23].

In these experimental models described above, only the effect of induction of BD on liver tissue was evaluated. Unfortunately, the other conditions (ischemia and reperfusion) that are present in the clinical practice of transplantation were not included. It is important to evaluate such conditions, since they negatively affect liver grafts already damaged by BD when these grafts, especially steatotic ones, are obtained from cadaveric donors.

Given the prevalence of hepatic steatosis in the population, this represents a large potential pool of donors. However, the clinical problem is still unresolved as steatotic livers are more susceptible to I/R injury and, when used, have poorer outcome than non-steatotic livers [6]. To date, only one experimental study has evaluated the effect of BD on optimal and steatotic liver grafts, which were subsequently subjected to cold ischemia and transplantation. In such research [1], authors have tested the influence of hepatic steatosis and BD separately and in combination in an experimental model of LT [1]. A balloon catheter was introduced through the drill hole in the extradural space with the tip pointing caudally. The intracranial pressure was increased by inflating the balloon for 1 min. The increase in intracranial pressure induced rapid brain injury, leading to immediate BD, simulating a condition comparable to acute isolated cerebral trauma in humans. The state of BD was confirmed by the absence of corneal reflexes and an apnea test and liver grafts were extracted from donors at 6 h after the induction of BD [1]. Steatotic and non-steatotic liver grafts were preserved during 6 h and then were transplanted and submitted to reperfusion for 4 h. Authors report for the first time that the injurious effects of BD in LT are exacerbated in the presence of hepatic steatosis and occur before liver grafts are retrieved from donors [1]. In addition, the mechanisms responsible for the detrimental effects of BD were different depending of the type of the liver, which would interfere with protective pharmacological or surgical strategies applied in liver grafts, avoiding its potential benefits [6]. In such a study, BD-induced dysfunction in the cholinergic anti-inflammatory pathway and prevented the benefits induced by ischemic preconditioning, a surgical strategy that shows benefits when it is applied in non-BD clinical situations. In fact, the study indicated that the combination of acetylcholine and ischemic preconditioning could be considered as a feasible and easy-to-perform intervention to reduce the adverse effects of BD and improve the quality of liver grafts. So authors propose that the time frame between the declaration of BD and organ retrieval provides an important window for cytoprotective intervention, which may counteract the detrimental effects of BD [1].

Table 1 summarizes the experimental models used in small animals to study the effect of BD on liver graft quality.

3.2. Experimental BD in large animals

In the baboon, BD is produced by creating intracranial hypertension. Under full inhalation anesthesia, a Foley catheter was introduced into the subdural space through a frontal burr hole in the skull and filled with 20–30 mL of saline, then BD occurred within 20 min [62, 63]. BD has been also induced in pigs by ligation of both brachiocephalic arteries, from which arise the carotid and vertebral arteries. Both experimental models of BD led to a series of major pathophysiological changes that may be collectively referred to as the autonomic storm. Though there was a brief initial period of excessive parasympathetic activity, evidenced by a marked bradycardia, most of the effects of this autonomic activity were brought about by the sympathetic nervous system [63].

Porcine BD models have been widely used in transplant surgery studies. A research group [64] performed a study with a lengthening of the induction phase to 60 min with gradual epidural balloon inflation up to 15 mL. Furthermore, they suggested that prolonged BD process might give the necessary preconditions to trigger a systemic inflammatory response that might contribute to organ dysfunction. Compared to the clinical situation, other authors [27] considered that 60 min was still a relatively short time. They therefore wanted to prolong the BD induction phase up to 200 min by stepwise increase of intracranial volume, followed by a 30-min observation period. Analysis of the monitoring results showed a classic intracranial pressure-volume relationship. Furthermore, intracranial compliance decreased gradually when intracranial pressure increased, which reflects a decreasing ability to compensate for added intracranial volume [27]. The described so-called Cushing response with arterial blood pressure increase, bradycardia, and respiratory irregularities was also demonstrated [27]. Authors believe that their model has the advantage of applying gradual progressive changes in intracranial pressure, cerebral perfusion pressure, and brain tissue oxygenation, leading to cellular injury in parenchymatous organs. Therefore, the model provides the possibility

Small animals

Article	Type of BD	Time of sustained BD	Support during BD	Cold ischemia
Ref. [1]	Sudden	6 h	Ventilation	6 h
Ref. [23]	Sudden	1 or 6 h	Ventilation	Not realized
Ref. [26]	Gradual	1 or 4 h	Ventilation Inotropic support	Not realized
Ref. [31]	Gradual and sudden	6 h	Ventilation	Not realized
Ref. [42]	Sudden	1 or 6 h	Ventilation Inotropic support	Not realized
Ref. [60]	Sudden	6 h	Ventilation	Not realized

Table 1. Experimental models in small animals used to study the effect of BD on liver graft quality.

of studying the effects of BD processes on organ quality and function as well as outcomes after transplantation. Furthermore, the model also may be used for explorative studies of brain injury mechanisms and for evaluating new neuromonitoring devices [27]. In another experimental model [65], BD has been induced by surgically placing an epidural balloon and gradually increasing the inflation to increase intracranial pressure to 15, 25, 35 and 45 mm Hg, maintaining each pressure level for 30 min, in piglets [65]. However, opposite results in comparison with the experimental model using a BD induction phase of 200 min [27] were observed, this means a decrease of the arterial blood pressure and tachycardia. The reason for this difference is unclear, but it is well-known from the clinical situation that a Cushing response is not always observed in patients with BD developing [27].

More recently, [66] have established a clinically relevant, reproducible, large animal model of BD in pigs, based on a controlled cerebral hemorrhage. To induce intracranial hemorrhage, a needle was inserted through a burr hole over the left hemisphere, and stereotaxically placed in the internal capsule at the level of the lateral ventricle. Blood was withdrawn from the central arterial catheter in a 10 ml unheparinized syringe and then was injected in the brain with a rate of 40 ml/h. The infusion of blood continued for 60 min to maintain an intracranial pressure sufficient to ensure BD. Pigs in the control group underwent surgical preparations similar to the BD group, including burr holes and tissue glue but without injection of blood. Computerized tomographic angiography was performed 120–180 min after BD [66]. Irreversible damage to the brain stem was validated by a negative atropine test, disappearance of corneal and pupillary light reflexes, and a negative cerebral perfusion pressure sustained for more than 60 min. The disappearance of intracranial pulse pressure waves supports the diagnosis, as this is a clinical parameter associated with BD [66].

Further investigations will be required to investigate whether all of these experimental models of BD above mentioned are adequate to study the effect of BD on a graft that also presents I/R injury and which one best simulates the conditions present in clinical practice.

Another experimental model of BD in large animals has been reported [67], which has been previously established and neuropathologically validated [19, 67]. In this model the effect of BD on liver grafts also undergoing cold preservation and transplantation was evaluated. BD was induced suddenly by the injection of 8–17 ml of normal saline solution into the catheter balloon over a period of 5–10 min using dogs as experimental animals. This produced a sudden rise in arterial blood pressure (systolic and diastolic) and heart rate, reflecting an explosive intracranial pressure increase and defined as the "Cushing reflex" [67]. Once the diagnosis of BD was established, the dog was monitored for 16 h before the liver was removed [67]. Livers were stored floating in 1000 ml of the UW preservation solution at 4°C for 24 h [67] and at the end of the preservation time, the livers were transplanted orthotopically using a modified technique with a sutured upper caval anastomosis and cuffed anastomoses for the infrahepatic vena cava and the portal vein [67]. Although not all the clinical scenario of BD could be replicated, this experimental model simulates the sudden rise in intracranial pressure caused by acute cerebrovascular lesions or traumatic brain injury [67]. As reflected by the hepatic enzyme release during the course of BD, no evidence of deterioration of function in livers retrieved from BD donors was found. These findings are different from rodent models. In addition, it should be borne in mind that in clinical practice it is well documented that BD negatively

Large animals				
Article	**Type of BD**	**Time of sustained BD**	**Support during BD**	**Cold ischemia**
Ref. [27]	Gradual	1 h	Ventilation	Not realized
Ref. [64]	Gradual	6 h	Ventilation	Not realized
Ref. [65]	Gradual	30 or 60 min	Not described	Not realized
Ref. [66]	Gradual	8 h	Not described	Not realized
Ref. [67]	Sudden	6, 12 and 16 h	Inotropic support	27 h

Table 2. Experimental models in large animals used to study the effect of BD on liver graft quality.

affects the function of liver grafts that are procured from a cadaveric donor and subsequently transplanted [68]. Therefore, to achieve a successful design of therapeutic strategies to protect liver grafts against harmful effects of BD, it is important to take into account only experimental models in which the negative effects of BD on the liver tissue have been demonstrated.

Table 2 summarizes the experimental models in large animals used to study the effect of BD on liver graft quality.

4. Conclusions

Most organs for transplantation originate from BD donors. Although the detrimental consequences of BD have been clinically described, the underlying mechanisms and their relevance in transplantation remain poorly understood. Indeed, few studies have evaluated the effect of BD on transplantation, and, as stated along this chapter, most of the experimental studies focused in the pathophysiological changes occurring during BD without transplantation. Moreover, these studies have been performed in the different sudden and gradual BD models, so dissimilar results on pathophysiological changes and treatments have been described.

Comparison of the results of animal studies and their extrapolation to human beings is feasible, but with limitations such as differences in BD and ischemia tolerance, anatomy of the liver of various species, surgical conditions used in clinical practice and those used in the experimental models. Importantly, studies performed in small animals are of limited applicability to human beings due to their different size and anatomy of the liver and their faster metabolism. Large animals exhibit greater similarity in their anatomy and physiology to humans; however, their use is restricted by serious logistical and financial difficulties, ethical concerns and limited availability of immunological tools for use in large animal species. In addition, in some cases, experimental models of BD in large animals did not mimic the clinical conditions in liver transplantation from BD. Despite the limitations of the experimental animal models, these are the best options to study hepatic I/R, especially considering that the progress of human studies is slow, the majority of human tissues are not routinely accessible for research, and there is very limited opportunity for interventional studies. The clinical application of strategies

Clinical effects	Sudden model		Gradual model	
	Small animals	Large animals	Small animals	Large animals
Release of catecholamines [7]	Observed [31]	Not described	Few [31]	Not described
Hemodinamic deterioring [16, 24, 28–31]	Acute [1, 18, 23, 42]	Observed [67]	Few [24, 26]	Observed [27] Not observed [65]
Hormonal alterations [33, 63]	Observed [1]	Not described	Not described	Not described
Inflammatory response [44]	Observed [60]	Observed [63]	Observed [26]	Few [64, 66]
Inotropic support [33]	Applied [1, 42]	Applied [67]	Not necessary [26, 31]	Not described

Table 3. Reproducible clinical effects of brain death in the different experimental models.

designed at benchside will depend on the use of experimental models of BD that resemble as much as possible the clinical conditions that happens in BD and LT [69]. **Table 3** summarizes the reproducible clinical effects of BD that happens in the different experimental models.

We recognize the complication, but future research in similar experimental models of transplantation using BD donors is required to understand the pathophysiology of BD and elucidate the consequences of BD, especially in sub-optimal liver grafts. Thus, multidisciplinary research groups should devote additional efforts to better understand the pathophysiology of BD to ultimately develop effectual therapeutic strategies aimed at improving graft viability, and at significantly increasing the organ donor pool.

Acknowledgements

This research was supported by the Ministerio de Economía y Competitividad (project grant SAF-2015-64857-R) Madrid, Spain; the European Union (FondosFeder, "unamanera de hacer Europa"); by CERCA Program/Generalitat de Catalunya; by the Secretariad'Universitats i Recerca (Grant 2017SGR-551) Barcelona, Spain; and the ConsejoNacional de Ciencia y Tecnología (CONACYT) (Fondo Sectorial de Investigaciónpara la Educación, Grant 257743), México. MECornide-Petronio has a Sara Borrell contract from the Instituto de Salud Carlos III (Grant CD15/00129), Madrid, Spain. MB Jiménez-Castro has a contract from the Programa de Promocióndeltalento y suempleabilidad from the Ministerio de Economía y Competitividad (Grant EMP-TU-2015-4167), Madrid, Spain.

Author details

Maria Eugenia Cornide-Petronio[1†], Araní Casillas-Ramírez[2,3†], Mónica B. Jiménez-Castro[4] and Carmen Peralta[1,5,6*]

*Address all correspondence to: cperalta@clinic.ub.es

1 Institut d'Investigacions Biomèdiques August Pi i Sunyer (IDIBAPS), Barcelona, Spain

2 Hospital Regional de Alta Especialidad de Ciudad Victoria "Bicentenario 2010", Ciudad Victoria, Mexico

3 Facultad de Medicina e Ingeniería en Sistemas Computacionales de Matamoros, Universidad Autónoma de Tamaulipas, Mexico

4 Transplant Biomedicals, S.L., Barcelona, Spain

5 Centro de Investigación Biomédica en Red de Enfermedades Hepáticas y Digestivas (CIBEREHD), Barcelona, Spain

6 Facultad de Medicina, Universidad International de Cataluña, Barcelona, Spain

†Both authors contributed equally to this work

References

[1] Jiménez-Castro MB, Meroño N, Mendes-Braz M, Gracia-Sancho J, Martínez-Carreres L, Cornide-Petronio ME, Casillas-Ramirez A, Rodés J, Peralta C. The effect of brain death in rat steatotic and non-steatotic liver transplantation with previous ischemic preconditioning. Journal of Hepatology. 2015;**62**:83-91. DOI: 10.1016/j.jhep.2014.07.031

[2] van der Hoeven JA, Lindell S, van Schilfgaarde R, Molema G, Ter Horst GJ, Southard JH, Ploeg RJ. Donor brain death reduces survival after transplantation in rat livers preserved for 20 hr. Transplantation. 2001;**72**:1632-1636

[3] van der Hoeven JA, Moshage H, Schuurs T, Nijboer M, Van Schilfgaarde R, Ploeg RJ. Brain death induces apoptosis in donor liver of the rat. Transplantation. 2003;**76**:1150-1154. DOI: 10.1097/01.TP.0000080983.14161.95

[4] Kotsch K, Francuski M, Pascher A, Klemz R, Seifert M, Mittler J, Schumacher G, Buelow R, Volk HD, Tullius SG, Neuhaus P, Pratschke J. Improved long-term graft survival after HO-1 induction in brain-dead donors. American Journal of Transplantation. 2006;**6**:477-486. DOI: 10.1111/j.1600-6143.2005.01208.x

[5] Wijdicks EF, Varelas PN, Gronseth GS, Greer DM. Evidence-based guideline update: Determining brain death in adults: Report of the Quality Standards Subcommittee of the American Academy of Neurology. Neurology. American Academy of Neurology. 2010;**74**:1911-1918. DOI: 10.1212/WNL.0b013e3181e242a8

[6] Jiménez-Castro MB, Gracia-Sancho J, Peralta C. Brain death and marginal grafts in liver transplantation. Cell Death & Disease. 2015;**6**:e1777. DOI: 10.1038/cddis.2015.147

[7] Berman M, Ali A, Ashley E, Freed D, Clarke K, Tsui S, Parameshwar J, Large S. Is stress cardiomyopathy the underlying cause of ventricular dysfunction associated with brain death? The Journal of Heart and Lung Transplantation. 2010;**29**:957-965. DOI: 10.1016/j.healun.2010.04.008

[8] Manara AR, Murphy PG, O'Callaghan G. Donation after circulatory death. British Journal of Anaesthesia. 2012;**108**(Suppl 1):i108-i121. DOI: 10.1093/bja/aer357

[9] Dziodzio T, Biebl M, Pratschke J. Impact of brain death on ischemia/reperfusion injury in liver transplantation. Current Opinion in Organ Transplantation. 2014;**19**:108-114. DOI: 10.1097/MOT.0000000000000061

[10] Cornide-Petronio ME, Negrete-Sánchez E, Mendes-Braz M, Casillas-Ramírez A, Bujaldon E, Meroño N, Martínez-Carreres L, Gracia-Sancho J, Rodés J, Jiménez-Castro MB, Peralta C. The effect of high-mobility group box 1 in rat steatotic and nonsteatotic liver transplantation from donors after brain death. American Journal of Transplantation. 2016;**16**:1148-1159. DOI: 10.1111/ajt.13560

[11] Uchiyama H, Yanaga K, Nishizaki T, Soejima Y, Yoshizumi T, Sugimachi K. Effects of deletion variant of hepatocyte growth factor on reduced-size liver transplantation in rats. Transplantation. 1999;**68**:39-44

[12] Selzner N, Selzner M, Tian Y, Kadry Z, Clavien PA. Cold ischemia decreases liver regeneration after partial liver transplantation in the rat: A TNF-alpha/IL-6-dependent mechanism. Hepatology. 2002;**36**:812-818. DOI: 10.1053/jhep.2002.35535

[13] Samstein B, Emond J. Liver transplants from living related donors. Annual Review of Medicine. 2001;**52**:147-160. DOI: 10.1146/annurev.med.52.1.147

[14] Franco-Gou R, Peralta C, Massip-Salcedo M, Xaus C, Serafín A, Roselló-Catafau J. Protection of reduced-size liver for transplantation. American Journal of Transplantation. 2004;**4**:1408-1420. DOI: 10.1111/j.1600-6143.2004.00532.x

[15] Emre S, Umman V. Split liver transplantation: An overview. Transplantation Proceedings. 2011;**43**:884-887. DOI: 10.1016/j.transproceed.2011.02.036

[16] Floerchinger B, Tilney NL, Tullius SG. Pathophysiology of brain death in small animal models. In: Novitzky D, Cooper DKC, editors. The Brain-Dead Organ Donor: Pathophysiology and Management. Springer Science+Business Media New York; 2013. pp. 55-64. DOI: 10.1007/978-1-4614-4304-9_6

[17] Pratschke J, Neuhaus P, Tullius SG. What can be learned from brain-death models? Transplant International. 2005;**18**:15-21. DOI: 10.1111/j.1432-2277.2004.00018.x

[18] Shivalkar B, Van Loon J, Wieland W, Tjandra-Maga TB, Borgers M, Plets C, Flameng W. Variable effects of explosive or gradual increase of intracranial pressure on myocardial structure and function. Circulation. 1993;**87**:230-239. DOI: 10.1161/01.CIR.87.1.230

[19] Bittner HB, Kendall SW, Campbell KA, Montine TJ, Van Trigt PA. Valid experimental brain death organ donor model. The Journal of Heart and Lung Transplantation. 1995;**14**:308-317

[20] Chen EP, Bittner HB, Kendall SW, Van Trigt P. Hormonal and hemodynamic changes in a validated animal model of brain death. Critical Care Medicine. 1996;**24**:1352-1359

[21] Herijgers P, Leunens V, Tjandra-Maga TB, Mubagwa K, Flameng W. Changes in organ perfusion after brain death in the rat and its relation to circulating catecholamines. Transplantation. 1996;**62**:330-335

[22] Okamoto S, Corso CO, Nolte D, Rascher W, Thiery J, Yamaoka Y, Messmer K. Impact of brain death on hormonal homeostasis and hepatic microcirculation of transplant organ donors. Transplant International. 1998;**11**(Suppl 1):S404-S407. DOI: 10.1111/j.1432-2277.1998.tb01168.x

[23] van der Hoeven JA, Ploeg RJ, Postema F, Molema I, de Vos P, Girbes AR, van Suylichem PT, van Schilfgaarde R, Ter Horst GJ. Induction of organ dysfunction and up-regulation of inflammatory markers in the liver and kidneys of hypotensive brain dead rats: A model to study marginal organ donors. Transplantation. 1999;**68**:1884-1890

[24] Pratschke J, Wilhelm MJ, Kusaka M, Laskowski I, Tilney NL. A model of gradual onset brain death for transplant-associated studies in rats. Transplantation. 2000;**69**:427-430

[25] Sawauchi S, Marmarou A, Beaumont A, Tomita Y, Fukui S. A new rat model of diffuse brain injury associated with acute subdural hematoma: Assessment of varying hematoma volume, insult severity, and the presence of hypoxemia. Journal of Neurotrauma. 2003;**20**:613-622. DOI: 10.1089/089771503322144536

[26] Kolkert JL, 'tHart NA, van Dijk A, Ottens PJ, Ploeg RJ, Leuvenink HG. The gradual onset brain death model: A relevant model to study organ donation and its consequences on the outcome after transplantation. Laboratory Animals. 2007;**41**:363-371

[27] Purins K, Sedigh A, Molnar C, Jansson L, Korsgren O, Lorant T, Tufveson G, Wennberg L, Wiklund L, Lewén A, Enblad P. Standardized experimental brain death model for studies of intracranial dynamics, organ preservation, and organ transplantation in the pig. Critical Care Medicine. 2011;**39**:512-517. DOI: 10.1097/CCM.0b013e318206b824

[28] Avlonitis VS, Wigfield CH, Kirby JA, Dark JH. The hemodynamic mechanisms of lung injury and systemic inflammatory response following brain death in the transplant donor. American Journal of Transplantation. 2005;**5**:684-693. DOI: 10.1111/j.1600-6143.2005.00755.x

[29] Atkinson C, Varela JC, Tomlinson S. Complement-dependent inflammation and injury in a murine model of brain dead donor hearts. Circulation Research. 2009;**105**:1094-1101. DOI: 10.1161/CIRCRESAHA.109.194977

[30] Paton JF, Dickinson CJ, Mitchell G. Harvey cushing and the regulation of blood pressure in giraffe, rat and man: Introducing 'Cushing's mechanism. Experimental Physiology. 2009;**94**:11-17. DOI: 10.1113/expphysiol.2008.043455

[31] Pomper G, Trescher K, Santer D, Hasun M, Baumgartner A, Adelmann K, Inci M, Dietl W, Zuckermann AO, Podesser BK. Introducing a mouse model of brain death. Journal of Neuroscience Methods. 2010;**192**:70-74. DOI: 10.1016/j.jneumeth.2010.07.019

[32] Novitzky D, Cooper DK, Morrell D, Isaacs S. Change from aerobic to anaerobic metabolism after brain death, and reversal following triiodothyronine therapy. Transplantation. 1988;**45**:32-36

[33] Floerchinger B, Oberhuber R, Tullius SG. Effects of brain death on organ quality and transplant outcome. Transplantation Reviews (Orlando, Fla.). 2012;**26**:54-59. DOI: 10.1016/j.trre.2011.10.001

[34] Vendemiale G, Grattagliano I, Caraceni P, Caraccio G, Domenicali M, Dall'Agata M, Trevisani F, Guerrieri F, Bernardi M, Altomare E. Mitochondrial oxidative injury and energy metabolism alteration in rat fatty liver: Effect of the nutritional status. Hepatology. 2001;**33**:808-815. DOI: 10.1053/jhep.2001.23060

[35] Jiménez-Castro MB, Casillas-Ramirez A, Massip-Salcedo M, Elias-Miro M, Serafin A, Rimola A, Rodes J, Peralta C. Cyclic adenosine 3′,5′-monophosphate in rat steatotic liver transplantation. Liver Transplantation. 2011;**17**:1099-1110. DOI: 10.1002/lt.22359

[36] Hers HG, Hue L. Gluconeogenesis and related aspects of glycolysis. Annual Review of Biochemistry. 1983;**52**:617-653

[37] Peralta C, Bartrons R, Riera L, Manzano A, Xaus C, Gelpí E, Roselló-Catafau J. Hepatic preconditioning preserves energy metabolism during sustained ischemia. American Journal of Physiology. Gastrointestinal and Liver Physiology. 2000;**279**:G163-G171. DOI: 10.1152/ajpgi.2000.279.1.G163

[38] Nogueira-Machado JA, Lima e Silva FC, Medina LO, Costa DC, Chaves MM. Modulation of the reactive oxygen species (ROS) generation mediated by cyclic AMP-elevating agents or interleukin 10 in granulocytes from type 2 diabetic patients (NIDDM): A PKA-independent phenomenon. Diabetes & Metabolism. 2003;**29**:533-537. DOI: 10.1016/S1262-3636(07)70068-X

[39] Olinga P, van der Hoeven JA, Merema MT, Freund RL, Ploeg RJ, Groothuis GM. The influence of brain death on liver function. Liver International. 2005;**25**:109-116. DOI: 10.1111/j.1478-3231.2005.01035.x

[40] Timek T, Vahl CF, Bonz A, Schäffer L, Rosenberg M, Hagl S. Triiodothyronine reverses depressed contractile performance after excessive catecholamine stimulation. The Annals of Thoracic Surgery. 1998;**66**:1618-1625. DOI: 10.1016/S0003-4975(98)00764-4

[41] Zhu C, Li J, Zhang G, Zhang Y, Zhai W, Shi J, Li Z, Li J, Zhang S. Brain death disrupts structure and function of pig liver. Transplantation Proceedings. 2010;**42**:733-736. DOI: 10.1016/j.transproceed.2010.02.028

[42] van der Hoeven JA, Ter Horst GJ, Molema G, de Vos P, Girbes AR, Postema F, Freund RL, Wiersema J, van Schilfgaarde R, Ploeg RJ. Effects of brain death and hemodynamic status on function and immunologic activation of the potential donor liver in the rat. Annals of Surgery. 2000;**232**:804-813. DOI: 10.1097/00000658-200012000-00009

[43] Toyama H, Takada M, Suzuki Y, Kuroda Y. Brain death-induced expression of ICAM-1 and VCAM-1 on rat hepatocytes. Hepato-Gastroenterology. 2003;**50**:1854-1856

[44] Barklin A, Hvas CL, Toennesen E. The inflammatory response to brain death. In: Novitzky D, Cooper DKC, editors. The Brain-Dead Organ Donor: Pathophysiology and Management. Springer Science+Business Media. New York; 2013. pp. 107-119. DOI: 10.1007/978-1-4614-4304-9_9

[45] Lentsch AB, Kato A, Yoshidome H, McMasters KM, Edwards MJ. Inflammatory mechanisms and therapeutic strategies for warm hepatic ischemia/reperfusion injury. Hepatology. 2000;**32**:169-173. DOI: 10.1053/jhep.2000.9323

[46] Saikumar P, Dong Z, Weinberg JM, Venkatachalam MA. Mechanisms of cell death in hypoxia/reoxygenation injury. Oncogene. 1998;**17**:3341-3349. DOI: 10.1038/sj.onc.1202579

[47] Kusaka M, Pratschke J, Wilhelm MJ, Ziai F, Zandi-Nejad K, Mackenzie HS, Hancock WW, Tilney NL. Activation of inflammatory mediators in rat renal isografts by donor brain death. Transplantation. 2000;**69**:405-410

[48] Kusaka M, Pratschke J, Wilhelm MJ, Ziai F, Zandi-Nejad K, Mackenzie HS, Hancock WW, Tilney NL. Early and late inflammatory changes occurring in rat renal isografts from brain dead donors. Transplantation Proceedings. 2001;**33**:867-868. DOI: 10.1016/S0041-1345(00)02355-1

[49] Li C, Jackson RM. Reactive species mechanisms of cellular hypoxia-reoxygenation injury. American Journal of Physiology. Cell Physiology. 2002;**282**:C227-C241. DOI: 10.1152/ajpcell.00112.2001

[50] Diepenhorst GM, van Gulik TM, Hack CE. Complement-mediated ischemia-reperfusion injury: Lessons learned from animal and clinical studies. Annals of Surgery. 2009;**249**:889-899. DOI: 10.1097/SLA.0b013e3181a38f45

[51] Omura T, Ishikura H, Nakajima Y, Kimura J, Ito K, Isai H, Tamatani T, Miyasaka M, Yoshiki T, Uchino J. The expression of LFA-1/ICAM-1 in liver transplantation in rats. Transplantation Proceedings. 1992;**24**:1618-1619

[52] Wakabayashi H, Miyauchi A, Karasawa Y, Hamamoto I, Maeba T, Tanaka S. Effect of warm ischemia and reperfusion injury on inducing major histocompatibility complex antigens on hepatocytes and nonparenchymal cells in the rat liver. Transplantation Proceedings. 1993;**25**:3205-3207

[53] Steinhoff G, Behrend M, Schrader B, Duijvestijn AM, Wonigeit K. Expression patterns of leukocyte adhesion ligand molecules on human liver endothelia. Lack of ELAM-1 and CD62 inducibility on sinusoidal endothelia and distinct distribution of VCAM-1, ICAM-1, ICAM-2, and LFA-3. The American Journal of Pathology. 1993;**142**:481-488

[54] Hoffmann MW, Wonigeit K, Steinhoff G, Herzbeck H, Flad HD, Pichlmayr R. Production of cytokines (TNF-alpha, IL-1-beta) and endothelial cell activation in human liver allograft rejection. Transplantation. 1993;**55**:329-335

[55] Steinhoff G, Brandt M. Adhesion molecules in liver transplantation. Hepato-Gastroenterology. 1996;**43**:1117-1123

[56] Jassem W, Koo DD, Cerundolo L, Rela M, Heaton ND, Fuggle SV. Leukocyte infiltration and inflammatory antigen expression in cadaveric and living-donor livers before transplant. Transplantation. 2003;**75**:2001-2007. DOI: 10.1097/01.TP.0000061605.30685.03

[57] Catania A, Lonati C, Sordi A, Gatti S. Detrimental consequences of brain injury on peripheral cells. Brain, Behavior, and Immunity. 2009;**23**:877-884. DOI: 10.1016/j.bbi.2009.04.006

[58] Weiss S, Kotsch K, Francuski M, Reutzel-Selke A, Mantouvalou L, Klemz R, Kuecuek O, Jonas S, Wesslau C, Ulrich F, Pascher A, Volk HD, Tullius SG, Neuhaus P, Pratschke J. Brain death activates donor organs and is associated with a worse I/R injury after liver transplantation. American Journal of Transplantation. 2007;**7**:1584-1593. DOI: 10.1111/j.1600-6143.2007.01799.x

[59] Wilhelm MJ, Pratschke J, Beato F, Taal M, Kusaka M, Hancock WW, Tilney NL. Activation of the heart by donor brain death accelerates acute rejection after transplantation. Circulation. 2000;**102**:2426-2433. DOI: 10.1161/01.CIR.102.19.2426

[60] Takada M, Nadeau KC, Hancock WW, Mackenzie HS, Shaw GD, Waaga AM, Chandraker A, Sayegh MH, Tilney NL. Effects of explosive brain death on cytokine activation of peripheral organs in the rat. Transplantation. 1998;**65**:1533-1542

[61] Morariu AM, Schuurs TA, Leuvenink HG, van Oeveren W, Rakhorst G, Ploeg RJ. Early events in kidney donation: Progression of endothelial activation, oxidative stress and tubular injury after brain death. American Journal of Transplantation. 2008;**8**:933-941. DOI: 10.1111/j.1600-6143.2008.02166.x

[62] Novitzky D, Wicomb WN, Cooper DKC, Rose AG, Fraser RC, Barnard CN. Electrocardiographic, haemodynamic and endocrine changes occurring during experimental brain death in the Chacma baboon. The Journal of Heart Transplantation. 1984;**4**:63-69

[63] Novitzky D, Wicomb WN, Cooper DKC. Pathophysiology of brain death and effects of hormonal therapy in large animal models. In: Novitzky D, Cooper DKC, editors. The Brain-Dead Organ Donor: Pathophysiology and Management. Springer Science+Business Media; New York; 2013. pp. 65-90. DOI: 10.1007/978-1-4614-4304-9_7

[64] Barklin A, Larsson A, Vestergaard C, Koefoed-Nielsen J, Bach A, Nyboe R, Wogensen L, Tønnesen E. Does brain death induce a pro-inflammatory response at the organ level in a porcine model? Acta Anaesthesiologica Scandinavica. 2008;**52**:621-627. DOI: 10.1111/j.1399-6576.2008.01607.x

[65] Bauer R, Walter B, Torossian A, Fritz H, Schlonski O, Jochum T, Hoyer D, Reinhart K, Zwiener U. A piglet model for evaluation of cerebral blood flow and brain oxidative metabolism during gradual cerebral perfusion pressure decrease. Pediatric Neurosurgery. 1999;**30**:62-69. DOI: 10.1159/000028765

[66] Hvas CL, Nielsen TK, Barklin A, Sørensen JC, Pedersen M, Andersen G, Tønnesen E. Brain death induced by cerebral haemorrhage—A new porcine model evaluated by

CT angiography. Acta Anaesthesiologica Scandinavica. 2012;**56**:995-1005. DOI: 10.1111/j.1399-6576.2012.02682.x

[67] Compagnon P, Wang H, Lindell SL, Ametani MS, Mangino MJ, D'Alessandro AM, Southard JH. Brain death does not affect hepatic allograft function and survival after orthotopic transplantation in a canine model. Transplantation. 2002;**73**:1218-1227

[68] Pratschke J, Wilhelm MJ, Kusaka M, Basker M, Cooper DK, Hancock WW, Tilney NL. Brain death and its influence on donor organ quality and outcome after transplantation. Transplantation. 1999;**67**:343-348

[69] Gracia-Sancho J, Casillas-Ramírez A, Peralta C. Molecular pathways in protecting the liver from ischaemia/reperfusion injury: A 2015 update. Clinical Science (London). 2015;**129**: 345-362. DOI: 10.1042/CS20150223

12

Cardiovascular Diseases in Patients with Renal Transplantation

Daniela Loncar and Selma Hodzic

Abstract

Kidney transplantation has become the primary method of treating severe chronic renal failure. The first successful kidney transplant was performed in 1954 in Boston, the graft was in function for 7 years, and patient died because of the heart disease. Cardiovascular disease is the leading cause of death in patients with a transplanted kidney. Despite the fact that patients with a transplanted kidney are highly susceptible to infections and have an increased tendency to develop malignant diseases, these patients die mainly of cardiovascular disease. Patients with a transplanted kidney are exposed to atherogenic risk which is associated with previous dialysis treatment and the use of immunosuppressive drugs. An excessive risk of developing cardiovascular disease in patients with a transplanted kidney is due to the high frequency and accumulation of atherogenic risk factors before and after transplantation. Pre-transplant cardiovascular disease is a major risk factor for the development of post-transplant cardiovascular disease. Risk factors for the development of cardiovascular diseases in patients with a transplanted kidney are divided into traditional and nontraditional. Traditional risk factors such as immutable (age, gender, and inheritance) and variable (smoking, hyperlipidemia, hypertension, obesity, diabetes mellitus, physical activity, stress). Nontraditional risk factors such as risk factors related to the status of transplantation and its treatment and risk factors associated with chronic regression in allograft function. The most common cardiovascular diseases in patients after kidney transplantation are as follows: ischemic heart disease, congestive heart failure and left ventricular hypertrophy. Of all cardiovascular complications, ischemic heart disease is by far the most common cause of mortality (more than 50%) in patients with a transplanted kidney. Frequency of left ventricular hypertrophy ranges from 50 to 70% in patients with a transplanted kidney. Early detection of high-risk patients for the development of cardiovascular diseases allows timely application of an appropriate therapeutic strategy that ensures high survival rates for patients with a transplanted kidney.

Keywords: kidney transplantation, risk factors, traditional risk factors, nontraditional risk factors, cardiovascular disease

1. Introduction

1.1. History of transplantation

Organ transplantation is one of the greatest achievements in history of medicine in the twentieth century. Kidney transplantation has become the primary method of treating severe chronic renal failure. The first successful kidney transplant was performed in 1954 in Boston, the graft was in function for 7 years, and patient died because of the heart disease. Over the past decades, organ transplantation has achieved incredible proportions through the development of surgical techniques, organ preservation methods, new diagnostic procedures, but, in particular, through discovery of powerful immunosuppressants.

1.2. Kidney transplant recipients

1.2.1. Becoming a kidney recipient

Kidney transplantation has become the primary method of treating severe chronic renal failure. After kidney transplantation, life is better, more quality and longer than during dialysis. It is recommended that all patients in end-stage kidney disease should be considered as potential kidney transplant recipients no matter of absolute contraindications. Because of the lack of available organs for transplant and all possible risks of immunosupresive drugs, careful consideration and adequate preparation of patients are indispensable. All studies related to the preparation of the transplant patient are covered by a protocol that includes detailed medical history, physical examination, system review including an examination by a psychologist. To be considered as transplant recipient, patient should be put on the transplant program's waiting list. To select recipients from a deceased donor in our country, we use the prescribed criteria. Among these criteria, an important place includes a blood type, match between the recipient and the donor, tissue typing, length of time on the dialysis and sensibility of the recipient [1].

1.2.2. Contraindications for kidney transplantation in the recipient

Contraindications for kidney transplantation in the recipient may be absolute, relative and temporary. Absolute contraindications: contraindications for general anesthesia or surgery, metastatic malignancy, refractory cardial decompensation, chronic respiratory insufficiency, advanced coronary or cerebrovascular disease, coagulopathy, chronic infection, mental retardation, psychosis, alcoholism, drug addiction. Relative contraindications: frequent respiratory infections, heart failure with frequent exacerbations, frequent digestive bleeding, previous malignancy, primary renal disease with a high degree of postoperative recurrence.

Temporary contraindications: tuberculosis and other chronic infections, bleeding, unexplained focal infection, unresolved bladder anomalies, arterial hypertension with complications, pronounced secondary hyperparathyroidism.

1.3. Kidney transplant donors

The kidney can be transplanted from deceased-donor (cadaveric transplantation) or from living-donors: genetically related (living-related) or nonrelated (living-unrelated) transplants, depending on whether a biological relationship exists between the donor and recipient. The basic prerequisite is for the donor to be mentally and physically healthy and willing to give the kidney. Numerous studies have shown that there are no proteinuria, hypertension or renal insufficiency in the carefully selected donors at 10 and 20 years after the kidneys in relation to the healthy population.

1.4. Pre-emptive kidney transplant

A pre-emptive kidney transplant (before kidney function deteriorates to the point of needing dialysis) should be offered to all candidates for transplantation who have a potential live donor. Earlier kidney transplants from a cadaveric donor can be offered to all potential recipients, but of particular importance are for children and patients with diabetes mellitus. To do the preemptive kidney transplantation, two conditions must be fulfilled: the patient must have irreversible and progressive renal impairment and the creatinine clearance must be less than 15 ml/min. Numerous studies have shown that survival of patients and calves after pre-emptive kidney transplantation was the same or even better than the transplantation done after the dialysis began [2].

1.5. Surgical procedures in kidney transplantation

Transplantation of the kidneys is a surgical procedure where the donor's kidney is placed in the lower part of the abdominal cavity of the recipient. The renal artery and veins connect to the large pelvic artery and vein of the recipient. The urinary tract of the transplanted kidney is attached to the recipient's bladder.

1.6. Immunosuppressive therapy

Renal transplantation is an important form of treatment for patients with terminal renal insufficiency. However, an obstacle to the success of the greatest number of transplants represents the immune response of a recipient directed against the transplanted kidney.

Due to the constant immunological response to renal allograft, permanent immunosuppressive therapy is carried out to prevent graft rejection. Theoretically, it should not be used only on identical twins. The basis of immunosuppression is a calcineurin inhibitor that is combined with corticosteroids and mycophenolate mofetil (Cellcept). Immunosuppressive drugs have enabled the success of organ transplantation, but they do not only act to prevent rejection of the transplanted organism but also they have numerous side effects on the body. Important side effects of immunosuppressants are the increased risk of infection and the atherogenic effect of immunosuppressive therapy.

1.7. Transplantation complications

The early period after kidney transplantation relates to the first 2 months after the surgery [3]. Acute surgical complications (bleeding, thrombosis of the transplanted kidney) are common in first few days after surgery, other clinical and immunological complications occur later.

Reactions of graft rejections are classified into four types based on the clinical picture, but differ in pathogenesis, histomorphological picture, and reactions own flow [4]. Those are hyperactivity, acceleration, acute and chronic rejection. Hyperacute rejection occurs in the first minutes or hours after kidney transplantation. Accelerating rejection begins 5–7 days after kidney transplantation and is demonstrated by rapid deterioration of the graft function. Acute rejection usually occurs from the fifth day to the end of the third month after kidney transplantation, but it can occur later on. Chronic graft rejection signifies the process in which transplanted kidney progressively deteriorates for several months and years, although the transplantation was successful in the first place. Other complications after kidney transplant are: urological complications, cardiovascular diseases, infections, gastrointestinal tract and liver diseases, malignant tumors, skin, bone and muscle diseases [4].

2. Risk factors for cardiovascular disease after kidney transplantation

Risk factors for the development cardiovascular diseases in patients with a transplanted kidney are more common than the risk factors in the general population.

They include traditional risk factors, such as arterial hypertension, diabetes mellitus, hyperlipidemia, and nontraditional risk factors associated with reduced glomerular filtration, such as anemia, hyperhomocysteinemia, or factors typical for transplantation, including direct effects of immunosuppression or rejection [5].

Patients with a transplanted kidney are exposed to atherogenic risk which is associated with previous dialysis treatment and the use of immunosuppressive drugs. An excessive risk of developing cardiovascular disease in patients with a transplanted kidney is due to the high frequency and accumulation of atherogenic risk factors before and after transplantation. Pre-transplant cardiovascular disease is a major risk factor for the development of post-transplant cardiovascular disease [6].

Cardiovascular diseases represent the most frequent cause of morbidity and mortality in patients at the end stage of renal diseases. Left ventricle hypertrophy occurs in 75% of patients treated by chronic dialysis. The prevalence of coronary heart disease in patients who are treated by chronic hemodialysis is 40%. The frequency of congestive heart failure in patients undergoing hemodialysis is 46%. Cardiac diseases represent the leading cause of death of dialyzed patients of which sudden cardiac death is the most frequent that is responsible for around 25% of all deadly outcomes. The rate of cardiovascular mortality in patients undergoing chronic dialysis is nearly 9% per annum. In patients treated by chronic dialysis, the risk of development of CVD is 10–20 times higher than in general population. Uremic milieu contributes to occurrence of atherosclerosis and atherosclerotic cardiovascular complications and often the development of accelerated, galloping atherosclerosis is present. The patients undergoing chronic dialysis are exposed to traditional and nontraditional risk factors for the development of cardiovascular complications. Nontraditional risk factors are the consequences of the uremic milieu and are related with the dialysis technique itself, and they are divided into hemodynamic and metabolic risk factors. Hemodynamic risk factors are anemia, retention of sodium and water, arteriovenous (AV) fistula, while the metabolic risk factors are hyperhomocysteinemia, hypoalbuminemia, oxidative stress, microinflammation and secondary hyperparathyroidism.

Risk factors for cardiovascular diseases in patients with a transplanted kidney are divided into traditional and nontraditional [5]: traditional risk factors are: immutable (age, gender, and inheritance), variable (smoking, hyperlipidemia, hypertension, obesity, diabetes mellitus, physical activity, and stress); and nontraditional risk factors are: risk factors related to the status of transplantation and its treatment (immunosuppressive agents, graft rejection, and viral infection —cytomegalovirus) and risk factors associated with chronic regression in allograft function (anemia, volume load, hyperhomocysteinemia, oxidative stress, secondary hyperparathyroidism, and microinflammation).

2.1. Traditional risk factors

Smoking is not only a risk factor for the development of cardiovascular diseases, but is also associated with the risk of developing chronic kidney disease defined as a reduction in glomerular filtration to <45 ml/min/1.73 m^2. Long-term smoking of more than 20 cigarettes per day is associated with 1.52 times higher relative risk of chronic kidney disease [7]. For comparison, smoking and obesity are associated with a 1.77 times higher relative risk of chronic kidney disease. These risks are more conspicuous in men than in women. Smoking begins and improves the process of atherosclerosis in the blood vessels. In various studies, it has been shown that smoking leads to cardiovascular complications, reduces survival of the patient and graft, and its effect on patient survival is similar to the same one on patients with diabetes mellitus [8]. Smoking cigarette is an independent risk factor for the development of cardiovascular events in patients with a transplanted kidney. In the population of patients with transplanted kidney, the prevalence of smoking is 25%, and the smoking cessation includes pharmacological therapy—NRT (nicotine replacement therapy).

Risks of cardiovascular diseases increase with increasing body weight because it increases the blood pressure, serum lipids, and glucose intolerance. A particularly harmful factor is the central obesity characterized by an increase in intra-abdominal fat tissue. Central obesity (waistline >88 cm for women and >102 cm for men) is a risk factor for declining allograft function in patients with a transplanted kidney. Obesity fosters the development of the insulin resistance, diabetes mellitus, ischemic heart disease, and reduces survival of allograft [9].

A cohort study by Adabag of 14,941 men and women, aged 45–64 years, showed that obesity was associated with an increased risk of sudden cardiac death [10]. According to research by Chan, obesity is a risk factor for the development of cardiovascular disease following kidney transplantation [11]. Although the role of obesity in the pre-transplant period is uncertain, after kidney transplantation, obesity increases the risk of graft failure and mortality.

Weight loss reduces and changes other risk factors for the development of cardiovascular disease [12]. Metabolic syndrome is a risk factor for the development of cardiovascular disease in patients with a transplanted kidney. It is characterized by obesity (central type of obesity), physical inactivity, hypertension (arterial blood pressure greater than 130/80 mmHg), hyperlipidaemia (triglycerides greater than 1.7 mmol/l, HDL cholesterol less than 1.0 mmol/l in men and less than 1.3 mmol/l in women) and systemic insulin resistance (fasting blood sugar greater than 6.5 mmol/l). Six years after kidney transplantation, 63% of patients have criteria for metabolic syndrome, reduced survival of allograft and an increased number of cardiovascular incidents [9].

Diabetes mellitus is one of the most common causes of renal disease, this disease independent and in itself increases the risk of cardiovascular disease. The results of two large clinical studies, Framingham Study and Multiple Risk Factor Intervention Trial (MRFIT) show that diabetes mellitus doubles the possibility of coronary artery disease in men and triples the risk of coronary artery disease in women [13]. Diabetes mellitus is a relatively common complication after kidney transplantation and is defined as a fasting glucose greater than 7 mmol/l. The incidence of diabetes mellitus is between 3.6 and 18% and depends mainly on immunosuppressive therapy. Kidney transplantation can lead to the deterioration of existing diabetes mellitus or to the development of "de novo" diabetes mellitus. The most common cause of post-transplantation diabetes mellitus is corticosteroid therapy, and it depends on immunosuppressive therapy. The two main mechanisms by which corticosteroids cause diabetes mellitus are inducing insulin resistance and increasing body weight [14]. Immunosuppressive drugs can lead to the development of diabetes. The prevalence of post-transplant diabetes in patients treated with cyclosporin ranges from 2.5 to 20%. The treatment of diabetes in hospitalized transplant recipients requires attention to a multitude of factors that can impact glycemic control and influence the risk for adverse effects. Methods to manage hyperglycemia vary among transplant centers and also vary according to whether the patient is immediately post-transplant or is being admitted in the post-transplant setting for another issue. Immediately after transplantation in post-transplant we use frequently require IV insulin infusion protocol. Once iv requirements are established and stable, switch to insulin every 8 h plus fast-acting correction insulin every 4–6 h.

The prevalence of post-transplant hypertension is between 60 and 85%. Causes of hypertension in patients with a transplanted kidney are as follows: stenosis of graft renal artery, presence of native kidneys, immunosuppressive therapy, graft dysfunction, genetic predisposition of donors and recipients. Native kidneys and pre-transplant hypertension have been described as independent factors associated with post-transplant hypertension. Native kidney of recipient can cause systemic hypertension through the renin-angiotensin system. Immuno suppressive drugs are also responsible for the appearance of hypertension in patients with a transplanted kidney. It is believed that corticosteroids aggravate hypertension through hemodynamic and hormonal disorders as well as retention of salt and water. The role of cyclosporin in the development of hypertension in the transplantation of the heart, liver and bone marrow, as well as in patients with uveitis and diabetes mellitus, has been demonstrated, while its role in kidney transplantation is controversial. On the one hand, cyclosporin can cause hypertension with its nephrotoxic effect, and on the other hand, if cyclosporin prevents chronic rejection, it may delay the occurrence of hypertension. In two large retrospective studies with a follow-up period of 2 and 3 years, the prevalence of hypertension remained stable over time, but in the group of patients treated with ciclosporin, the prevalence of hypertension increased by 25% compared to patients treated with azathioprine [15]. Tacrolimus therapy causes hypertension, whose mechanism is probably similar to cyclosporin-induced hypertension. It is a general opinion that the main cause of hypertension after renal transplantation is chronic graft dysfunction or chronic graft nephropathy. Hypertension is often the first clinical sign of chronic rejection. It is known that arterial hypertension is a risk factor for cardiovascular disease in the general population. In a retrospective analysis, Ponticelli and associates have found a higher number of cardiac infarcts after kidney transplantation in patients with hypertension than in normotensive patients [16]. Arterial hypertension correlates with cardiovascular disease after transplantation [17]. In most cases for treatment post-transplant hypertension, routine antihypertensive treatment is effective. We can use ACE inhibitors, beta blockers and calcium channel blockers.

Hyperlipidemia is known as the traditional risk factor for the development of cardiovascular diseases, both in the general population and in the population of patients with terminal stage of renal failure. Several observational studies have shown that total cholesterol and low-density lipoproteins (LDL) are one of the most important independent factors of cardiovascular morbidity and mortality [18]. Patients with renal function impairment have significant changes in the metabolism of lipoproteins, whose exact role in the pathogenesis of atherosclerosis in these patients is still controversial [19]. Hyperlipidemia can occur already after 3 months of transplantation and does not resolve spontaneously, and in most patients, it can persist for a very long, even 10 or more years after kidney transplantation [20]. Patients with a transplanted kidney usually have an increased total cholesterol, LDL cholesterol and triglycerides, while HDL cholesterol is usually normal or even high, although its composition may be pathological [21]. Immunosuppressive drugs such as corticosteroids, cyclosporin, tacrolimus and, in particular, sirolimus contribute to the development of post-transplant hyperlipidemia, usually depending on the dose of medicine [22]. Many epidemiological studies of patients with a transplanted kidney showed a correlation between elevated total cholesterol, triglyceride, LDL and incidence of cardiovascular diseases, the same as a low level of HDL is associated with an increase in cardiovascular risk [23]. Hyperlipidemia in patients with a transplanted kidney may affect the progression of chronic graft nephropathy. Based on data about the prevention of cardiovascular disease, it is known that the reduction of LDL-cholesterol by 1 mmol/l over 4–5 years reduces the risk of coronary and cerebrovascular incidents by 25%. Extrapolation from general population studies and some data in kidney transplant patients support the view that the assessment and treatment of dyslipidemias should be part of routine post-renal transplant care. For treating hyperlipidemia in kidney transplant patient, we use statins.

2.2. Risk factors related to the status of transplantation and its treatment

In patients who at the moment of transplantation have no signs of atherosclerosis, reduced graft function and immunosuppressive therapy may cause hypertension, dyslipidemia, diabetes mellitus, and proteinuria, which can lead to myocardial infarction, stroke, or peripheral vascular disease.

Allograft function disorder is a risk factor for the development of cardiovascular disease [24]. A year after renal transplantation, chronic allograft disease at stage 3 (glomerular filtration <60 ml/min/1.73 m^2) has 60%, and in stage 4 (glomerular filtration value <30 ml/min/1.73 m^2) has 15% of patients [25]. With the decline in the allograft function, nontraditional risk factors appear. They occur when the glomerular filtration value falls below 60 ml/min/1.73 m^2, and especially when it is below 45 ml/min/1.73 m^2.

Reduced function of transplanted kidney in transplant recipient is an independent and important risk factor for the development of cardiovascular diseases due to adverse effects on hypertension, anemia, dyslipidemia, hyperhomocysteinemia [26]. The American National Kidney Foundation (NKF) reported that the value of glomerular filtration (GFR) measured or estimated is a better parameter of renal function than serum creatinine only [27]. The prevalence of left ventricular hypertension is inversely proportional to the level of glomerular filtration. In one study, the frequency of left ventricular hypertension was 45, 31 and 27% in patients with creatinine clearance <25, 25–50, and >50 ml/min [28].

2.3. Risk factors relating to chronic decline in graft function

With an increased risk of cardiovascular complications, homocysteine, infection, pathological coagulation and fibrinolysis are associated.

Anemia is a risk factor for the development of cardiovascular disease in patients with a transplanted kidney. The American Society of Transplantation (AST) defines anemia as a hemoglobin concentration lower than 120 g/l in men and lower than 110 g/l in women [29]. Anemia occurs in 20–60% of patients with a transplanted kidney, and its prevalence is the highest in the early post-transplant period (6–12 months after kidney transplantation). The main causes of its development in the early post-transplant period are: blood loss due to surgery, abrupt termination of erythropoietin administration, iron deficiency, bone marrow suppression caused by induction therapy, increased erythropoietin resistance due to infection (viral infection) and/or inflammatory status caused by systemic immune response on the presence of alloantigens, the use of drugs (mycophenolate mofetil). Reduced production of endogenous erythropoietin due to loss of allograft function, erythropoietin resistance due to secondary hyperparathyroidism and chronic microinflammatory disease are the main causes of anemia in late post-transplantation [30].

Post-transplantation anemia (a hemoglobin less than 110 g/l 3 months after renal transplantation) was associated with the development of congestive heart failure, a lower survival rate of allograft and patient, and a higher rate of acute rejection [31]. The relative risk for the cardiovascular incident was 1.32 with a decrease in hemoglobin by 0.5 g/dl, which is just slightly less than the relative risk of 1.37 related to an increase in systolic pressure of 15 mmHg. Anemia together with hypertension leads to left ventricular hypertrophy.

Treatment of patients with transplanted kidney and post-transplant anemia should be started with erythropoietin, when the hemoglobin concentration is less than 110 g/l and the target hemoglobin level should be 110–120 g/l.

Homocysteine concentration is an independent risk factor for cardiovascular disease after kidney transplantation [32]. In patients with a transplanted kidney, the concentration of homocysteine decreases compared to patients treated with dialysis but is higher than the concentration of homocysteine in healthy population, so hyperhomocysteinemia is common in patients after kidney transplantation [33]. For the treatment of hyperchomocysteinemia, we use folate and Vitamin B (12).

There is clear evidence that elevated levels of fibrinogen, factor VII, and von Willebrand factor in the general population are associated with an increased risk of acute insult or coronary disease [34]. These factors have also been elevated in patients following kidney transplantation, in more patients with cardiovascular disorders than in patients who do not have them.

Secondary hyperparathyroidism is a risk factor for the development of cardiovascular disease in patients with a transplanted kidney [35]. After transplantation of the kidney, hyperparathyroidism is maintained in 50% of patients, characterized by hypercalcaemia, hyperphosphatemia and increased parathormone concentration [36]. Secondary hyperparathyroidism in post-transplantation may also occur new, as a consequence of the decline in the function of the allograft and the lack of calcitriol. The disorder of metabolism of calcium and phosphate results in calcification of peripheral arteries, including coronary artery calcification. Cinacalcet may be useful in the treatment of persistent hyperparathyroidism after kidney transplant.

The effect of local inflammatory stimulus such as products of the oxidation process, the end products of glycosylation and chronic infectious processes alter the blood vessel in terms of the development of atherosclerosis. Microinflammation is a risk factor for the development of atherosclerotic cardiovascular diseases in patients with a transplanted kidney [24]. These patients have a low level of microinflammation as a consequence of a systemic immune response to the presence of all antigens but also because of chronic infections [25]. C-reactive protein (>5 mg/l > 0.5 mg/dl) is associated with an increased risk of developing cardiovascular events in the population of patients with a transplanted kidney.

Proteinuria occurs in one-third of post-transplant patients and is a risk factor for the development of cardiovascular disease in patients with a transplanted kidney [37].

3. Cardiovascular disease in patients with transplanted kidney

Thanks to the progress in histocompatibility testing and better immunosuppressive therapy, graft survival has increased, so that the leading cause of graft loss after transplantation has been the death of a patient with functional graft. Cardiovascular disease is the leading cause of death in patients with a transplanted kidney [38]. Despite the fact that patients with a transplanted kidney are highly susceptible to infections and have an increased tendency to develop malignant diseases, these patients die mainly of cardiovascular disease. Although kidney transplantation, in contrast to dialysis, reduces the risk of cardiovascular disease by restoring kidney function, it also brings new risk factors related to the status of transplantation and its treatment and risk factors related to the chronic decline in the function of the allograft. The increased incidence of cardiovascular diseases in patients with transplanted kidney is a consequence of the high prevalence of risk factors for the development of cardiovascular diseases in these patients. The incidence of cardiovascular disease in patients with a transplanted kidney is three to five times higher than in the general population [39]. A cardiovascular event with congestive heart failure or coronary heart disease was manifested in almost 40% of patients 36 months after kidney transplantation [9]. Cardiovascular disease is the most common cause of death in transplanted patients, accounting for 35–50% of all causes of death, and occurs at least two times more often than in the general population [40]. Most kidney recipients die with functional graft and half of these patients die due to ischemic heart disease or other vascular diseases [41].

The most common cardiovascular diseases in patients after kidney transplantation are as follows: ischemic heart disease, congestive heart failure and left ventricular hypertrophy [6]. Of all cardiovascular complications, ischemic heart disease is by far the most common cause of mortality (more than 50%) in patients with a transplanted kidney [41]. Frequency of left ventricular hypertrophy ranges from 50 to 70% in patients with a transplanted kidney [42]. Left ventricular hypertrophy is associated with an increased degree of ventricular arrhythmias. In Europe, cardiovascular disease account for 36% of the total mortality of patients with a transplanted kidney [43]. In the United States, the annual mortality rate of cardiovascular diseases in these patients is 0.54% and is approximately twice as high (0.28%) than in the general population [39].

Ischemic heart disease causes 53% of deaths in patients with transplanted kidney and preserved graft function. The risk of mortality from ischemic heart disease is 6.4 times higher in nondiabetic transplanted renal patients, 8.6 times higher in dialysis patients and 20.8 times higher in transplanted renal patients with diabetes than in the general population [41]. Diagnostic strategy for early detection of patients with an increased risk of developing asymptomatic disorders of the systolic and diastolic function of the left ventricle should include: echocardiographic examination, tests for coronary artery disease and tests for the determination of myocardial function (BNP, Tt-pro BNP). In a study of Aakhus and associates on cardiovascular diseases in patients with a transplanted kidney, involving 406 patients with a transplanted kidney, the mean annual mortality was 4.4, and 74% of them were cardiovascular causes of mortality [44].

3.1. Left ventricular hypertrophy

The most significant risk factors for the development of left ventricular hypertrophy are as follows: hypertension, arteriosclerosis, secondary aortic stenosis and anemia.

Left ventricular hypertrophy is a risk factor for the unfavorable outcome of patients with a transplanted kidney. The selection of patients with an increased risk of left ventricular hypertrophy, the timely application of appropriate treatment, the achievement and maintenance of the target values of risk factors, lead to decrease of the development and regression of existing left ventricular hypertrophy, reduction in the rate of cardiovascular morbidity and mortality, and improve the quality of life of patients with a transplanted kidney.

Left ventricular hypertrophy is present in most patients who begin treatment by replacing renal function and are associated with poor outcome. Time spent on dialysis can also affect the development of left ventricular hypertrophy. Transplantation of the kidneys leads to the withdrawal of left ventricular hypertrophy together with the normalization of blood pressure. The regression of left ventricular hypertrophy continues during the first 2 years after transplantation. Older age and hypertension can slow down this process [45].

The presence of left ventricular hypertension as well as the weak systolic function of the left ventricle before transplantation are related to an increased mortality after renal transplantation during 7.5-year follow-up, while other traditional risk factors such as hypertension, hyperlipidemia and smoking did not show such a connection. On cardiography of the heart made 4 months after transplantation, only left ventricular hypertension had a strong association with poor prognosis during monitoring [46].

3.2. Heart failure

Heart failure is a clinical syndrome characterized by reduced tolerance of physical activity and overload volume. The incidence of congestive heart failure in patients with a transplanted kidney is two to five times higher than the incidence in the general population [47]. The incidence of congestive heart failure in patients with a transplanted kidney was 10.2% 12 months after transplantation and 18.3% 36 months after transplantation [48].

In a study of Higashi and associates, 11 out of 190 (5.8%) kidney recipients, with preserved left ventricular systolic function and the presence of diastolic left ventricular dysfunction, developed a postoperative edema of the lungs [49].

Diastolic left ventricular dysfunction is present in 45% of patients with a transplanted kidney.

The clinical presentation is the same as in all other patients with cardiac insufficiency. The following symptoms are reported: difficulty breathing, intolerance of physical activity, edema of the lower extremities and stomach.

Treatment: the first measure is to reduce physical activity and reduce salt intake. If this is not enough, medication therapy is started with a combination of diuretics, ACE inhibitors and digitalis.

3.3. Ischemic heart disease

Ischemic heart disease (IHD) is the most common disease in the large group of all cardiovascular diseases. The prevalence of ischemic heart disease in patients with a transplanted kidney is five times higher than in the general population. The main cause of ischemic heart disease is atherosclerosis of the coronary arteries, and in patients with transplanted kidney there are many risk factors that contribute to atherosclerosis: elevated arterial blood pressure, lipid metabolism disorder, microinflammation, hyperhomocysteinemia, oxidative stress and secondary hyperparathyroidism.

In patients with a transplanted kidney, there is a high risk of sudden cardiac death. The main causes are coronary arterial heart disease, left ventricular hypertrophy, and reduced coronary perfusion. In patients with a transplanted kidney, the prevalence of coronary heart disease is five times higher than the general population [6].

In all patients with ischemic heart disease, the following should be done: detailed anamnesis and physical examination, ECG at rest, blood biochemical analysis (lipids, glucose, creatinine, urea, hepatogram, complete blood count, uric acid, fibrinogen, hsCRP, etc.) echocardiographic examination, ergometric testing. In patients with transplanted kidney, the risk factors for the development of atherosclerosis should be controlled in the primary prevention and prevention of coronary artery disease development. In clinical practice, patients with acute myocardial infarction with elevation of ST connectors are using modern reperfusion therapy (thrombolysis or percutaneous coronary intervention). Medical treatment implies the use of anti-aging therapy, statins and beta blockers.

3.4. Valvular heart disease, heart rhythm disorders, and pericardial disease

Valvular heart disease is common in patients with chronic dialysis. Current knowledge of heart valve disease (the evolution of pre-dialysis disease or the emergence of de novo diseases of the heart valve) in patients following kidney transplantation is scarce. In the literature, there are few data about heart rhythm disorders in patients with transplanted kidney. In a study by Sever and associates on the frequency of pericarditis in patients following kidney transplantation, an incidence of 2.4% was observed [50].

The development of pericarditis in patients with a transplanted kidney may contribute to the use of immunosuppressive therapy as it increases the risk of infection [51].

4. Assessment of the risk of cardiovascular disease in asymptomatic patients with a transplanted kidney

Cardiovascular diseases are the main cause of morbidity and mortality in post-transplant patients [52]. The risk assessment of cardiovascular disease in asymptomatic patients with a transplanted kidney is of great practical importance because it allows the identification of patients at high risk for cardiovascular events, which further allows timely intervention before the disease develops. To assess the risk of cardiovascular disease in asymptomatic patients with a transplanted kidney, we can apply the scores used for assessment of cardiovascular risk in general population. The scores for the general population are the Systematic Coronary Risk

Age	Sistolni krvni pritisak	ŽENE Nepušači 4	5	6	7	8	ŽENE Pušači 4	5	6	7	8	MUŠKARCI Nepušači 4	5	6	7	8	MUŠKARCI Pušači 4	5	6	7	8
65	180	7	8	9	10	12	13	15	17	19	22	14	16	19	22	26	26	30	35	41	47
65	160	5	5	6	7	8	9	10	12	13	16	9	11	13	15	16	18	21	25	29	34
65	140	3	3	4	5	6	6	7	8	9	11	6	8	9	11	13	13	15	17	20	24
65	120	2	2	3	3	4	4	5	5	6	7	4	5	6	7	9	9	10	12	14	17
60	180	4	4	5	6	7	8	9	10	11	13	9	11	13	15	18	18	21	24	28	33
60	160	3	3	3	4	5	5	6	7	8	9	6	7	9	10	12	12	14	17	20	24
60	140	2	2	2	3	3	3	4	5	5	6	4	5	6	7	9	8	10	12	14	17
60	120	1	1	2	2	2	2	3	3	4	4	3	3	4	5	6	6	7	8	10	12
55	180	2	2	3	3	4	4	5	5	6	7	6	7	8	10	12	12	13	16	19	22
55	160	1	2	2	2	3	3	3	4	4	5	4	5	6	7	8	8	9	11	13	16
55	140	1	1	1	1	2	2	2	2	3	3	3	3	4	5	6	5	6	8	9	11
55	120	1	1	1	1	1	1	1	2	2	2	2	2	3	3	4	4	4	5	6	8
50	180	1	1	1	2	2	2	2	3	3	4	4	4	5	6	7	7	8	10	12	14
50	160	1	1	1	1	1	1	2	2	2	3	2	3	3	4	5	5	6	7	8	10
50	140	0	1	1	1	1	1	1	1	1	2	2	2	2	3	3	3	4	5	6	7
50	120	0	0	1	1	1	1	1	1	1	1	1	1	2	2	2	2	3	3	4	5
40	180	0	0	0	0	0	0	0	0	1	1	1	1	1	2	2	2	2	3	3	4
40	160	0	0	0	0	0	0	0	0	0	0	1	1	1	1	1	1	2	2	2	3
40	140	0	0	0	0	0	0	0	0	0	0	0	1	1	1	1	1	1	1	2	2
40	120	0	0	0	0	0	0	0	0	0	0	0	0	1	1	1	1	1	1	1	1

Holesterol mmol (4 5 6 7 8) — 150 200 250 300 mg/dl

Table 1. Heart score high risk map.

Evaluation SCORE system, the Prospective Cardiovascular Munster PROAM score system, and the National Cholesterol Education Program Adult Treatment Panel III NTEP ATP III [53].

The new risk assessment model is based on the Heart Score system (Systematic Coronary Risk Evaluation). The Heart Score Risk Card has been developed on the basis of large prospective studies in Europe and predicts the fatal outcomes of cardiovascular disease for 10 years. The assessment is based on the following risk factors: age, sex, smoking, systolic blood pressure, total cholesterol, or cholesterol/HDL ratio. A high risk threshold based on a fatal cardiovascular outcome is defined as more than or equal to 5%.

Early detection of high-risk patients for the development of cardiovascular diseases allows timely application of an appropriate therapeutic strategy that ensures high survival rates for patients with a transplanted kidney (**Table 1**).

Assessing the patient's risk of developing cardiovascular disease enables the identification of patients at high risk for the development of cardiovascular events, which allow the intervention before the disease develops. In asymptomatic patients, cardiovascular risk assessment should be carried out and preventive activates should be performed accordingly. Patients with established multifactorial risk should be subjected to preventive activities, and, if necessary to medication therapy.

Several studies have shown that the use of standard scores in the assessment of the degree of risk of cardiovascular disease in patients with renal disease is insufficient [54]. In these scores, we use the following data: age, gender, blood pressure, lipid level, without taking into account nontraditional risk factors for occurrence of cardiovascular diseases.

Nontraditional risk factors that are not included in these scores can play an important role in the insufficient assessment of the risk of cardiovascular disease in patients with a transplanted kidney. All these point should be consider by creating a new risk score that would include both traditional and nontraditional risk factors for cardiovascular disease. It is recommended that standard risk factors be enhanced with additional risk factors (e.g., homocystein, C-reactive protein). Additional risk factors are recommended for increasing the precision of risk assessment.

5. Conclusion

Cardiovascular disease is the leading cause of death in patients with a transplanted kidney. The incidence of cardiovascular disease in patients with a transplanted kidney is 3–5 times higher than in the general population. Risk factors for the development of cardiovascular diseases in patients with a transplanted kidney are divided into traditional and nontraditional. Traditional risk factors: immutable (age, gender, inheritance), variable (smoking, hyperlipidemia, hypertension, obesity, diabetes mellitus, physical activity, stress). Nontraditional risk factors: risk factors related to the status of transplantation and its treatment (immunosuppressive agents, graft rejection, viral infection - cytomegalovirus) and risk factors associated with chronic regression in allograft function (anemia, volume load, hyperhomocysteinemia, oxidative stress, secondary hyperparathyroidism, microinflammation). The most common cardiovascular diseases in patients after kidney transplantation are as follows: ischemic heart disease, congestive heart failure and left ventricular hypertrophy. Of all cardiovascular complications, ischemic heart disease is by far the most common cause of mortality (more than 50%) in patients with a transplanted kidney. Frequency of left ventricular hypertrophy ranges from 50 to 70% in patients with a transplanted kidney. The incidence of congestive heart failure in patients with a transplanted kidney is 2–5 times higher than the incidence in the general population. The incidence of congestive heart failure in patients with a transplanted kidney was 10.2% 12 months after transplantation and 18.3% 36 months after transplantation. The risk assessment of cardiovascular disease in asymptomatic patients with a transplanted kidney is of great practical importance because it allows the identification of patients at high risk for cardiovascular events, which further allows timely intervention before the disease develops. To assess the risk of cardiovascular disease in asymptomatic patients with a transplanted kidney, we can apply the scores used for assessment of cardiovascular risk in general population. Several studies have shown that the use of standard scores in the assessment of the degree of risk of cardiovascular disease in patients with renal disease is insufficient. It is recommended that standard risk factors be enhanced with additional risk factors (e.g., homocystein, C-reactive protein). Additional risk factors are recommended for increasing the precision of risk assessment. Assessing the patient's risk of developing cardiovascular disease enables the identification of patients at high risk for the development of cardiovascular events, which allow the intervention before the disease develops.

Author details

Daniela Loncar and Selma Hodzic*

*Address all correspondence to: hodzic_selma@live.com

Clinic for Internal Disease, University Clinical Center Tuzla, Bosnia and Herzegovina

References

[1] Tabaković M. Transplantacija bubrega: Faktori rizika nakon transplantacije bubrega U: Suada Mulić-Bačić. Interna medicina, I izdanje. OFF-SET Tuzla: Tuzla; 2011. pp. 355-378

[2] Asderakis A, Augustine T, Dyer P. Pre-emptive kidney transplantation: The attractive alternative. Nephrology, Dialysis, Transplantation. 1998;**13**:1799-1803

[3] Amend WJC, Vincenti F, Tomlanovich S. The first posttransplant months. In: Danovich GM, editor. Handbook of Kidney Transplantation. Ed Little, Brown and Comp; 1996

[4] Ležaić V, Stojković D. Rani period posle transplantacije bubrega U: Višnja Ležaić, Ljubica Đukanović. Transplantacija bubrega, I izdanje. Beograd: Zavod za udžbenike i nastavna sredstva; 2004. pp. 177-192

[5] Mark S, Andrew L, Anton CS, Josef C, et al. Kidney disease as a risk factor for development of cardiovascular disease. Circulation. 2003;**108**:2154-2169

[6] Radivojević D. Kardiovaskularne bolesti posle transplantacije bubrega U: Višnja Ležaić, Ljubica Đukanović. Transplantacija bubrega, I izdanje. Beograd: Zavod za udžbenike i nastavna sredstva; 2004. pp. 231-245

[7] Zoccali C. Tradicional and emerging cardiovascular and renal risk factors: An epidemiological perspective. Kidney International. 2006;**70**(1):26-33

[8] Arend SM, Mallat MJ, Wastendorp RJ. Patient survival after renal transplantation: More than 25 years follow-up. Nephrology, Dialysis, Transplantation. 1997;**12**:1672-1679

[9] Shirali AC, Bia MJ. Management of cardiovascular disease in renal transplant recipients. Clinical Journal of the American Society of Nephrology. 2008;**3**:491-504

[10] Adabag S, Huxley RR, Lopez FL, Chen LY, Sotoodehnia N, Siscovick D, Deo R, Konety S, Alonso A, Folsom AR. Obesity related risk of sudden cardiac death in the atherosclerosis risk in communities study. Heart. 2015;**101**(3):215-221

[11] Chan W, Bosch JA, Jones D, McTernan PG, Phillips AC, Borrows R. Obesity in kidney transplantation. Journal of Renal Nutrition. 2014;**24**(1):1-12

[12] Smith SC, Blair SN, Criqui MH, et al. AHA medical/scientific statement. Preventing heart attack and death in patients with coronary disease. Circulation. 1995;**92**:2

[13] Stamler J, Vaccaro O, Neaton JD, Wentworth D. Diabetes, other risk factors, and 12-yr cardiovascular mortality for men screened in the multiple risk intervention trial. Diabetes Care. 1993;**16**:434-444

[14] Jindal RM. Posttransplant diabetes mellitus. A review. Transplantation. 1994;**58**:1289-1298

[15] Schorn T. Cyclosporine-associated posttransplant hypertension. Incidence and effect on renal transplant function. Transplantation Proceedings. 1998;**20**(supl 3):610-614

[16] Ponticelli C, Montagnino G, Aroldi A. Hypertension after transplantation. American Journal of Kidney Diseases. 1993;**21**(Suppl 2):S73-S78

[17] Kasiske BL, Guijarro C, Massy ZA. Cardiovascular disease after renal transplantation. Journal of the American Society of Nephrology. 1996;**7**:158-165

[18] Lewington S, Whitlock G, Clarke R, Sherliker P, Emberson J, Halsey J. Blood cholesterol and vascular mortality by age, sex, and blood pressure: A meta-analysis of individual data from 61 prospective studies with 55,000 vascular deaths. Lancet. 2007;**370**:1829-1839

[19] Tsimihodimos V, Mitrogianni Z, Elisaf M. Dyslipidemia Associated with Chronic Kidney Disease. Open Cardiovascular Medicine Journal. 2011;**5**:41-48

[20] Markell MS, Armenti V, Dsnovitch G, Sumrani N. Hyperlipidemia and glucose intolerance in the post-renal transplant patient. Journal of the American Society of Nephrology. 1994;**4**:S37-S47

[21] Kobashigawa JA, Kasiske BL. Hyperlipidemia in solid organ transplantation. Transplantation. 1997;**63**:331-338

[22] Groth CG, Backman L, Morales JM. Sirolimus (rapamycin)-based therapy in human renal transplantation: Similar efficacy and different toxicity compared with cyclosporine. Sirolimus European renal transplant study group. Transplantation. 1999;**67**:1036-1042

[23] Drueke TB, Abdulmassih Z, Lacour B. Atherosclerosis and lipid disorders after renal transplantation. Kidney International. 1991;**39**(Supll 31):S24-S28

[24] Marcen R. Cardiovascular risk factors in renal transplantation-current controversies. Nephrology, Dialysis, Transplantation. 2006;**21**(Suppl 3):3-8

[25] Moreso F, Grinyo JM. Graft dysfunction and cardiovascular risk-an unholy alliance. Nephrology, Dialysis, Transplantation. 2007;**22**:699-702

[26] Liefeldt L, Budde K. Risk factors for cardiovascular disease in renal transplant recipients and strategies to minimize risk. Transplant International. 2010;**23**(12):1191-1204

[27] Levey AS, Coresh J, Balk E. National Kidney Foundation practice guidelines for chronic kidney disease: Evaluation, classification and stratification. Annals of Internal Medicine. 2003;**139**:137-147

[28] Levin A, Singer J, Thompson CR, et al. Prevalent left ventricular hypertrophy in the predialysis population: Identifying opportunities for intervention. American Journal of Kidney Diseases. 1996;**27**:347-354

[29] Blosser CD, Bloom RD. Posttransplant anemia in solid organ recipients. Transplantation Reviews. 2010;**24**:89-98

[30] Winkelmayer W, Chandraker A. Posttransplantation anemia: Management and rationale. Clinical Journal of the American Society of Nephrology. 2008;(Suppl 2):49-55

[31] Rihard B, Loucaidou M, Chusney G, Borrows S, Van Tromp J, Cairns T, Griffith M, Hakim N, McLean A, Palmer A, Papalois V, Taube D. Anaemia and congestive heart failure early post-renal transplantation. Nephrology, Dialysis, Transplantation. 2008;**23**:1728-1734

[32] Duclos D, Motte G, Challier B, Gibey R, Chalopin JM. Serum total homocysteine and cardiovascular disease occurrence in chronic stable renal transplant recipients: A prospective study. Journal of the American Society of Nephrology. 2000;**11**:134-137

[33] Arnadottir M, Hultberg B, Wahlberg J. Serum total homocysteine concentration before and after renal transplantation. Kidney International. 1998;**54**:1380-1384

[34] Frishman WH. Biologic markers as predictors of cardiovascular disease. The American Journal of Medicine. 1998;**104**:S18-S27

[35] Rosas SE, Mensah K, Weinstein RB, Bellamz SL, Rader DJ. Coronary artery calcification in renal transplant recipients. American Journal of Transplantation. 2005;**5**:1942-1947

[36] Chonchol M, Wuthrich RP. Potential future uses of calcmimetics in patients with chronic kidney disease. NDT Plus. 2008;**1**(Suppl 1):36-46

[37] Ibis A, Akgül A, Ozdemir N, Colak T, Sezer S, Arat Z, Haberal M. Posttransplant proteinuria is associated with higher risk of cardiovascular disease and graft failure in renal transplant patients. Transplantation Proceedings. 2009;**41**(5):1604-1608

[38] Ferreira SR, Moisés VA, Tavares A, Pacheco-Silva A. Cardiovascular effects of successful renal transplantation: a 1-year sequential study of left ventricular morphology and function, and 24-hour blood pressure profile. Transplantation. 2002;**74**(11):1580-1587

[39] Foley RN, Parfrey PS, Sarnak MJ. Clinical epidemiology of cardiovascular disease in chronic renal disease. American Journal of Kidney Diseases. 1998;**32**:S112-S119

[40] Ojo AO, Hanson JA, Wolfe RA. Long-termsurvival in renal transplant recipients with graft function. Kidney International. 2000;**57**:307-313

[41] Lindholm A, Albrechtsen D, Frodin L. Ischemic heart disease–major cause of death and graft loss after renal transplantation in Scandinavia. Transplantation. 1995;**60**:451-457

[42] Hernandez D, Lacalzada J, Rufino M, et al. Prediction of left ventricular mass changes after renal transplantation by polymorphism of the angiotensin-converting enzyme gene. Kidney International. 1997;**51**:1205-1211

[43] Raine AEG, Margreiter R, Brunner FP, et al. Report of management on renal failure in Eurpoe XXII. Nephrology, Dialysis, Transplantation. 1992;**7**(Suppl 2):7-35

[44] Aakhus S, Dahl K, Widerøe TE. Cardiovascular disease in stable renal transplant patients in Norway: Morbidity and mortality during a 5-yr follow-up. Clinical Transplantation. 2004;**18**(5):596-604

[45] Rigatto C, Foley RN, Kent GM. Long-termchanges in left ventricular hypertrophy after renal transplantation. Transplantation. 2000;**70**:570-575

[46] McGregor E, Stewart G, Rodger RS, Jardine AG. Early echocardiographic changes and survival following renal transplantation. Nephrology, Dialysis, Transplantation. 2000;**15**:93-98

[47] Rigatto C, Parfery P, Foley R, Negrijn C, Tribula C, Jeffery J. Congestive heart failure in renal transplant recipients: Risk factors, outcomes, and relationship with ischemic heart disease. Journal of the American Society of Nephrology. 2002;**13**:1084-1090

[48] Lentine KL, Schnitzler MA, Abbott KC, Li L, Burroughs TE, Irish W, Brennan DC. De novo congestive heart failure after kidney transplantation: A common condition with poor prognostic implications. American Journal of Kidney Diseases. 2005;**46**(4):720-733

[49] Higashi M, Yamaura K, Ikeda M, Shimauchi T, Saiki H, Hoka S. Diastolic dysfunction of the left ventricle is associated with pulmonary edema after renal transplantation. Acta Anaesthesiologica Scandinavica. 2013;**57**(9):1154-1160

[50] Sever MS, Steinmuller DR, Hayes JM, Streem SB, Novick AC. Pericarditis following renal transplantation. Transplantation. 1991;**51**(6):1229-1232

[51] Alpert MA, Ravenscraft MD. Pericardial involvement in end-stage renal disease. The American Journal of the Medical Sciences. 2003;**325**(4):228

[52] Montanaro D, Gropuzzo M, Tulissi P, Boscutti G, Risaliti A. Cardiovascular disease after renal transplantation. Giornale Italiano di Nefrologia. 2004;**21**(Suppl 26):S53-S66

[53] Smajić E, Kušljugić Z, Barakowić F. Hiperlipoproteinemije U: Kušljugić Z, Baraković F Kardiologija, I izdanje. Tuzla: PrintCom; 2006. pp. 81-207

[54] Sarnak MJ, Coronado BE, Greene T, et al. Cardiovascular disease risk factors in chronic renal insufficiency. Clinical Nephrology. 2002;**57**:327-335

13

Anaesthesia for Liver Transplantation

Gabriela Droc and Lavinia Jipa

Abstract

Liver transplantation is a high-risk surgery performed on a high-risk patient and is the only treatment for end-stage liver disease. Ever since the first successful liver transplant performed, patient survival increased due to improvement of surgical technique and anaesthetic management as well as the emergence of new generations of immunosuppressants. The pre-anaesthetic evaluation is mandatory and plays an important role in patient inclusion on the transplant list. Liver transplantation is performed under general anaesthesia, and the anaesthetic monitoring is very important for a successful liver transplantation as it can expose problems before irreversible damage occurs. Haemodynamic instability is common during surgery, requiring complex invasive haemodynamic monitoring. Continuous assessment of the patient's volemic status and the amount of perfused fluids represent the key to a successful liver transplantation. Inadequate fluid therapy can lead to pulmonary oedema, abnormal gas exchange, congestion, decrease in perfusion and oedema of the graft. Liver reperfusion takes place in the neohepatic phase and is the most unstable period during liver transplantation, representing a real challenge for the anaesthetist. It can have severe consequences due to a decrease in cardiovascular function with haemodynamic instability, abnormal acid base balance and metabolic abnormalities.

Keywords: liver transplant, cirrhotic cardiomyopathy, postreperfusion syndrome

1. Introduction

Liver transplantation is the only treatment for end-stage liver disease regardless of its aetiology as well as for other categories of liver failure. The procedure is performed on a high-risk patient with impairment of cardiovascular, pulmonary, renal and coagulation systems. Due to increasingly good results, transplant candidates are older and frequently have co-morbidities.

Since the first transplant interventions in the 1960s, postintervention morbidity rate decreased and patient survival increased. This is due to the improvement of surgical technique and anaesthetic management as well as the emergence of new generations of immunosuppressants. Medical care of pre-transplant patients has also experienced a favourable evolution.

The outcome of patients undergoing liver transplantation depends on the perioperative management. Dedicated and specialized teams for liver transplantation have a major role on the outcome of these patients.

2. Preoperative assessment

Liver transplantation is a high-risk surgery performed on a high-risk patient, the cirrhotic patient with end-stage liver disease. The pre-anaesthetic evaluation is mandatory and plays an important role in accepting the inclusion of the patient on the transplant list. Today, patients eligible for transplant are older and often associate co-morbidities.

2.1. Cardiac evaluation

2.1.1. Coronary artery disease (CAD)

The cirrhotic patient has long been considered to be protected from coronary artery disease (CAD) due to his/her haemodynamic profile associated to a low serum cholesterol level. However, recent studies show that CAD has the same prevalence in this group compared to the general population. Patients frequently associate risk factors for CAD such as obesity, diabetes and hypertension.

The incidence of CAD does not seem to be influenced by the aetiology of cirrhosis except for non-alcoholic steatohepatitis (NASH), in which case it is twice as high, NASH associating with the metabolic syndrome [1]. The importance of CAD detection is due to the haemodynamic high stress during liver transplant leading to exacerbation of the cardiac suffering during surgery or generating postoperative cardiac complications [2, 3]. Recognizing CAD is very important, but the best therapeutic approach in case of significant coronary stenosis is not well defined.

Coronary angioplasty may be recommended, but due to the need for heavy anti-aggregation, this may increase the risk of bleeding in the cirrhotic patient. When required, bare metal stents are preferred to pharmacologically active ones because of a shorter period of anti-aggregation. Surgical intervention for myocardial revascularization is not recommended due to a very high mortality risk in the cirrhotic patient [2, 4].

2.1.2. Cirrhotic cardiomyopathy

Cirrhotic patients have myocardial dysfunction secondary to hepatic impairment [5].

Regardless of the aetiology of cirrhosis, cardiomyopathy is characterized by

- increased cardiac output at baseline,
- impaired contractile reserve in response to stress; this is due to a lower density of beta adrenergic receptors as well as to the negative inotropic effect of excess nitric oxide production,

- diastolic dysfunction; it is more pronounced in patients with ascites,
- electrophysiological alterations like prolongation of the QT interval [3, 6].

The prolonged QT interval is associated with the severity of liver disease and the degree of portal hypertension as well as mortality [2]. A QTc interval of >440 ms correlates with an increased risk of ventricular arrhythmias [7].

Both diastolic and systolic dysfunction can be causes of postoperative pulmonary oedema. Right heart dysfunction, when present, has a higher predictive value for postoperative cardiac complications.

2.1.3. Other causes for cardiac impairment

Chronic consumption of ethanol may cause dilated cardiomyopathy; it is characterized by left ventricular dilatation with altered systolic function. In the initial stages of heart disease, abstinence from alcohol can significantly improve the symptoms.

In the case of haemochromatosis, excess iron will be deposited in the myocardium, leading to restrictive cardiomyopathy [2].

2.1.4. Steps of cardiac evaluation

Investigating a patient will begin with the existence of a history of heart disease as well as symptoms suggestive of cardiovascular events such as rhythm disorders or angina. Because of their low exercise capacity due to cirrhosis, the incidence of angina is low and frequently coronary heart disease can be underestimated.

The baseline assessment includes an electrocardiographic (ECG) recording at rest and an echocardiography.

The echocardiography evaluates the following [8]:

- measurements of cardiac chambers
- valvular characteristics and function
- evaluation of systolic function of the left ventricle (LV) expressed as ejection fraction; we must not forget that these values are obtained under the conditions of low blood pressure due to the vasodilatation of the cirrhotic patient, so they can underestimate the real ejection fraction
- evaluation of diastolic function of the left ventricle by measuring early and late diastolic velocities through the mitral valve to determine the E/A ratio (ventricular filling phases = initial E vs. tardive A); E/A < 1 reflects a diastolic dysfunction; diastolic dysfunction is more pronounced in patients with ascites [6]

If electrocardiogram and echocardiography are two mandatory pre-transplant investigations, the question is what other methods should be used in those patients who require additional methods.

According to AASLD (American Association for the Study of Liver Disease), AHA (American Heart Association) and ACCF (American College of Cardiology Foundation), additional investigations should be undertaken for patients who have three or more associated risk factors of the following: diabetes, left ventricular hypertrophy, history of CAD, age > 60 years, smoking, hypertension, dyslipidaemia and obesity [4, 9].

Several types of investigations have been proposed:

- stress echocardiography using dobutamine, adenosine or dipyridamole,
- myocardial perfusion scintigraphy,
- computerized cardiac tomography which allows calculating the calcium score; this is a rapid and non-invasive way to measure calcium deposits in the coronary vessel wall as an expression of coronary stenosis; results are measured in Ca scores: a Ca of >100 score carries a moderate risk of cardiac events and a score of >400 a high risk [10].

Valvular dysfunctions in the cirrhotic patient on the transplant list are poorly studied. The evaluation of such a patient should include the severity of the valve dysfunction, either stenosis or regurgitation, the degree of alteration of myocardial contractility and the clinical presence of signs of insufficient cardiac output. Several cases of simultaneous liver transplantation and aortic valve replacement for tight aortic stenosis were reported in the cirrhotic patient [6].

2.2. Pulmonary system

Chronic liver disease can affect both the pleural space and the pulmonary parenchyma. The two pulmonary conditions characteristic of the cirrhotic patient are hepatopulmonary syndrome and pulmonary hypertension. The two syndromes exclude each other, and their pathophysiology depends on predominant vasodilator or vasoconstrictor elements resulting from liver dysfunction.

Portopulmonary hypertension is a pulmonary hypertension syndrome with vascular obstruction, coexisting with portal hypertension. The portopulmonary syndrome has important haemodynamic consequences with minor changes in blood gases.

All patients proposed for transplantation should be screened for portopulmonary hypertension as the postoperative evolution depends on it. It might be suspected in the case of a right branch block on ECG. Echocardiography can detect pulmonary hypertension and can evaluate it, but correct values are obtained by right heart catheterization. Depending on the mean pressure in the pulmonary artery (PAPm), hypertension is classified in mild (PAPm 25–34 mmHg), moderate (PAPm 35–44 mmHg) and severe (PAPm >45 mmHg).

Severe pulmonary hypertension excludes the patient from liver transplantation; moderate form may benefit from vasodilator drug treatment in pre-transplant [4]. Decision to perform liver transplant in this case depends on the response to therapy and is taken by the transplant team on an individual basis.

Hepatopulmonary syndrome is characterized by hypoxemia secondary to intrapulmonary shunt due to vascular dilation. In contrast with pulmonary hypertension that may be aggravated by surgery for liver transplant, the hepatopulmonary syndrome's evolution is extremely favourable post transplantation with net amelioration or even complete resolution.

The cirrhotic patient might develop **pleural effusions**. The hydrothorax appears most frequently on the right side and generally accompanies ascites. It is due to an anatomical defect in the right hemidiaphragm. Sometimes, it might need drainage prior to surgery [11–13].

The cirrhotic patient may suffer from any other pulmonary disease not related to the chronic liver failure. Chronic obstructive pulmonary disease may be associated with cirrhosis, especially in smoker patients, resulting in obstructive respiratory insufficiency, which together with restrictive ascites dysfunction may greatly compromise respiratory function. Patients will be evaluated by a pneumologist for treatment and encouraged to quit smoking.

Since the necessary immunosuppression after transplantation may lead to reactivation of a dormant latent tuberculosis, it is mandatory to test transplant candidates for latent tuberculosis. This is done either with the tuberculin skin test or with the quantiferon TB test, a cell immune response assay using a *Mycobacterium tuberculosis*-like protein substrate.

Depending on the lung's status, investigations will be limited to a chest X-ray or will go further to pulmonary ultrasound or computed tomography (CT) scan of the thorax [14, 15].

2.3. Evaluation of renal function

Renal dysfunction in the cirrhotic patient is due to a decreased blood volume due to vasodilation, with a decrease in glomerular filtration. It may not be reflected correctly in serum creatinine levels; the end-stage liver disease patient often has a less muscle mass and a low creatinine production. Higher sensitivity tests are cystatin C or NGAL (neutrophil gelatinase-associated lipocalin).

Two types of kidney dysfunction are related to cirrhosis: hepatorenal syndrome is type 1 with rapid deterioration in renal function (doubling serum creatinine or increasing it to >2.5 mg/dl in less than 2 weeks) and a type 2 with slower evolution.

The occurrence of renal dysfunction can be precipitated by haemorrhage and infection [4, 16]. Preoperative renal dysfunction increases the risk of adverse development of postoperative complications.

2.4. Coagulation status

Coagulation abnormalities are caused by reduced concentrations of vitamin K-dependent factors and an imbalance between procoagulant and anticoagulant factors. Standard coagulation tests do not reflect rebalanced haemostasis and must not be used to predict the risk of bleeding. Procoagulant factors must not be administered unless signs of bleeding are present [17].

The Guidelines of the European Society of Anaesthesia regarding cirrhotic patients do not recommend routine preoperative correction of international normalized ratio (INR) (1.5–5) using fresh-frozen plasma but advise correction through point of care tests: rotational thromboelastometry or thromboelastography [18].

3. Conduct of anaesthesia

Despite recent advances, liver transplantation remains a major challenge to the anaesthetist due to the important cardiovascular changes throughout surgery: important changes in preload, afterload, arrhythmias, hypotension and hyperkalaemic events. All these increase the chances of severe cardiac dysfunction.

Liver transplantation is characterized by haemodynamic instability and various complications that can arise throughout the three important surgical phases: preanhepatic, anhepatic and neohepatic.

- Preanhepatic: dissection and liver mobilization takes place; usually massive bleeding can occur that can lead to hypovolaemia and haemorrhagic shock.
- Anhepatic: between clamping hepatic inflow and before graft reperfusion; consists of clamping of the inferior vena cava (IVC); significant decrease in cardiac output (CO) occurs.
- Neohepatic: characterized by liver reperfusion, reappearance of flow in the vena cava and vena porta, blood volume goes back to normal; can be complicated by reperfusion syndrome or bleeding from vascular anastomosis (hepatic artery, portal vein).

3.1. Patient monitoring during liver transplantation

Liver transplantation is performed under general anaesthesia, and the anaesthetic monitoring plays an important part in a successful liver transplantation as it can expose problems before irreversible damage occurs.

Haemodynamic instability is common during liver transplantation, and that is why the anaesthetic monitoring is complex, being divided into standard monitoring, haemodynamic (invasive and non-invasive), neurologic and neuromuscular monitoring.

3.1.1. Standard monitoring

According to the American Society of Anaesthesia (ASA) protocols, standard monitoring applies to all patients during all types of anaesthesia with the aim of increasing patients' quality of care. Trained personnel must be present in the operating room during the entire surgery, while continuous monitoring of the oxygenation, ventilation, circulation and temperature is mandatory [19].

Oxygenation: gas monitoring as the level of inspired oxygen (FiO_2) and the level of expired CO_2 ($ETCO_2$ capnography) and blood oxygenation in a continuous form as peripheral capillary oxygen saturation (SpO_2 pulsoxymetry).

Ventilation: chest movements and lung auscultation but also the volume of expired gas and capnography.

Circulation: continuous electrocardiogram (ECG) for rhythm, frequency, signs of ischaemia (ST segment), QT interval and measurement of blood pressure in a non-invasive way before induction of anaesthesia.

Temperature: central temperature is the blood temperature which bathes the vital organs (heart and brain). Important sites of measurement are the following: tympanic membrane, nasopharynx, distal oesophagus, blood, urinary bladder and rectum [20].

3.1.2. *Haemodynamic monitoring*

Patients with chronic liver disease usually present many other systemic complications including portal hypertension, ascites, coagulopathy, hyperdynamic circulatory syndrome (high cardiac index and low systemic vascular resistance) and cirrhotic cardiomyopathy. Due to all these changes, advanced haemodynamic monitoring is necessary. Monitoring parameters and normal values are shown in **Table 1** [21].

3.1.2.1. *Invasive blood pressure*

Invasive arterial pressure monitoring represents standard practice during liver transplantation. The arterial catheter is usually inserted in the radial artery and is being used for continuous pressure monitoring, blood gas analysis and other blood tests. Due to variations of radial artery pressure which may sometimes underestimate aortic pressure in hypotensive states, when high dose vasopressors are used and after reperfusion of the liver, some anaesthetists prefer using the femoral artery. Despite all these, the mean central and peripheral arterial pressures are usually the same [22]. An important problem when deciding the sites for catheter insertion is the cirrhotic coagulopathy which can lead to important puncture site bleeding. The number and sites of line insertion vary according to the transplant centre and experience.

3.1.2.2. *Central venous pressure*

Central venous pressure (CVP) monitoring is essential during liver transplantation. Central venous pressure is measured via a central catheter inserted in the superior vena cava system. Maintaining a low CVP in a normovolaemic patient can reduce the risk of bleeding but can increase the risk of vital organ hypoperfusion in case of a hypovolaemic patient or a massive bleeding [23].

3.1.2.3. *Cardiac output and pulmonary artery pressures*

Since its discovery, the pulmonary artery flotation catheter (Swan Ganz) has been considered the gold standard for cardiac output measurement. Swan Ganz catheters are still used routinely in some transplant centres around the world. A pulmonary artery catheter is mandatory if pulmonary hypertension is diagnosed or suspected.

Pulmonary artery pressures, cardiac output measurements and mixed venous oxygen saturation help in the diagnosis and management of haemodynamic instability during surgery. The new modified Swan Ganz catheters help anaesthetists with continuous cardiac output measurements and right ventricular end-diastolic volume as a more accurate parameter of preload.

Despite the massive use in the last 40 years, its high cost and patient safety have led to question its utility [24].

Parameter	Abbreviation	Formula	Normal value
Median arterial pressure	MAP	SBP+(2 × DBP)/3	75–105 mmHg
Arterial oxygen concentration	CaO_2	(0.0138 × Hb × SaO_2) + 0.003 × PaO_2	16–22 ml/dl
Venous oxygen concentration	CvO_2	(0.0138 × Hb × SvO_2) + 0.003 × PvO_2	15 ml/dl
Peripheral capillary oxygen saturation	SpO_2	Measurement	95–100%
Arteriovenous oxygen difference	$C(a\text{-}v)O_2$	CaO_2-CvO_2	4–6 ml/dl
Stroke volume	SV	CO/HR × 1000	60–100 ml/beat
Stroke volume index	SVI	CI/HR × 1000	33–47 ml/m^2/beat
Cardiac output	CO	HR × SV/1000	4–8 l/min
Cardiac index	CI	CO/BSA	2.5–4 l/min/m^2
Central venous pressure	CVP	Measurement	2–6 mmHg
Central venous oxygen saturation	$ScvO_2$	Measurement	70–80%
Extravascular lung water	EVLW	CO × DSt-0.25GEDV	
Extravascular lung water index	EVLWI	EVLW/PBW	0–7 ml/kgc
Global ejection fraction	GEF	SV × 4/GEDV	>20%
Global end-diastolic volume	GEDV	CO × MTt × f(S1/S2)	
Global end-diastolic volume index	GEDI	CI × MTt × f(S1/S2)	650–800 ml/kgc
Intrathoracic blood volume	ITBV	1.25 × GEDV	
Intrathoracic blood volume index	ITBI	1.25 × GEDI	850–1000 ml/m^2
Left ventricular stroke work	LVSW	SI × MAP×0.0144	8–10 g/m^2/beat
Left ventricular stroke work index	LVSWI	SVI× (MAP-PAOP) × 0.0136	50–62 g/m^2/beat
Mean pulmonary artery pressure	MPAP	PASP+(2 × PADP)/3	9–18 mmHg
Oxygen consumption	VO_2	$C(a\text{-}v)O_2$ × CO × 10	200–250 ml/min
Oxygen delivery	DO_2	CaO_2 × CO × 10	950–1150 ml/min
Pulmonary artery occlusion pressure	PAOP	Measurement	6–12 mmHg
Pulmonary artery systolic pressure	PASP	Measurement	15–30 mmHg
Pulmonary artery diastolic pressure	PADP	Measurement	8–15 mmHg
Pulmonary vascular resistance	PVR	80× (MPAP-PAOP)/CO	<250 dynes/s/cm^5
Pulmonary vascular resistance index	PVRI	80× (MPAP-PAOP)/CI	255–285 dynes/s/cm^5/m^2
Stroke volume variation	SVV	SVmax-SVmin/SVmean×100	10–15%
Systemic vascular resistance	SVR	80× (MAP-RAP)/CO	800–1200 dynes/s/cm^5
Systemic vascular resistance index	SVRI	80× (MAP-RAP)/CI	1970–2390 dynes/sec/cm5/m2

Table 1. Haemodynamic parameters.

3.1.2.4. Other ways of measuring cardiac output

The pulse contour analysis is useful for continuous monitoring of cardiac output and needs frequent calibration via thermodilution technique:

- PiCCO system (Pulse-induced Contour Cardiac Output): this consists of a thermistor catheter placed in the femoral artery and can estimate stroke volume. A central venous catheter inserted in the superior vena cava circulation is needed for the pulmonary calibration which must be done every 8 h in a haemodynamic stable patient and more frequent for unstable patients [25].
- LiDCO: it uses the same algorithm for stroke volume monitoring. Lithium chloride is used for transpulmonary calibration and can be injected into a peripheral vein.
- Transoesophageal echocardiography gives continuous information on ventricular function and volume status and allows immediate diagnosis of air or thrombus embolization. It also provides information regarding contractility, valvular function, pericardial or pleural effusion. Its main advantage is the ease of continuous use during surgery due to the anaesthetized and intubated patient [26].
- Thoracic bioimpedance: it estimates cardiac output and other haemodynamic parameters based on the electric properties of the thorax produced by blood movements during cardiac cycle; rarely used in liver transplantation.

3.1.3. Neurologic monitoring

- Bispectral index: Fourier analysis of a fronto-parietal electroencephalogram (EEG). It varies between 0 (coma) and 10 (normal cortical activity) with an adequate value between 40 and 60 in an anaesthetized patient [27].
- Transcranial Doppler echography can diagnose vasospasm, intracranial hypertension and cerebral death.
- Oxygen saturation in the jugular bulb ($SjvO_2$): continuous monitoring of venous oxygen saturation via a central catheter inserted in the internal jugular vein that shows the balance between oxygen intake and consumption. Values below 50% show ischaemia while values above 75% show cerebral hyperaemia.
- Transcerebral cranial oximetry: resembles $SjvO_2$.
- Electroencephalogram: rarely used for continuous monitoring during surgery; requires a trained anaesthetist who must differentiate pathological changes from normal changes in a cerebral activity during anaesthesia.

3.1.4. Neuromuscular monitoring

Residual neuromuscular block after the use of neuromuscular blockade agents can have a detrimental effect in patients after surgery causing inadequate hypoxic ventilatory response, depressed pharyngeal tonus leading to an increased risk of airway obstruction and death.

Peripheral nerve stimulation and depth of block can be assessed using single twitch, train of four, tetanic stimulation and double burst stimulation.

3.1.5. Other parameters monitored during liver transplantation

Other parameters monitored during liver transplantation include the following:

- hourly diuresis,
- haemoglobin and haematocrit,
- electrolytes,
- base excess and lactate,
- coagulation parameters via rotational thromboelastometry (ROTEM).

3.2. Haemodynamic management during the three phases of liver transplantation

3.2.1. Volemic resuscitation

Ever since the first successful liver transplantation in 1960, the surgery has been associated with significant bleeding and an increased amount of blood products transfused [28]. Blood products used during liver transplantation have declined significantly in the last 20 years. Even if bleeding risk has decreased over time, it still can induce a volemic stress.

Clamping of the inferior vena cava during the second phase (anhepatic) of the liver transplantation leads to an important decrease in preload, CO and arterial pressure which need a quick diagnosis and management. Normal response of right ventricle (RV) and left ventricle (LV) to stress does not take place due to all the substances released from the liver in the anhepatic phase.

Continuous assessment of patient's volemic status and the amount of perfused fluids represent the key to a successful liver transplantation. This can be done using dynamic measurements of CVP and pulmonary capillary wedge pressure (PCWP), but these parameters do not correlate with changes in CO [29]. Another way of assessing fluid responsiveness is the use of stroke volume variation (SVV) and global end-diastolic volume index (GEDI). Inadequate fluid therapy can lead to pulmonary oedema, abnormal gas exchange, congestion, a decrease in perfusion and oedema of the graft [30].

This study does not offer an answer for the ideal monitoring system and guiding of fluid therapy [31]. In our clinic, the guidance of fluid management is done with the pulmonary thermodilution technique and pulse contour wave analysis via the PiCCO system.

Using adequate vasoactive substances, which protect the brain, heart and kidney, led to a greater haemodynamic stability, adequate CO and renal perfusion [31]. The CVP can also be correlated with the severity of the post-reperfusion syndrome [32].

Specific fluid management during liver transplantation can be described according to the three surgical phases:

- Preanhepatic phase: cirrhotic patients usually have variate quantities of ascites; the anaesthetist must try and compensate it in order to reach normovolaemia and avoid hypovolaemia during the next phase (anhepatic) when clamping the inferior vena cava. Albumin of 20 or 5% is used for volemic resuscitation.

- Anhepatic phase: fluid restriction is the best solution in this phase while maintaining adequate arterial pressure with the help of vasopressors. The vasopressor of choice is noradrenaline, and the parameters measured with the PiCCO system can guide us to using inotopes such as dobutamine.

- Neohepatic phase: in this stage, the patient needs adequate volemic resuscitation guided by the PiCCO parameters; an important decrease in vasopressors takes place.

Albumin determines the oncotic pressure that keeps fluids in the intravascular space. Cirrhotic patients usually have low albumin levels [32]. Studies have shown that the use of albumin during liver transplantation decreases the amount of intraoperative fluids used and the frequency of pulmonary oedema in cardiac and noncardiac surgery [33]. It has also been proved that albumin decreases mortality in cirrhotic patients, decreases the incidence of post-reperfusion syndrome and the use of vasopressor agents [34].

The use of Hetastarch is not recommended as it affects platelet aggregability and increases the risk of bleeding by decreasing the concentration of coagulation factor 8 [33]. Gelatines can have numerous side effects: anaphylactic reactions, a decrease in thrombin generation and worsening of fibrinolysis which is specific in the anhepatic phase [35].

Manitol can be used in the anhepatic phase before clamping of the IVC (0.5 g/kgc) in order to avoid blood congestion in the liver and intraabdominal organ oedema [36].

PiCCO monitoring has a number of advantages: accurate CO calculations and guiding fluid management. ITBV is an accurate parameter of preload even when IVC is clamped [37]. We can also use SVV in order to predict fluid responsiveness [38].

Fluid management is done using PiCCO parameters determined during the three phases of the liver transplantation. This guidance of fluid therapy decreases the post-anaesthesia care unit stay and mortality [39]. The decisional tree regarding fluid management is presented in **Table 2**.

TOE can also be helpful in high-risk patients with various cardiac problems. It has the advantage of direct assessment of cardiac contractility and assesses response to inotropes and volemic status. It can diagnose embolic complications and cardiac tamponade [40].

The use of different monitoring techniques is the key to successful management of haemodynamic instability and fluid guidance during liver transplantation.

3.2.2. Vasoactive substances and inotropes

There are a variety of substances that can be used when haemodynamic instability takes place during liver transplantation. Noradrenaline is most often used, followed by adrenaline and dobutamine. Indications are shown in **Table 3**.

CI < 3 l/min/m²			
GEDI <700 ml/m² or ITBI <850 ml/m²		GEDI >700 ml/m² or ITBI >850 ml/m²	
ELWI <10	ELWI >10	ELWI <10	ELWI >10
Administer fluids	Administer fluids (limited) Vasopressor	Vasopressor	Vasopressor Fluid restriction
CI > 3 l/min/m²			
GEDI <700 ml/m² or ITBI <850 ml/m²		GEDI >700 ml/m² or ITBI >850 ml/m²	
ELWI <10 ml/m²	ELWI >10 ml/m²	ELWI <10 ml/m²	ELWI >10 ml/m²
Administer fluids	Administer fluids	No measure	Fluid restriction

Table 2. Fluid therapy decisional tree.

3.2.3. Postreperfusion syndrome

Liver reperfusion takes place in the neohepatic phase and is the most unstable period during liver transplantation, representing a real challenge for the anaesthetist. The postreperfusion syndrome is defined as a 30% decrease in the mean arterial pressure that lasts for at least a minute and appears in the first 5 min after the unclamping of the inferior vena cava (IVC) [41].

It can have severe consequences due to a decrease in cardiovascular function with haemodynamic instability, abnormal acid base balance and metabolic abnormalities. Haemodynamic instability is the consequence of severe vasodilation, negative inotropic effects and massive bleeding which may appear during surgery. Graft reperfusion can have fatal consequences such as severe arrhythmias or asystole [42].

The incidence of PRS varies between 5.9 and 60% due to different surgical techniques, haemodynamic intraoperative differences and geographic factors (in some countries, the number of reduced donors led to marginal graft use-expanded criteria donors) [43].

Causes of PRS are not yet clear, but there are several theories. Dyselectrolytemia, cold solutions used for graft preservation and severe vasodilation due to NO release may contribute to PRS. Unclamping of the inferior vena cava leads to vasoactive pro-inflammatory substance released from Kupffer cells and which are the result of the postischaemic graft [44].

Substance	Indications	Dose
Noradrenaline	Arterial hypotension	0.2–1 μg/kgc/min
Adrenaline	Asystole, severe arterial hypotension	0.01–0.5 μg/kgc/min
Dobutamine	Cardiogenic shock	2.5–10 μg/kgc/min
Ephedrine	Arterial hypotension Before unclamping IVC	5–25 mg i.v. bolus every 10 min

Table 3. Main indications of inotropes during liver transplantation.

One of the most important elements released from the graft is potassium as a result of the portal venous congestion. All these substances can contribute to postoperative ischaemia and reperfusion lesions [45]. Another theory is represented by the pro-inflammatory cytokines (IL 1B, IL 2, IL 8, TNF-α) produced by ischaemia and released during the reperfusion of the graft leading to a marked inflammatory response and cellular death. They also have vasodilation and negative inotropic effect. The amount of pro-inflammatory cytokines released does not correlate with the duration of cold ischaemia time (CIT) [46].

Factors that may predict PRS are the following:

- donor-related: age, obesity, hypernatraemia (>155 mEq), hepatic steatosis, prolonged intensive care unit (ICU),
- intraoperative factors: duration of the surgery,
- cold ischaemia time exceeding 6 h.

Risk factors include

- patient's volemic status before reperfusion,
- myocardial depression (due to cold solutions released in circulation, abnormal acid base status),
- severity of metabolic acidosis.

Studies have shown that patients who had PRS have a higher risk of postoperative renal dysfunction and 15 days of mortality [43].

Postreperfusion syndrome leads to

- a decrease in arterial pressure and SVR,
- a decrease in CO,
- a moderate increase in PAP,
- frequent malignant arrhythmias.

Therapeutic options include the following:

- optimizing volemic status,
- adequate haemodynamic management,
- adequate graft perfusion; vasodilators are rarely used (calcium channel blockers, prostaglandins),
- liver graft wash with flush fluid of albumin 5% before IVC unclamping,
- correction of hypocalcaemia and hyperkalaemia,
- give ephedrine bolus 5 min before unclamping of the IVC in order to obtain a MAP of 85–100 mmHg [47].

3.3. Coagulation management

Cirrhotic patients have been regarded as having a high risk of bleeding due to standard coagulation test abnormalities caused by cirrhotic coagulopathy. Recent studies have shown that bleeding episodes are caused by vascular abnormalities and portal hypertension [48].

Standard coagulation tests (prothrombin time, INR and activated partial thromboplastin time (aPTT)) reveal the deficit of procoagulant factors without showing the status of the anticoagulant factors.

In order to have an optimal view regarding cirrhotic coagulopathy, global coagulation tests (viscoelastic tests) are recommended [49].

Intraoperative blood transfusion has a negative impact on patient outcome. Intraoperative packed red cells and platelet transfusion are independent predictors of 1 year mortality [50].

There are a few measures that can decrease the need of blood transfusion:

- maintaining a low CVP,
- use of antifibrinolytic agents,
- use of recombinant activated factor 7,
- use of point of care tests for transfusion guidance.

The most important coagulation problems that can appear during the three transplant phases are specific for each phase:

- Preanhepatic phase: bleeding occurs due to extensive dissection, collateral circulation and portal hypertension. Maintaining a normal volemic status may lead to dilutional coagulopathy and thrombocytopaenia [51]. A low CVP must be maintained in this phase. Cell saver can also be used after evacuation of ascites and before biliary anastomosis.
- Anhepatic phase: between clamping hepatic inflow and before graft reperfusion. Usually, minimal bleeding takes place here, but the risk exists. Platelets and coagulation factors are low due to loss and consumption from the previous phase. Synthesis and liver clearance do not exist. An increase in the release of tPA from endothelial cells and the absence of hepatic clearance can lead to hyperfibrinolysis and bleeding. Viscoelastic tests are mandatory for the diagnosis and management of hyperfibrinolysis.
- Neohepatic phase: bleeding can occur due to surgical problems or haemostatic abnormalities. Usually, hypothermia, metabolic acidosis and hypocalcaemia must be corrected before any further decision is taken. Platelets are seized in the liver graft after reperfusion causing important thrombocytopaenia. Some platelets are partially activated in the liver graft and released in the circulation as inefficient.

Hyperfibrinolysis can often appear during liver transplantation, but is self-limited as long as the liver graft is viable.

Antifibrinolytic agents can be used when diffuse bleeding occurs or when point of care tests show hyperfibrinolysis. In case of diffuse bleeding, the anaesthetist must correct hypothermia, acidosis, hypocalcaemia, treat hyperfibrinolysis and then administer fibrinogen 24 mg/kgc and platelets.

4. Conclusion

Anaesthesia for liver transplantation is one of the most difficult anaesthesias. This is due to the haemodynamic problems that can occur in the intraoperative, related both to the status of the patient (cardiomyopathy of the cirrhosis, etc.) and to the surgical moments (bleeding and reperfusion syndrome) as well as to the blood coagulation pattern of the patient.

A good understanding of the pathophysiology of the cirrhotic patient is very important for best decision making. Adequate perioperative management is extremely important for a successful liver transplantation with a good outcome.

Author details

Gabriela Droc* and Lavinia Jipa

*Address all correspondence to: gabidroc@gmail.com

Fundeni Clinical Institute, University of Medicine and Pharmacy "Carol Davila", Bucharest, Romania

References

[1] Gologorsky E, Pretto Jr EA, Fukazawa K. Coronary artery disease and its risk factors in patients presenting for liver transplantation. Journal of Clinical Anesthesia. 2013;**25**:618-623

[2] Ripoll C, Yotti R, Bermejo J, Banares R. The heart in liver transplantation. Journal of Hepatology. 2011;**54**:810-822

[3] Martinez-Palli G, Cardenas A. Preoperative cardio pulmonary assessment of the liver transplant candidate. Annals of Hepatology. 2011;**10**:421-433. https://www.hindawi.com/journals/ccrp/2012/539412/cta/

[4] Martin P, DiMartini A, Feng S, Brown Jr S, Fallon M. Evaluation for liver transplantation in adults: 2013 practice guideline by the AASLD and the American Society of Transplantation. Hepatology. 2014;**59**:1144-1165

[5] Figueiredo A, Romero-Bermejo F, Perdigoto R, Marcelino P. The end-organ impairment in liver cirrhosis: Appointments for critical care. Critical Care Research and Practice. 2012. DOI: 10.1155/2012/539412

[6] Garg A, Armstrong W. Echocardiography in liver transplant candidates. JACC: Cardiovascular Imaging. 2013;**6**:105-119

[7] Raval Z, Harinstein M, Skaro A, Erdogan A, DeWolf A, Shah S, et al. Cardiovascular risk assessment of the liver transplant candidate. Journal of the American College of Cardiology. 2011;**58**:223-231

[8] Chen Y, Chan A, Chan SC, Chok SH, Sharr W, Fung J, et al. A detailed evaluation of cardiac function in cirrhotic patients an its alteration with or without liver transplantation. Journal of Cardiology. 2016;**67**:140-146

[9] Lentine K, Costa S, Weir M, Robb J, Fleisher L, Kasiske B, et al. Cardiac disease evaluation and management among kidney and liver transplantation candidates. A scientific statement from the American Heart Association and the American College of Cardiology Foundation. Circulation. 2012;**126**:617-663. DOI: 10.1161/CIR.0b013e31823eb07a

[10] Mandell MS, Lindenfeld JA, Tsou MY, Zimmerman M. Cardiac evaluation of liver transplant candidates. World Journal of Gastroenterology. 2008;**22**:3445-3451

[11] Cartin-Ceba R, Krowka M. Preoperative assessment and management of liver transplant candidates with portopulmonary hypertension. Advances in Pulmonary Hypertension. 2013;**2**:60-67

[12] Bozbas SS, Yilmaz EB, Dogrul I, Ergur FO, Savas N, Eyuboglu F, Haberal M. Preoperative pulmonary evaluation of liver transplant candidates: Results from 341 adult patients. Annals of Transplantation. 2011;**16**:88-96

[13] Dalal A. Anesthesia for liver transplantation. Transplantation Reviews. 2016;**30**:51-60

[14] Bozbas SS, Eyuboglu F. Evaluation of liver transplant candidates: A pulmonary perspective. Annals of Thoracic Medicine. 2011;**6**:109-114

[15] Jafri SM, Singal A, Kaul D, Fontana RJ. Detection and management of latent tuberculosis in liver transplant patients. Liver Transplantation. 2011;**17**:306-314

[16] Weber M, Ibrahim H, Lake J. Renal dysfunction in liver transplant recipients: Evaluation of the critical issues. Liver Transplantation. 2012;**18**:1290-1301

[17] Westerkamp AC, Lisman T, Porte RJ. How to minimize blood loss during liver surgery in patients with cirrhosis. HPB: The Official Journal of the International Hepato Pancreato Biliary Association. 2009;**11**(6):453-458

[18] Kozek-Langenecker SA, Afshari A, Albaladejo P, Santullano CAA, De Robertis E, Filipescu DC, et al. Management of severe perioperative bleeding: Guidelines from the European Society of Anaesthesiology. European Journal of Anaesthesiology. 2013; **30**(6):270-382

[19] Anaesthesiologists ASo [Internet]. 2015. Available from http://www.asahq.org/quality-and-practice-management/standards-guidelines-and-related-resources/standards-for-basic-anesthetic-monitoring [Accessed: 2018-01-05]

[20] Anaesthesia UK. Temperature measurement sites [Internet]. 2005. Available from: http://www.frca.co.uk/article.aspx?articleid=100352 [Accesed: 2018-01-05]

[21] Liu H, Gaskari SA, Lee SS. Cardiac and vascular changes in cirrhosis: Pathogenic mechanisms. World Journal of Gastroenterology: WJG. 2006;**12**(6):837-842. DOI: 10.3748/wjg.v12.i6.837

[22] Dorman T, Breslow MJ, Lipsett PA, Rosenberg JM, Balser JR, Almog Y, Rosenfeld BA. Radial artery pressure monitoring underestimates central arterial pressure during vasopressor therapy in critically ill surgical patients. Critical Care Medicine. 1998;**26**(10): 1646-1649

[23] Jones RM, Moulton CE, Hardy KJ. Central venous pressure and its effect on blood loss during liver resection. The British Journal of Surgery. 1998;**85**(8):1058-1060

[24] Marik PE, Baram M, Vahid B. Does central venous pressure predict fluid responsiveness? A systematic review of the literature and the tale of seven mares. Chest. 2008;**134**(1):172-178. DOI: 10.1378/chest.07-2331

[25] Alhashemi JA, Cecconi M, Hofer CK. Cardiac output monitoring: An integrative perspective. Critical Care. 2011;**15**(2):214

[26] De Pietri L, Mocchegiani F, Leuzzi C, Montalti R, Vivarelli M, Agnoletti V. Transoesophageal echocardiography during liver transplantation. World Journal of Hepatology. 2015;**7**(23):2432-2448

[27] The bispectral index (BIS) [Internet]. 2005. Available from http://www.frca.co.uk/article.aspx?articleid=100502 [Accessed: 2018-01-05]

[28] Starzl TE, Iwatuski S, VanThiel DH, et al. Evolution of liver transplantation. Hepatology. 1982;**2**:614-636

[29] Lucey MR. Liver transplantation in patients with alcoholic liver disease. Liver Transplantation. 2011;**56**:751-759

[30] Feltracco P, Barbieri S, Galligioni H, Michieletto E, Carollo C, Ori C. Intensive care management of liver transplanted patients. World Journal of Hepatology. 2011;**3**(3):61-71

[31] Feltracco P, Biancofiore G, Ori C, Saner FH, Della Rocca G. Limits and pitfalls of hemodynamic monitoring systems in liver transplantation surgery. Minerva Anestesiologica. 2012;**78**:1372-1384

[32] Abdel MM, Brakat AR, Tawfeek TA, Eid EA, Osman M. Effect of albumin administration prior to graft reperfusion on the severity of reperfusion syndrome during living related liver transplantation. AJAIC. 2005;**3**(8):46-50

[33] Haynes G, Navickis R, Wilkes M. Albumin administration- what is the evidence of clinical benefit? A systematic review of randomized controlled trails. European Journal of Anaesthesiology. 2003;**20**:771-793

[34] Goldwasser P, Feldman J. Association of serum albumin and mortality risk. Journal of Clinical Epidemiology. 1997;**50**:693-703; (Abstract)

[35] Hartmut J. Molecular mechanisms of hepatic ischemia-reperfusion injury and preconditioning. Gastrointestinal and Liver Physiology. 2003;**248**:G15-G26

[36] Vater Y, Levy A, Martay K, et al. Adjuvant drugs for end-stage liver failure and transplantation. Medical Science Monitor. 2004;**10**:RA 77-RA 88

[37] Della Roca G, Brondani A, Costa MG. Intraoperative hemodynamic monitoring during organ transplantation: What is new? Current Opinion in Organ Transplantation. 2009;**14**:291-296

[38] Ferrario M, Pala S, Aletti F, Toschi N, Canichella A, Guerrisi M, et al. Fluid responsiveness in liver surgery:Comparisons of different indices and approaches. Jounal of Computational Surgery. 2014;**1**(6):1-13

[39] Marik PE. Noninvasive cardiac output monitors: A state of the art review. Journal of Cardiothoracic and Vascular Anesthesia. 2013;**27**:121-134

[40] Robertson AC, Eagle SS. Transesophageal echocardiography during orthotopic liver transplantation: Maximizing information without the distraction. Journal of Cardiothoracic and Vascular Anesthesia. 2014;**28**:141-154

[41] Fukazawa K, Pretto EA. The post-reperfusion syndrome (PRS): Diagnosis, incidence and management. In: Liver Transplantation-Basic Issues. 2012 Available from http://intechopen.com/books/liver-transplantation-basicissues/the-post-reperfusion-syndrome-prs-diagnosis-incidence-and-management

[42] Zhen-Dong X, Hai-Tao X, Hong-Bin Y, Zhang H, Rui-Hua J, Zui Z, et al. Postreperfusion syndrome during orthotopic liver transplantation: A single-center experience. Hepatobiliary Pancreas Diseases International. 2012;**11**:34-39

[43] Bukowicka B, Akar RA, Olszewska A, Smoter P, Krawczyk M. The occurrence of postreperfusion syndrome in orthotopic liver transplantation and its significance in terms of complications and short-term survival. Annals of Transplantation. 2011;**16**:26-30

[44] Ijtsma AJC, Van der Hilst CS, et al. The clinical relevance of the anhepatic phase during liver transplantation. Liver Transplantation. 2009;**15**:1050-1055

[45] Paugam-Burtz C, Kavafyan J, et al. Postreperfusion syndrome during liver transplantation for cirrhosis: Outcome and predictors. Liver Transplantation. 2009;**15**:522-529

[46] Bezinover D, Kadry Z, McCullough P, McQuillan PM, Uemura T, Welker K, et al. Release of cytokines and hemodynamic instability during the reperfusion of a liver graft. Liver Transplantation. 2011;**17**:324-330

[47] Fayed NA, Murad WS. Goal directed preemptive ephedrine attenuates the reperfusion syndrome during adult living donor liver transplantation. Egyptian Journal of Anaesthesia. 2014;**30**:187-195

[48] Lisman T, Caldwell SH, Burroughs AK, Northup PG, Senzolo M, Stravitz RT, et al. Hemostasis and thrombosis in patients with liver disease: The ups and downs. Journal of Hepatology. European Association for the Study of the Liver. 2010;**53**(2):362-371

[49] Gatt A, Riddell A, Calvaruso V, Tuddenham EG, Makris M, Burroughs AK. Enhanced thrombin generation in patients with cirrhosis-induced coagulopathy. Journal of Thrombosis and Haemostasis. 2010;**8**(9):1994-2000

[50] De Boer MT, Christensen MC, Asmussen M, Van der Hilst CS, Hendriks HGD, Slooff MJH, et al. The impact of intraoperative transfusion of platelets and red blood cells on survival after liver transplantation. Anesthesia and Analgesia. 2008;**106**(1):32-44

[51] Gorlinger K. Coagulation management during liver transplantation. Hämostaseologie. 2006;**26**(3 Suppl 1):S64-S76

Permissions

All chapters in this book were first published in ODTCSFC, by InTech Open; hereby published with permission under the Creative Commons Attribution License or equivalent. Every chapter published in this book has been scrutinized by our experts. Their significance has been extensively debated. The topics covered herein carry significant findings which will fuel the growth of the discipline. They may even be implemented as practical applications or may be referred to as a beginning point for another development.

The contributors of this book come from diverse backgrounds, making this book a truly international effort. This book will bring forth new frontiers with its revolutionizing research information and detailed analysis of the nascent developments around the world.

We would like to thank all the contributing authors for lending their expertise to make the book truly unique. They have played a crucial role in the development of this book. Without their invaluable contributions this book wouldn't have been possible. They have made vital efforts to compile up to date information on the varied aspects of this subject to make this book a valuable addition to the collection of many professionals and students.

This book was conceptualized with the vision of imparting up-to-date information and advanced data in this field. To ensure the same, a matchless editorial board was set up. Every individual on the board went through rigorous rounds of assessment to prove their worth. After which they invested a large part of their time researching and compiling the most relevant data for our readers.

The editorial board has been involved in producing this book since its inception. They have spent rigorous hours researching and exploring the diverse topics which have resulted in the successful publishing of this book. They have passed on their knowledge of decades through this book. To expedite this challenging task, the publisher supported the team at every step. A small team of assistant editors was also appointed to further simplify the editing procedure and attain best results for the readers.

Apart from the editorial board, the designing team has also invested a significant amount of their time in understanding the subject and creating the most relevant covers. They scrutinized every image to scout for the most suitable representation of the subject and create an appropriate cover for the book.

The publishing team has been an ardent support to the editorial, designing and production team. Their endless efforts to recruit the best for this project, has resulted in the accomplishment of this book. They are a veteran in the field of academics and their pool of knowledge is as vast as their experience in printing. Their expertise and guidance has proved useful at every step. Their uncompromising quality standards have made this book an exceptional effort. Their encouragement from time to time has been an inspiration for everyone.

The publisher and the editorial board hope that this book will prove to be a valuable piece of knowledge for researchers, students, practitioners and scholars across the globe.

List of Contributors

Cristina Baleriola
South Eastern Area Laboratory Service, Prince of Wales Hospital, Sydney, Australia

William D Rawlinson
South Eastern Area Laboratory Services, Microbiology, Prince of Wales Hospital, Sydney, Australia

Maria Grazia Bocci, Alessia Prestifilippo, Ciro D'Alò, Alessandro Barelli, Massimo Antonelli, Alessandra Tersali, Alessandra Ionescu Maddalena and Roberta Barelli
Department of Anesthesiology and Intensive Care Medicine, Catholic University of the Sacred Heart, Rome, Italy

Emiliano Cingolani
UOSD Shock and Trauma, San Camillo Forlanini Hospital, Rome, Italy

Chih-Che Lin and Chao-Long Chen
Department of general surgery and liver transplant center, Chang Gung Memorial Hospital, Kaohsiung, Taiwan

Ahmed Mohammed Abdel Aziz Elsarawy
Liver transplant center, Chang Gung Memorial Hospital, Kaohsiung, Taiwan

Seema Naik, Hong Zheng and Kevin Rakszawski
Department of Medicine, Division of Hematology/Oncology, Penn State Cancer Institute, Milton S. Hershey Medical Center, Hershey, PA, USA

Clare Sample and Jeff Sample
Department of Immunology, Penn State College of Medicine, Milton S. Hershey Medical Center, Hershey, PA, USA

Michael Bayerl
Department of Pathology, Penn State College of Medicine, Milton S. Hershey Medical Center, Hershey, PA, USA

Kanmani Job and Anooja Antony
Amrita College of Nursing, Amrita Vishwa Vidyapeetham, Kochi, India

Bulang He
Medical School, The University of Western Australia, Sir Charles Gairdner Hospital, Nedlands, Perth, Australia

Xiuwu Han
Beijing Chaoyang Hospital (West Campus), Capital Medical University, Beijing, China

Michael A. Fink
Department of Surgery/Austin Health, Medicine Dentistry and Health Sciences, The University of Melbourne, Austraila

Pedro Ventura-Aguiar and Maria José Ricart
Nephrology and Kidney Transplant Department, Hospital Clinic Barcelona, Spain

Joana Ferrer-Fábrega
Hepato Bilio Pancreatic Surgery and Liver and Pancreas Transplantation Department, ICMDiM, Hospital Clínic Barcelona, Spain

Alyssa Green
Department of Research and Innovation, St. Luke's University Health Network, Bethlehem, PA, USA

Stanislaw P. Stawicki
Department of Research and Innovation, St. Luke's University Health Network, Bethlehem, PA, USA
Regional Level I Trauma Center, St. Luke's University Health Network, Bethlehem, PA, USA

Peter G. Thomas and Rebecca Wilde-Onia
Regional Level I Trauma Center, St. Luke's University Health Network, Bethlehem, PA, USA

Scott J. Kohler and Joan D. Sweeney
Center for Neurosciences, St. Luke's University Health Network, Bethlehem, PA, USA

Deborah M. Stahlnecker
Section of Pulmonary and Critical Care, Department of Medicine, St. Luke's University Health Network, Bethlehem, PA, USA

Young-Nam Roh
Keimyung University, Dongsan Medical Center, Daegu, South Korea

Sean Stevens
Synthetic Genomics, Inc., La Jolla, CA, USA

Maria Eugenia Cornide-Petronio
Institut d'Investigacions Biomèdiques August Pi Sunyer (IDIBAPS), Barcelona, Spain

Araní Casillas-Ramírez
Hospital Regional de Alta Especialidad de Ciudad Victoria "Bicentenario 2010", Ciudad Victoria, Mexico
Facultad de Medicina e Ingeniería en Sistemas Computacionales de Matamoros, Universidad Autónoma de Tamaulipas, Mexico

Mónica B. Jiménez-Castro
Transplant Biomedicals, S.L., Barcelona, Spain

Carmen Peralta
Institut d'Investigacions Biomèdiques August Pi Sunyer (IDIBAPS), Barcelona, Spain
Centro de Investigación Biomédica en Red de Enfermedades Hepáticas y Digestivas (CIBEREHD), Barcelona, Spain
Facultad de Medicina, Universidad International de Cataluña, Barcelona, Spain

Daniela Loncar and Selma Hodzic
Clinic for Internal Disease, University Clinical Center Tuzla, Bosnia and Herzegovina

Gabriela Droc and Lavinia Jipa
Fundeni Clinical Institute, University of Medicine and Pharmacy "Carol Davila", Bucharest, Romania

Index

A

Acute Rejection, 109, 113-115, 124-125, 128-129, 132-133, 196, 208, 213, 217

Allograft, 1-2, 9, 11, 19, 21, 76-77, 82, 87, 108, 135-137, 184, 207, 209-210, 212, 214-215, 217-219, 223

þÿ A l p h a f e t o P r o t e i n , 46, 48 Anastomosis, 50-51, 112, 121-124, 130, 133, 136, 200, 233, 241

Arterial Anastomosis, 50, 122

Autograft, 81

B

Biopsy, 46, 48, 56-57, 61, 96, 113, 132

Blood Product Transfusion, 6

Blood-borne Pathogens, 2

C

Cirrhosis, 3, 21, 41, 51, 54, 60, 65, 229-230, 232, 242-246

Cold Ischaemia Time, 10, 240

Cytokines, 55, 71, 176-178, 182, 194, 196, 207, 240, 246

Cytomegalovirus, 1, 3, 125, 214, 223

D

Diagnostic Markers, 68-69

Domino Transplant, 82

Donation After Brain Death, 95, 162, 166, 168, 171

Donation After Cardiac Death, 9-10, 83, 148, 151, 153, 156-157

Donor Assessment, 2

Donor-derived Infection, 1

Duodenum, 96, 98, 100-101, 103-104, 120-123, 136

E

End-stage Organ Failure, 81, 143

Endemic Infections, 2

Epstein-barr Virus, 1, 3, 66, 68-71, 74, 76-78

Eurotransplant Region, 10, 22

G

Gerota's Fascia, 104-105

Glycemia, 131-132, 149

Glycosylated Hemoglobin, 131-132

Graft Failure, 10, 22, 133, 137, 215, 226

H

Hematopoietic Stem Cell Transplant, 66-67

Hepatectomy, 44-45, 47, 50-51, 55

Hepatocellular Carcinoma, 40, 57-65

Histopathological Analysis, 44

I

Imaging, 43, 47, 51, 53, 61, 117, 127-128, 140, 147, 197, 243

Immunoglobulin, 8, 13, 77, 87

Immunosuppression, 54, 66, 68, 72-75, 87, 109-110, 114-115, 123, 126, 128-129, 131-134, 142-143, 153, 183, 212-213, 232

Intimal Dissection, 52, 64

Islet Transplantation, 111, 119, 133-135, 138

Isograft, 82

L

Lamivudine, 8, 21

Live Donors, 82, 91, 145

Liver Resection, 40-41, 44, 50, 52, 54, 59, 64, 244

Liver Transplantation, 10, 17, 21-22, 40-42, 45-52, 54, 56, 58-65, 80, 93-94, 154, 156, 189, 193, 201, 203-204, 206-208, 228-229, 231, 233-234, 236-239, 241-246

þÿ L o c o r e g i o n a l T h e r a p y , 44-45, 48-49, 52

Lymph Node Metastases, 51

Lymphadenectomy, 51, 63

M

Morphological Selection, 56

Multi-organ Procurement, 95-97, 100, 107-108

N

Nodal Disease, 43, 51, 73

Nondestructive Lesions, 71, 75

Nonmalignant Cases, 41-42, 44, 47, 51, 53

O

Omentum, 51-52, 98

Organ Transplantation, 1-2, 6, 8, 11-12, 18-19, 23, 68, 73, 76, 78-81, 84, 87, 89, 92-93, 95-96, 106-108, 111, 118, 129-130, 134, 136-137, 142, 146, 158-159, 162, 167, 170-172, 190, 194, 211-212, 225, 245

P

Pathological Necrosis, 45, 50

Pathological Spectrum, 66-67

Peritoneum, 51, 97, 123

Polyomavirus, 3

Portal Vein, 44, 98, 102, 106, 120, 122, 125, 133, 200, 233

Post-transplant Surveillance, 2, 15

Posttransplant Lymphoproliferative Disorder, 66, 71, 76, 78

Posttransplant Period, 68, 71

Preoperative Evaluation, 47

Pretransplantation, 43, 50

Psychosocial, 79-81, 87-88, 91, 93-94, 160

R

Relative Risk, 10, 214, 217-218
Renal Vein, 98, 102-105, 120
Risk Assessment, 1-2, 5, 10, 15-16, 221-224, 243
Risk Management, 1-2
Risk Mitigation, 1, 7, 15
Rituximab, 67, 74-76, 87, 191

S

Safety Margin, 51
Serology, 3-8, 96
Serum Bilirubin, 10
Serum Creatinine, 10, 217, 232
Solid Organ Transplant, 23, 66-67, 69
Split Transplant, 82

T

Tumor Biology, 49, 55
Tumor Burden, 41, 44, 47-49
Tumor Necrosis, 50, 59
Tumor Progression, 49-50, 53, 55

W

Window Period, 4

X

Xenograft, 82, 175-176, 189-191

www.ingramcontent.com/pod-product-compliance
Lightning Source LLC
LaVergne TN
LVHW080930210926
848485LV00004B/767